SCANNING ELECTRON MICROSCOPY of NORMAL and ABNORMAL HUMAN SKIN

by

Walter H. Wilborn, Ph.D.
Professor of Anatomy and Director of the Electron Microscopy Center

Barbara M. Hyde, M.T.A.
Electron Microscopy Specialist and Research Associate

Leopoldo F. Montes, M.D.
Adjunct Professor of Anatomy and Dermatology Research

from the

Electron Microscopy Center
University of South Alabama
College of Medicine
Mobile, Alabama 36688

VCH

ABOUT THE AUTHORS

Each author has contributed his/her special expertise*to produce this first book on the SEM of human skin. The fact that the authors have different backgrounds permitted each to play an essential role in the preparation of this volume. All three authors share an intense interest in the knowledge of cutaneous structure and function.

Walter Wilborn is Professor of Anatomy and Director of the Electron Microscopy Center, College of Medicine, University of South Alabama, Mobile, Alabama. He received his anatomical training at St. Louis University and the University of Tennessee in Memphis. Dr. Wilborn helped to pioneer the application of SEM to problems in Skin Biology, and for five years co-organized the Annual Symposium on SEM in Dermatology.

Barbara Mill Hyde acquired her degree in Medical Technology in Hamburg, West Germany. For 15 years, she has worked as an Electron Microscopist in Germany, Sweden, and the United States. Her skill and commitment to the science and art of Electron Microscopy were paramount for obtaining the high quality illustrations in this volume.

Leopoldo Montes is a Dermatologist and Dermatopathologist who obtained his undergraduate medical education in Argentina and his graduate training in the United States. Dr. Montes has a long, distinguished career in Academic and Clinical Dermatology. He is a well-known scholar with many scientific contributions, and he was the founder of the Journal of Cutaneous Pathology. He practices Dermatology in Buenos Aires and is a Professor at the University of South Alabama, Mobile, the University of Alabama Medical School, Birmingham, and Auburn University in Auburn, Alabama.

Acknowledgements

The authors wish to thank the many physicians who supplied specimens with clinical and histopathological information for this book. Special appreciation is extended to Dr. Stewart Carrington, Dr. Hugh Reynolds, Dr. Charles Behlen, Dr. Harold Hawkins, Dr. Fred Bodie, and Dr. Earl Eggers.

We thank Mrs. Wendy Hill of Design Graphics for making the drawings for this volume. We thank Paula Scott of Scott Graphics for working with us and the publisher to achieve the best possible arrangement of pictures and text.

We gratefully acknowledge and give special thanks to Richard Rose of Electron Optics Publishing Group for his cooperation, enthusiasm, and patience during the preparation of this book.

PREFACE

This book, the first on the scanning electron microscopy of human skin, is intended for dermatologists, pathologists, skin biologists, and students of medicine, biology, and electron microscopy.

A major goal has been to try to accurately present the most significant information that is currently available on the topographical microanatomy of human skin. The text and micrographs are based on our careful study of more than 1,000 human skin specimens (normal and abnormal) by correlative scanning electron microscopy (SEM), light microscopy (LM), and transmission electron microscopy (TEM). It required a continuum of effort during about seven years to obtain, prepare, photograph, and study the material included in this volume.

The SEM in this book reveals new information on the structure and function of the integumentary system and provides original information on some common skin lesions. We have used SEM to obtain topographical views of specimens and to complement and broaden the reliable and established information that has been obtained through the years by LM and TEM.

This volume consists of eleven chapters. The first introduces the reader to the methods and techniques of SEM. The second and third chapters describe both the fetal and the adult skin. The balance of the book is concerned with acne, psoriasis and the various cutaneous tumors that occur most frequently. Each chapter begins with a synopsis of the topic. The synopsis is followed by select references and labeled illustrations with accompanying text that enable the reader without a detailed knowledge of cutaneous ultrastructure to quickly gain visual and verbal insights into the topic. The references are key sources for excellent additional reading on the topic.

Topics are limited to those that we have studied thoroughly and have been able to reach some definitive conclusions. The topics do not represent all the lesions that we have studied from among the approximately 2,000 different types of cutaneous lesions. We are continuing our studies and plan to make additional volumes available as sufficient numbers of other lesions can be obtained, studied, and the results reported with confidence.

We believe this book will give the practicing *dermatologist* another view of the skin and its diseases, contribute to continuing education, and provide new insights into the basis for selecting modes of treatment. Of special interest to the *dermatopathologist* is the new information on the histogenesis and surface topography of tumors. It would require the preparation and study of hundreds of serial histological sections of a single lesion to obtain the information available in one scanning electron micrograph. Most *medical specialists* should appreciate the information in this book. They are recurrently confronted with the skin diseases shown here, because the skin, unlike deep organs, is exposed for examination with the unaided eye. *Students* will benefit from this book because it shows the skin's microscopy in a natural, unique manner that elicits respect for the largest organ of the body. The student is provided a basic foundation for acquiring additional knowledge on the subject.

Lastly, we hope this book will serve to deepen and make more meaningful the microanatomical knowledge of human skin.

TABLE OF CONTENTS

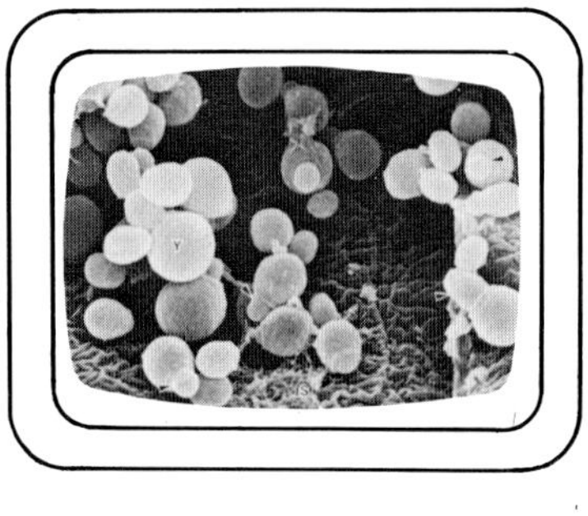

Distribution of hardcover edition:
VCH Verlagsgesellschaft, P.O. Box 1260/1280, D-6940 Weinheim (Federal Republic of Germany)
USA and Canada: VCH Publishers, 303 N.W. 12th Avenue, Deerfield Beach, FL 33442-1705 (USA)

ISBN 0-89573-277-7 (VCH Publishers) ISBN 3-527-26531-7 (VCH Verlagsgesellschaft)

Library of Congress Catalog Number: 84-082408

Printed in the United States of America

INTRODUCTION 1

With the naked or unaided eye, man can resolve structures no smaller than about 0.1 millimeter (mm). His desire to view living and non-living matter at higher magnification has led to the development of the light microscope (LM), the transmission electron microscope (TEM), and the scanning electron microscope (SEM). Figure 1–1 compares the three types of microscopes.

Resolving power or resolution is the capability of a microscope to separate images of objects that are close together. It is the capability to distinguish adjacent objects as separate objects. The resolving power of the LM, TEM, and SEM is about 200 nm, 0.2 nm, and 2 nm, respectively (nm = nanometer). Table 1–1 lists some standard units of measurement and their symbols.

Although the TEM permits the organelles and inclusions of the cell to be magnified many hundreds of thousands times their original size, the TEM does not give a three-dimensional image of the object. SEM provides this type of image and permits the viewing of surface details of large, unsectioned specimens at useful magnifications ranging from 10× to 50,000×. Although higher magnification can be achieved with the SEM, it is not practical for general use.

Since the SEM first became commercially available in 1965, advances have followed in the instrument itself and in the techniques of tissue processing that have permitted the application of SEM to a broad spectrum of biological problems. Consequently, significant new information has been generated on the three-dimensional microanatomy of all the body's tissues and organs.

With the technology available today, it is possible to almost totally characterize a specimen with the SEM. For example, one can (1) study the surface features of whole or fractured, quick-frozen specimens, (2) microdissect and examine specimens while in the microscope, (3) microanalyze specimens to reveal the elemental composition of the sample, and (4) map the distribution of enzymes and antigens on the surfaces of cells prepared by appropriate cytochemical and immunological techniques.

The variety of information that can be obtained with the SEM is made possible by the several different types of electrons that result when the primary electron beam strikes the specimen (Figure 1–2). These electrons and their uses are discussed more completely in textbooks of electron microscopy (see references). Only secondary electrons from the specimens were used to record the images included in this volume.

A modern scanning electron microscope (Philips 501 SEM) used in our laboratory for research and diagnostic purposes is shown in Figure 1–3. Figure 1–4 illustrates some of the equipment needed to prepare specimens for observation in the SEM. The two large items in the pictures are the critical point drying apparatus and the stereomicroscope. Their uses are described in the legends that accompany the pictures.

The number of skin biopsies and the types of lesions evaluated by SEM in this volume are shown in Table 1–2. The authors have studied much additional material by LM and TEM, but only the specimens used for SEM are tabulated.

The procedure for processing a skin biopsy is outlined in Table 1–3. The biopsy is divided so that one part can be used for histology (LM), and the other part for SEM and TEM. The portion for histology is fixed 12 or more hours in 10% phosphate buffered formalin in the conventional manner, dehydrated in a graded series of ethyl alcohols, embedded in paraffin, and sectioned at 6 μm. The sections are mounted on glass slides and stained with hematoxylin and eosin (H&E) or with a special stain to demonstrate a particular tissue component (e.g., elastic fibers, melanin, or keratin). Finally, a dermatopathologist examines the slides and reports the results.

An abbreviated processing procedure for SEM specimens can be completed in about 4 hours. In comparison, it takes 24 hours to routinely process a skin biopsy for LM or TEM. Although it is possible to prepare and examine specimens by SEM within 4 hours from the time of the biopsy, we usually take longer to process our specimens.

Table 1–3 does not give specific times for the steps of the processing procedure because the intervals are dependent on specimen size. The time required for each step is best learned through experience. Most SEM or TEM specimens of skin should be fixed a minimum of 1 hour in buffered glutaraldehyde. A postfixation time of about 1 hour in osmium tetroxide is necessary for skin samples to increase their conductivity and to preserve lipids. Dehydration for SEM requires about 2 hours. If dehydration is inadequate, the image is faulty due to outgasing when the specimen is placed under vacuum in an electron beam. Liquid carbon dioxide is used in our laboratory for the critical point drying of specimens. The procedure requires about 2 hours. Mounting the specimen, allowing the adhesive to dry, and sputter coating takes an additional 30 minutes.

We handle tissues carefully and with respect throughout all stages of processing for LM, TEM, and SEM. We attempt to preserve the skin's normal and abnormal architecture as closely as possible to its appearance in the "living state" and to record these features in our micrographs.

References

Abraham, J. L. Scanning electron microscopy as an aid in diagnosis — An overview. Scanning Electron Microscopy, Vol. II, 1977, SEM Inc., Chicago, IL, pp. 121–128.

Anderson, T. F. Electron microscopy of micro-organism. *In:* Physical Techniques in Biological Research. A. W. Pollister (ed). Academic Press, New York, NY, 1966, Vol. 3, Part A, 2nd edition, pp. 178–181.

Carteaud, J. B. Scanning electron microscopy in skin pathology. Scanning Electron Microscopy, Vol. III, 1973, SEM Inc., Chicago, IL, pp. 629–636.

DeNee, P. B., J. L. Abraham, and P. A. Williard. Histochemical stains for the scanning electron microscope — Qualitative and semi-quantitative aspects of specific silver stains. Scanning Electron Microscopy, Vol. I, 1974, SEM Inc., Chicago, IL, pp. 259–266.

Fawcett, D. W. The Cell. W. B. Saunders Co., Philadelphia, PA, 2nd edition, 1981.

Fujita, T., J. Tokunaga, and H. Inoue. Atlas of Scanning Electron Microscopy in Medicine. Elsevier Publishing Co., New York, NY, 1971.

Galle, P., J. B. Berry, and R. Lefevre. Microanalysis in biology and medicine. A review of results obtained with three microanalytical methods. Scanning Electron Microscopy, Vol. II, 1979, SEM Inc., Chicago, IL, pp. 703–710.

Hayat, M. A. Fixation for Electron Microscopy. Academic Press, New York, NY, 1981.

Hollenberg, M. J., and A. M. Erickson. The scanning electron microscope: Potential usefulness to biologists. A review. J. Histochem. Cytochem. 21: 109–130, 1973.

Hoyer, L. C., J. C. Lee, and C. Bucana. Scanning immunoelectron microscopy for identification and mapping of two or more antigens on cell surfaces. Scanning Electron Microscopy, Vol. III, 1979, SEM Inc., Chicago, IL, pp. 629–636.

Kessel, R. G., and R. H. Karden. Tissues and Organs: A Text-Atlas of Scanning Electron Microscopy. W. H. Freeman & Co., San Francisco, CA, 1979.
Kessel, R. G., and C. Y. Shih. Scanning Electron Microscopy in Biology. A Students' Atlas on Biological Organization. Springer-Verlag, New York, NY, 1974.
Papa, C. M., and B. Farber. Direct scanning electron microscopy of human skin. Arch. Dermatol. 104: 262–270, 1971.
Yoshi, Z., J. Tokunaga, and J. Tawara. Atlas of Scanning Electron Microscopy in Microbiology. The Williams & Wilkins Co., Baltimore, MD, 1976.

Units of Measurements, Symbols, and Definitions

Unit	Symbol and Definition
Micrometer (micron)	1 μm = 0.001 mm = 10,000 Å 1 μm = 1×10^{-3} mm
Nanometer (millimicron)	1 nm = 0.001 m = 10 Å 1 nm = 10^{-6} mm
Ångstrom	1 Å = 0.1 nm = 0.001 μm 1 Å = 1×10^{-7} mm

Table 1–1

SKIN BIOPSIES EXAMINED BY SEM

	No. of Specimen	No. of Patients	Age
Fetal Skin	32	—	7–32 weeks
Control Skin	21	15	21–77 years
Acne	150	20	18–30 years
Psoriasis	6	6	25–73 years
Seborrheic Keratosis	15	15	40–77 years
Capillary Hemangioma	5	5	16–39 years
Basal Cell Epithelioma	32	30	58–81 years
Squamous Cell Carcinoma	12	12	50–71 years
Keratoacanthoma	18	17	37–75 years
Pigmented Nevus	32	24	26–64 years

Table 1–2

SKIN BIOPSY

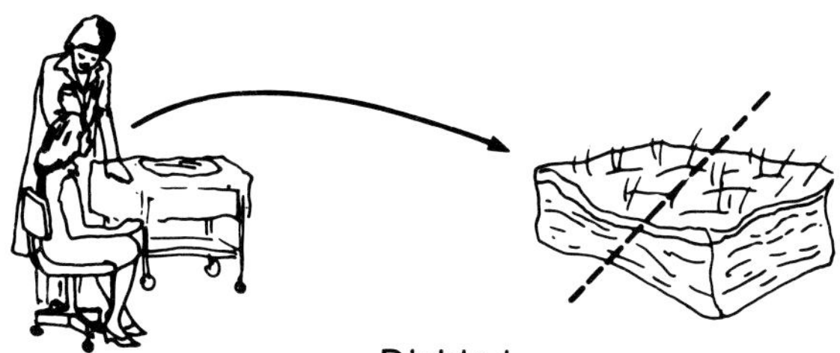

Divided

Histology

↓

Fix in 10% Neutral Buffered Formalin

↓

Process Tissue and Prepare Histological Slides

↓

Dermatopathologist Reads Slides and Reports Diagnosis

SEM & TEM

↓

Fix in 2% Glutaraldehyde in Millonig's Phosphate Buffer, pH 7.2

↓

Divide Sample for SEM and TEM

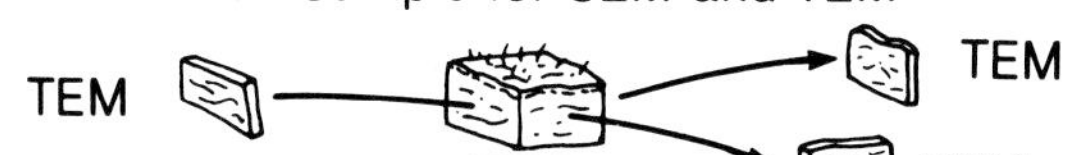

Rinse in Millonig's Buffer

↓

Postfix in 1% phosphate buffered OsO_4

↓

Rinse in Millonig's Buffer

↓

Dehydrate in Graded Ethanol

SEM	TEM
Amyl Acetate	Acetone
Critical Point Dry	Embed in Plastic
Mount Sample	Make 1 μm Sections (Stain with Toluidine Blue Examine with LM)
Sputter Coat	Ultrathin Sections
Examine by SEM	Stain with Uranyl Acetate and Lead Citrate
	Examine by TEM

Table 1–3

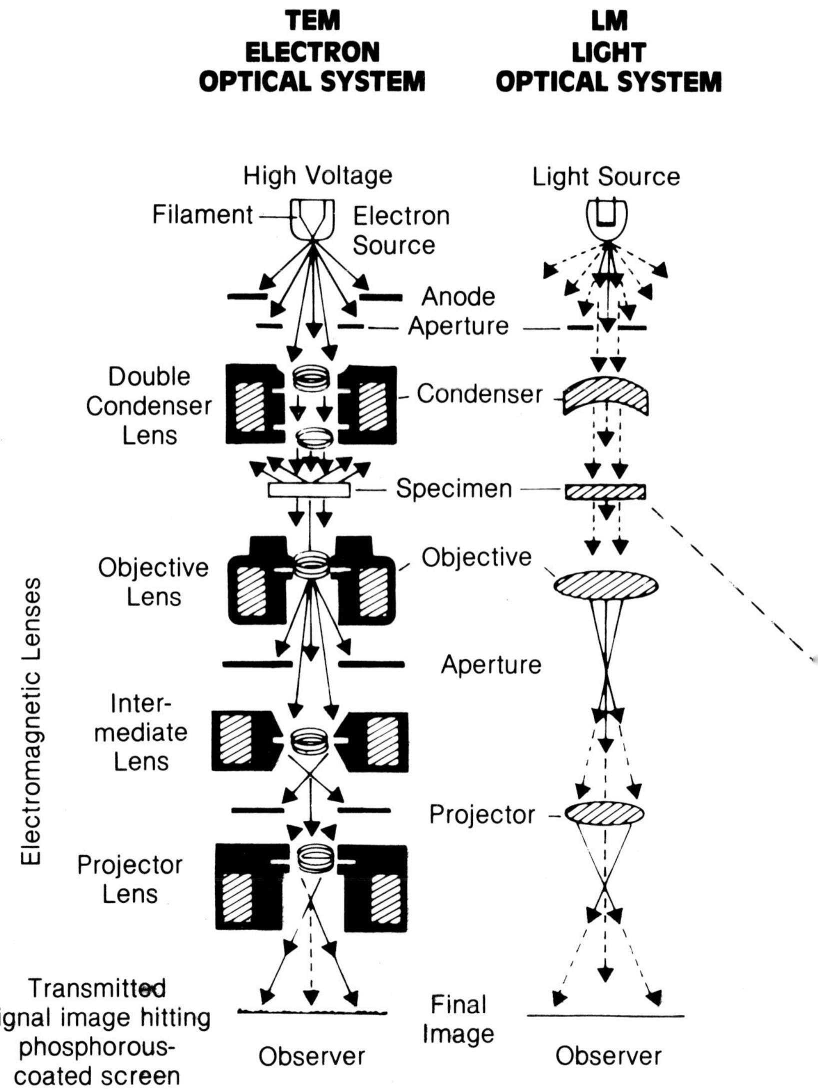

Figure 1–1. Schematic outline of basic differences in the formation of images with the transmission electron microscope (TEM), light microscope (LM), and scanning electron microscope (SEM).

The light source for the LM is a light bulb. Light passes through the sectioned specimen that is usually stained. The image is enlarged by a system of glass lenses. The resolution of the LM is about 0.2 μm and is limited by the wavelength of visible light rays.

In the TEM, the electron beam is from a filament connected to a high voltage source. Plastic embedding is required to support the specimens that must be cut into ultrathin sections in order to be penetrable by electrons. The image of biological specimans can be enhanced by staining with heavy metal salts, such as uranyl acetate, to impart electron density. The electron beam is controlled by electromagnetic lenses as it passes down the microscope column and through the specimen. The image can be magnified about 500,000 ×. Resolution is about 2 Å and is limited by the wavelength of the electron beam. The image is visualized on a phosphorus-coated screen.

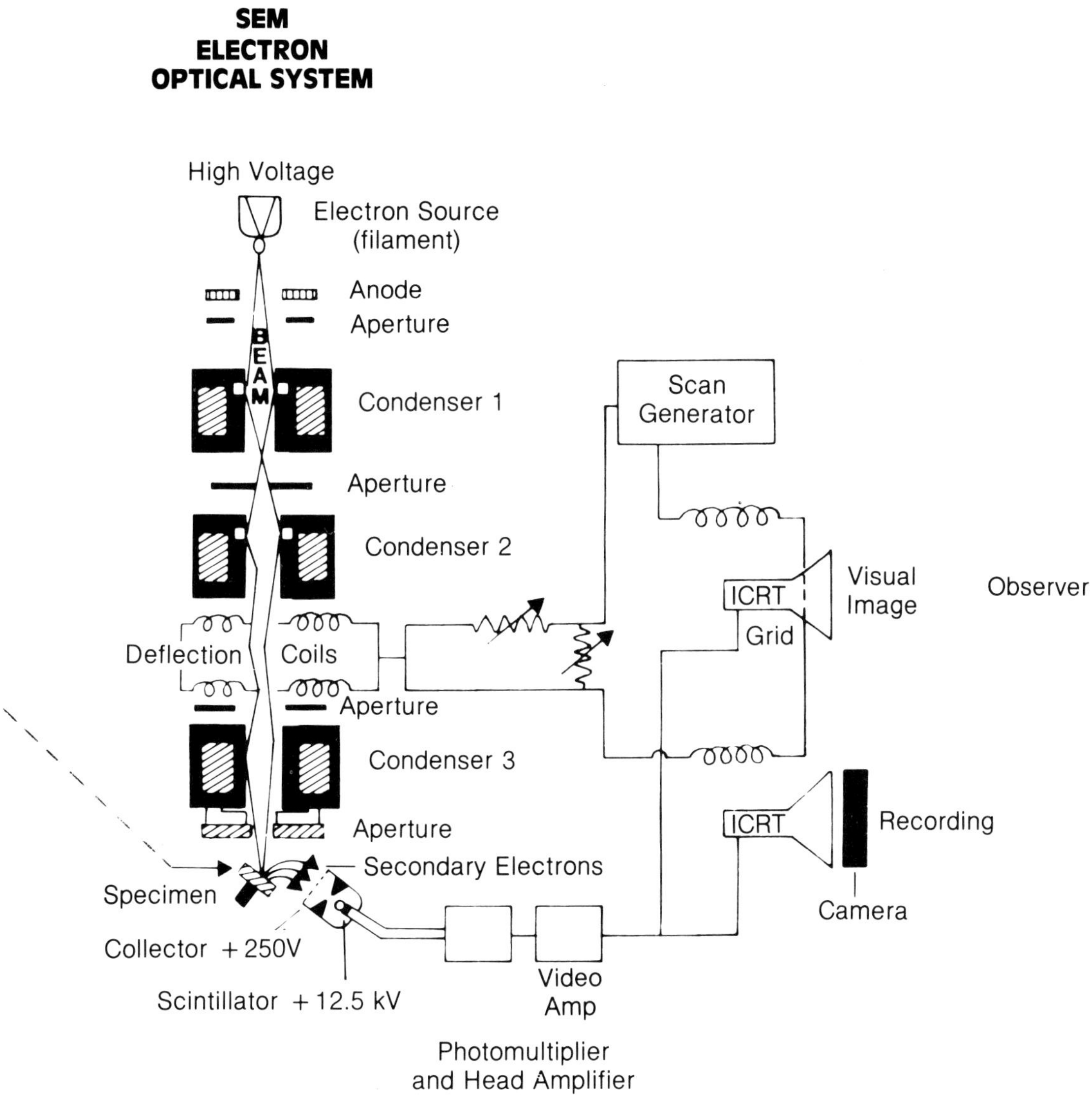

In the SEM, the image is obtained by an indirect method. Most biological specimens are less than 1 inch in diameter, but larger specimens can be studied in appropriately equipped microscopes. Natural or artificial surfaces of any dehydrated specimen can be viewed. The specimen must be either naturally conductive (e.g., metallic as is the case of some non-biological specimens) or coated with a conductive layer (e.g., gold or gold palladium for biological samples). As the primary electron beam scans the surface of the specimen, it results in several different types of emissions (see Figure 1–2). The secondary electrons are collected, transformed into photoelectrons, amplified, and the image visualized on a cathode ray tube (CRT) which is very similar to a black and white television screen. The SEM and TEM contain photographic negatives. The image is recorded photographically by exposing the emulsion to electrons.

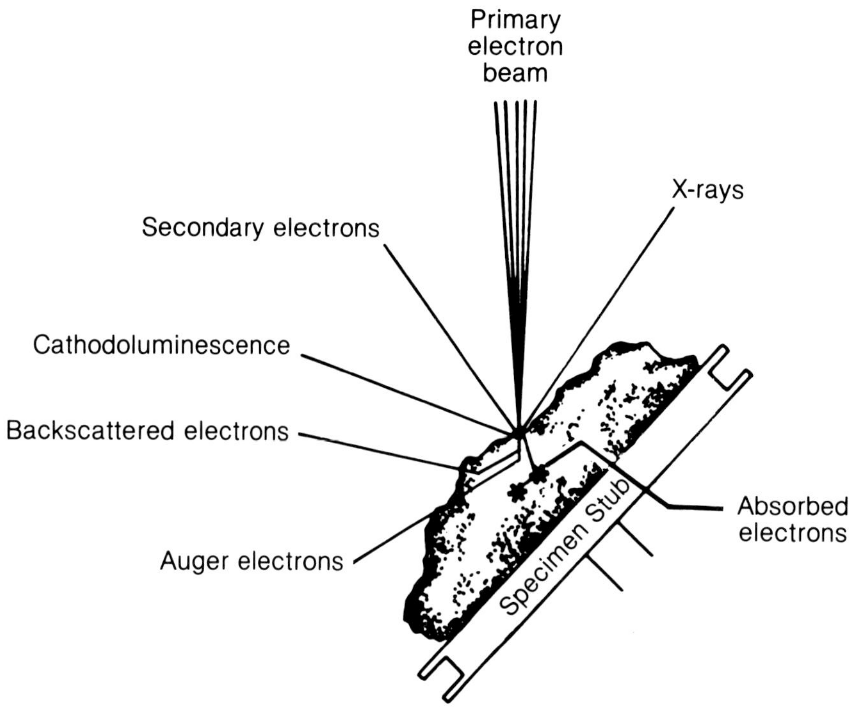

Figure 1–2. This diagram illustrates the types of emissions that are produced when the specimen is struck by the primary electron beam. The depth of penetration depends on the energy (kV) of the beam. Each type of emission can be used for obtaining important information regarding the specimen. X-rays are used to analyze the chemical composition of the sample; backscattered electrons provide information about the subsurface features of the specimen, and secondary electrons reveal the surface topography of the specimen. Only secondary electrons were employed for the micrographs in this volume.

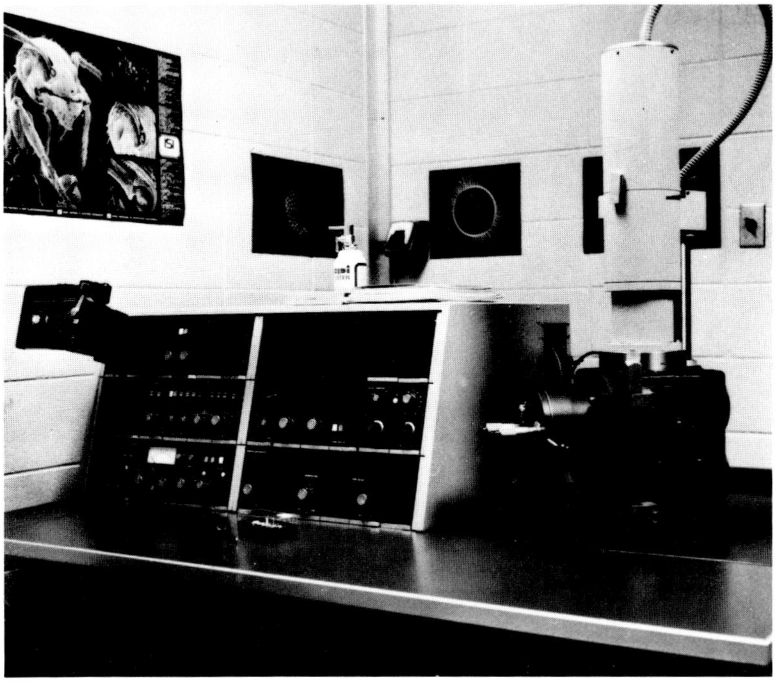

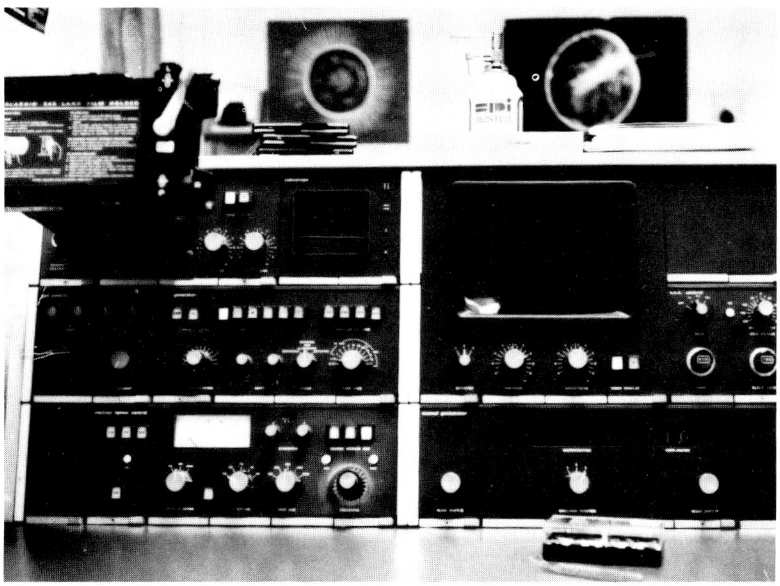

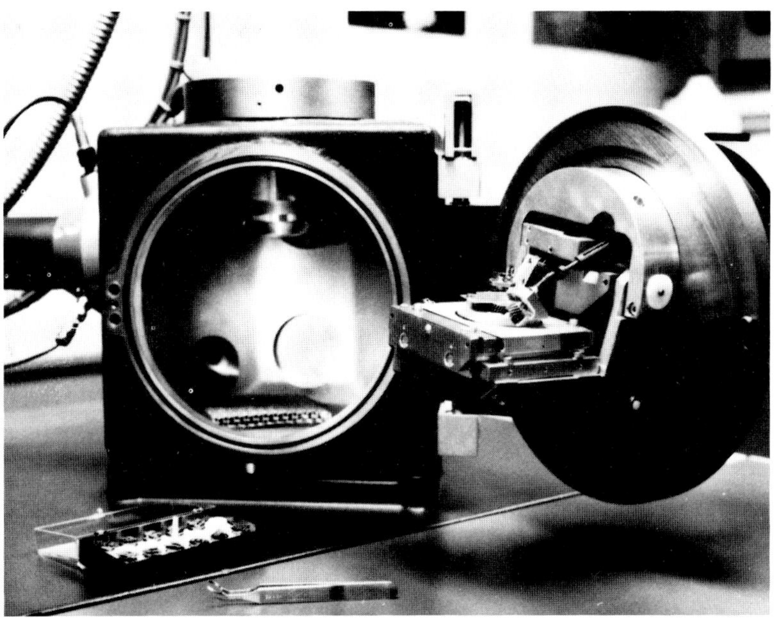

Figure 1–3. These photographs show a scanning electron microscope that was used for recording images in this volume. The upper picture is a view of the whole SEM. The control panel is depicted in the middle picture. The lower picture provides a view of the chamber and the stage that is mounted to the open door. A specimen from the box in the foreground is placed on the stage, the door is closed, and the column is pumped to high vacuum. When the door is closed, the specimen is directly beneath the center of the column at a 45° angle to the collector. The latter is located at the upper left on the inside of the chamber.

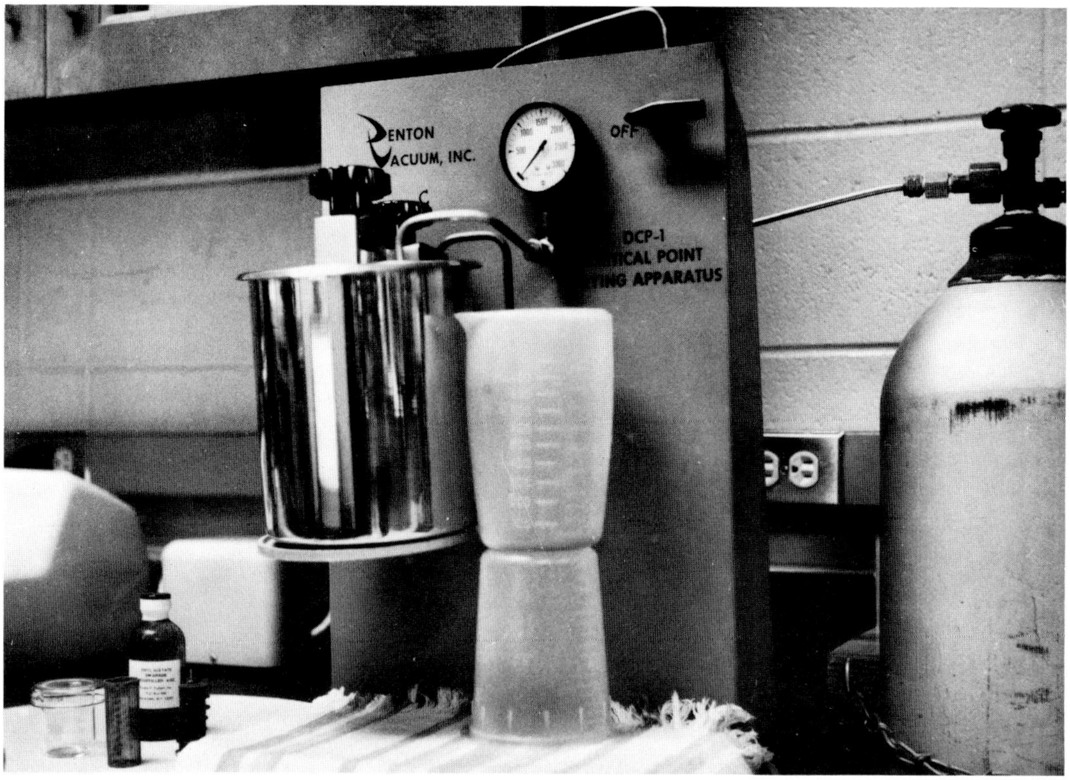
ENTON
ACUUM, INC.
OFF
DCP-1
TICAL POINT
YING APPARATUS

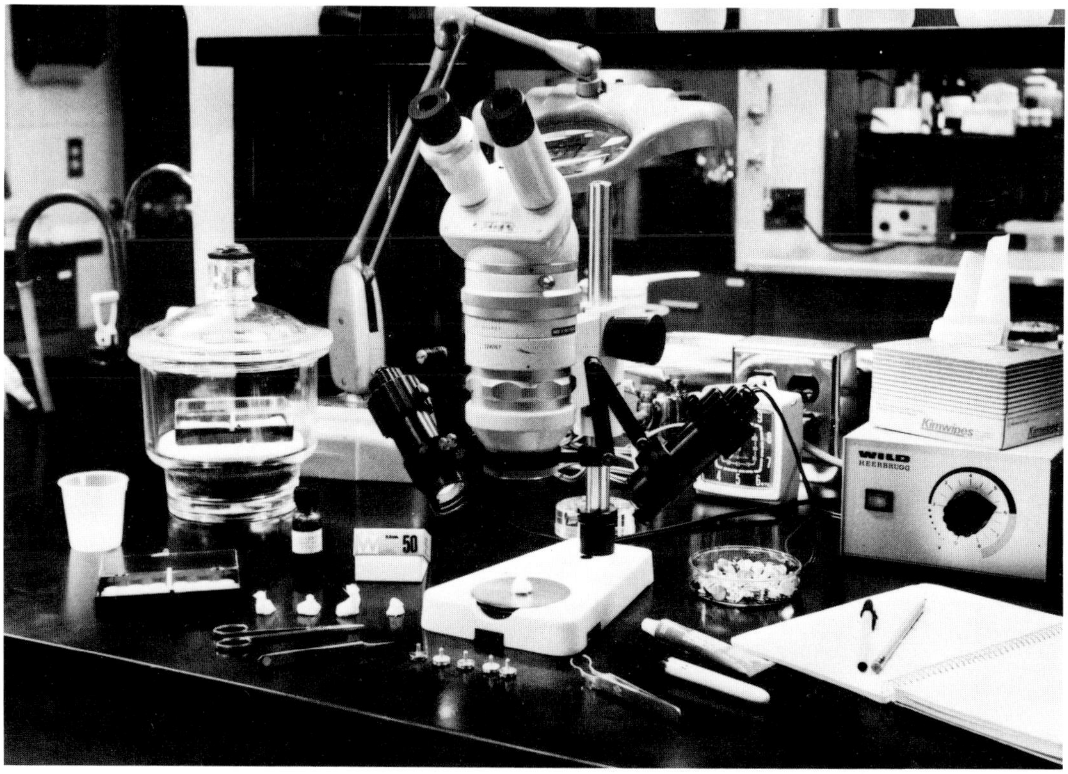
50
Kimwipes
WILD
HEERBRUGG

Figure 1–4. The upper photograph shows a critical point drying apparatus. On the right is a tank that contains liquid carbon dioxide (CO_2). It is connected to the specimen pressure chamber which is inside the stainless steel container where it is hidden from view. Wet specimens that are soaked with amyl acetate are placed inside the specimen pressure chamber, and the seal is locked. The stainless steel container is filled with ice and placed as an ice bath about the specimen pressure chamber. The ice cools the specimen pressure chamber to about 4° C. Liquid CO_2 is allowed to enter the specimen pressure chamber and the specimens become immersed in the liquid. By repeated flushings and reimmersions, the amyl acetate inside the tissues is replaced with liquid CO_2. Critical point drying is achieved by exchanging the ice in the stainless steel container for hot water which causes the pressure inside the specimen pressure chamber to rise above 1600 PSI. The process is closely monitored with the pressure gauge on the critical point drying apparatus. At the critical point, liquid CO_2 is changed instantaneously from the liquid phase to the gas phase. This change renders the tissues dry without creating significant artifacts. The pressure is then released gradually so that specimens can be removed and mounted.

In the lower photograph, dry specimens are shown ready to be mounted on stubs with the aid of a stereomicroscope. The tissues are inside the tiny bags of lens paper at the left where they rest on small pieces of numbered index cards. Each number is written on the bottom of the appropriate stub that will be used for mounting the tissue specimen. Three stubs are visible in the center of the picture immediately in front of the microscope base. As the bags are opened, each piece of tissue is carefully oriented and mounted on the stub with glue or conductive silver paint. Samples are handled with extreme care to avoid mechanical damage to their surfaces. Mounted specimens are placed inside the vacuum dessicator, such as the one visible in the left background, where the solvent from the adhesive is allowed to evaporate. Before the specimens are viewed in the SEM, a sputter coater is used to coat their surfaces with a thin conductive layer of evaporated metal (e.g., gold or gold palladium).

FETAL SKIN 2

Prior to birth, human skin is surrounded by germ-free amniotic fluid, maintained at constant temperature and pressure, protected from light and against infection, and buffered from shock. This situation changes abruptly at birth when the skin of the newborn is subjected to temperature fluctuations, dry air, light, shock and friction, microorganisms, chemicals, clothing, and innumerable other new onslaughts. The neonate could not survive if the skin had not developed mechanisms *in utero* to cope with the new and hostile conditions posed by extrauterine life.

The following account describes and shows pictorially the prenatal development of human skin. Knowledge of skin development is essential for appreciating the structure and function of normal adult skin, interpreting skin pathology in the adult and neonate, determining fetal age and blood type from cells and secretions in the amniotic fluid, and diagnosing diseases through the study of fetal skin biopsies.

Material for this study was obtained from 3 embryos and 29 fetuses. Gestational ages were based on the last menstrual period and ultrasound data. Ages of specimens were 6.5, 7, 8, 12, 14, 15, 16, 16.5, 24, 26, 28, 30, 31, and 32 weeks. Specimens were collected over a period of several years at times when it was necessary to perform hysterectomies for medical reasons.

The skin of each specimen was examined grossly and microscopically and found to be normal. Samples of skin were taken from the head, trunk, and limbs of each embryo or fetus. In some cases, an entire limb was sufficiently small to be examined *in toto* in the scanning electron microscope. About equal numbers of samples were fixed initially in 10% phosphate buffered formalin (pH 7.2) or in 1% to 2% glutaraldehyde buffered with sodium cacodylate buffer (pH 7.3) or phosphate buffer (pH 7.3). Both methods of fixation provided adequate preservation of cutaneous structures for SEM. Postfixation for SEM and TEM was carried out in 1% osmium tetroxide in cacodylate buffer. Standard methods were followed for dehydrating and embedding specimens for TEM, and for critical point drying and sputter coating samples for SEM. Some tissues from each formalin-fixed specimen were dehydrated, embedded in paraffin, sectioned, and stained by different methods for histochemical evaluation.

The skin of the embryo and fetus is usually described as having two layers, epidermis and dermis, derived from ectoderm and mesoderm, respectively. The earliest epidermis is represented by a single layer of cells. During the 4th week, the epidermis becomes bilaminar, consisting of an inner stratum basale (stratum germinativum) and an outer periderm. An intermediate layer or stratum intermedium is added in the 3rd month. It arises through mitotic activity of the stratum basale and eventually becomes several layers thick. The multilayered epidermis of fetal skin illustrates the tendency of ectoderm to stratify.

Glycogen is the chief component of undifferentiated epidermal cells and is present in the primordial cells of hair follicles and eccrine sweat glands. In contrast, adult epidermis contains little glycogen, although large amounts appear after injury and in skin grafts. The quantity of glycogen in cells of the fetal epidermis reflects their degree of cellular proliferation and differentiation. Glycogen is an energy source that is depleted as the epidermis differentiates, keratinizes, and specializes. It diminishes or disappears from epidermal cells in the following order and under the condition noted: (1) basal cells as they proliferate, (2) primordial germ cells as they differentiate, (3) periderm cells as they regress, and (4) intermediate cells as they differentiate. Glycogen is synthesized from glucose that is absorbed from amniotic fluid at a time when the glucose concentration is high in the fluid and the periderm cells contain the enzyme, alkaline phosphatase, that aids in glucose absorption. The enzyme, amylophosphorylase, catalyzes glycogen synthesis by the epidermal cells.

There are regional differences in the time of onset and rate of skin development. It is no longer accurate to state that epidermal development is always more advanced cephalically than caudally and that development procedes ventrally from the midaxillary line. Instead, the epidermis of the digits and head definitely show the most advanced development, and only hair follicle differentiation and hair eruption have a wave-like cephalocaudal progression. It is uncertain if regional differences exist in dermal differentiation. The dermis, however, profoundly influences the epidermis, and without the dermis, the epidermis does not divide, differentiate, or maintain its normal orientation.

The periderm is the transient, outermost layer of the epidermis which appears in the 1st month and is retained until the 7th month when it is shed into the amniotic fluid. This epithelium that is unique to fetal development arises from cells of the stratum basale. Once formed, the cells are self-sustaining through mitotic activity of their own until they begin to regress in the 6th month. Although regional differences are encountered, the cells are flat in the 1st month and somewhat elevated in the 2nd month. A single protrusion usually occupies the center of each cell in the 3rd month and part of the 4th month; multiple protrusions are frequently present on individual cells during the 4th, 5th and 6th months.

The free surface of periderm cells in contact with the amniotic fluid is lined by microvilli and coated with acid carbohydrates (glycosaminoglycans). The cells are glycogen-rich but contain few organelles, and these are usually restricted to the peripheral and perinuclear cytoplasm. Keratohyaline granules are absent. Periderm cells are attached to each other and to cells of the intermediate layer through numerous desmosomes.

The periderm reaches its highest degree of morphological development in the 16th week. The main function of the periderm is believed to be for the exchange of substances between the fetus and amniotic fluid. Many other functions have been postulated. The periderm begins to regress when epidermal differentiation intensifies with the eruption of lanugo hair and the formation of the stratum corneum. The periderm then undergoes atypical cornification to become a layer of flattened squames with a filamentous internal structure. The fact that intact periderm cells can be identified in amniotic fluid as late as term gives an idea of the continued structural stability of these cells after they have regressed and have been cast-off.

The stratum intermedium arises through mitotic activity of cells in the stratum basale and is present as a single layer of cells in the 2nd month. Additional cell layers appear in the 3rd and 4th months. They contain tonofilaments which are particularly abundant in the peripheral cytoplasm near the numerous desmosomal attachments. Because of the paucity of organelles, the cytoplasm would appear empty if it were not packed with glycogen. Glycogen is retained longer in cells of the stratum intermedium than in cells of the periderm or stratum basale. The intermediate layer gives rise to the strata spinosum, granulosum, and corneum.

The stratum corneum consists of dead cells produced by keratinization, a process that is similar in the fetus and adult. Signs of keratinization are present about the 20th week with the appearance of the stratum granulosum. Development of the stratum corneum is preceded by keratinization of the hair canals in that region. Hair canals of the scalp are the first to keratinize (15th week) and the process then continues in a cephalocaudal direction. A thin stratum corneum is present on much of the fetal epidermis by the 7th month and persists until birth as 4–6 layers of cornified cells. The stratum corneum is watertight and provides most of the mechanical strength for the epidermis. The viable strata of the epidermis by comparison are relatively permeable and mechanically weak. The stratum corneum protects the newborn against dessication.

The stratum basale gives rise to the periderm, stratum intermedium, and epithelial germ cells for hair follicles and eccrine sweat glands. Hair and sweat gland primordia are first recognizable as circumscribed proliferations of basal cells that grow into the dermis. Each primordium is a biological unit which grows by mitoses of its own cells and penetrates downward through the dermis and upward through the epidermis to the surface. An interaction of ectoderm and mesoderm is necessary for growth and differentiation of each epithelial germ. Cells of the stratum basale and the basal cells that give rise to the epithelial germs are the first epidermal cells to deplete most of their glycogen and to attain mature features similar to those in corresponding cells of adult skin. These features are manifested near the end of the 1st trimester when the basal cells begin to give rise to the epithelial germs for hair follicles.

The hair germ (pilar complex) begins as a proliferation of basal cells which soon extends into the mesenchyme. Each hair germ is the primordium for a hair follicle, sebaceous gland, and, in some instances, an apocrine sweat gland. The hair germ also provides the attachment site for the arrector pili muscle of the pilosebaceous unit. The glands and attachment site for the muscle are first represented as cellular bulges on the hair follicle (apocrine gland, sebaceous gland, and muscle named in order from highest to lowest on the hair follicle). Hair germs first appear in the 9th week in the regions of the eyebrows, upper lip, and chin, and grow obliquely as "hair pegs" downward into the dermis. General development of hair begins in the 4th month on the face and scalp and then extends caudally over the remainder of the body. Hair follicles are arranged in patterns, usually in groups of three. Their density decreases as body surface area increases, but postnatally there is no large-scale destruction of hair follicles or formation of new follicles.

"Anlagen" of sebaceous glands are first represented by solid, hemispherical extensions on the posterior surfaces of the hair pegs. The glands develop in all areas of the skin except the palms, soles, and dorsum of the feet. Sebaceous glands differentiate, enlarge, acquire the enzymes for lipid synthesis, and become functional in the fetus of 13–15 weeks of gestation. The duct of each gland forms where the gland takes origin from the hair follicle. In this area, the central cells degenerate and the peripheral cells become the stratified squamous epithelium that lines the duct.

Secretions of fetal sebaceous glands constitute a significant part of the vernix caseosa, defined as that variably adherent fetal skin surface film consisting of lipid from the sebaceous glands, lanugo hairs, epidermal cells, water, and other substances from the amniotic fluid. Sebaceous glands continue to be large and active in the newborn until the influence of maternal androgens have subsided. The glands then involute to their childhood state of immaturity and remain quiescent with only meager secretory activity until puberty.

Acne neonatum or infantile acne occasionally develops in infants and appears to result from hormonal stimulation of sebaceous glands that have not yet involuted. The retention of sebaceous material and keratin in the pilosebaceous units of the newborn causes milia, which appears as papules on the face of 40–50% of all infants. The papules disappear spontaneously and require no therapy.

Eccrine sweat gland germs develop in the palms and soles in the 4th month, in the axillae in the first part of the 5th month, and elsewhere in the latter part of the 5th month. They are smaller than hair germs. As the ends of eccrine germs reach the future junction of the dermis and subcutaneous connective tissue, they form secretory coils. The remainder of each germ is a solid eccrine duct rudiment, two layers thick, which forms its lumen by two methods. The intraepidermal portion of the duct is formed by the coalescence of groups of intracytoplasmic cavities within the inner layer of cells. The lumen in the intradermal portion of the duct is formed by the dissolution of desmosomes between the inner layer of cells. Eccrine secretory coils and ducts are patent by the end of the 2nd trimester. Eccrine glands do not produce sweat *in utero* or before 1 to 18 days postnatally; the inability of the newborn to dissipate heat by sweating is well-known. Failure to produce sweat at birth is probably due to the immaturity of the autonomic nerves to the glands. Apocrine sweat glands, unlike eccrine glands, are not well developed structurally in the neonate and do not undergo maximal development until after puberty.

The dermis (corium) is derived from the mesenchyme beneath the surface ectoderm, and the dermis and epidermis are mutually dependent for growth, differentiation, and function. Before the 3rd month, the dermis consists mostly of mesenchymal cells, ground substance, and plexuses of blood vessels. During the 3rd month, mesenchymal cells differentiate into active fibroblasts that produce ground substance and small collagenous fibers that are known as reticular fibers. Most of the small fibers increase in number and thickness to become bundles of collagenous fibers. Fibroblasts also produce the elastic fibers which appear in the reticular layer of the dermis about the 22nd week. Most elastic fibers, however, develop after birth.

Due to differences in size and arrangement of the collagenous fibers, the dermis in the 5th month can be divided into papillary and reticular layers. As in adult skin, the papillary layer is just beneath the epidermis. It is more cellular and vascular and consists of smaller collagenous fibers than found in the deeper and larger reticular layer of the dermis.

In addition to active fibroblasts, there are other cell types in the dermis, all of which can be identified by the 14th week. These include inactive fibroblasts, macrophages, mast cells, Langerhans cells, melanocytes and melanoblasts, Merkel cells, Schwann cells, and pericytes. Schwann cells are associated with nerves, and pericytes with blood vessels. Mesenchymal cells give rise to pericytes and endothelial cells, and in the 4th month to fat cells. Some macrophages in the fetal dermis are derived from monocytes.

Three cell types in the dermis pass into the epidermis where they reside as immigrant cells. These cells are the dendritic melanocytes and Langerhans cells, and the non-dendritic Merkel cells. Both types of dendritic cells are present in the epidermis at 6 weeks. A great influx of dendritic cells occurs in the latter part of the first trimester with melanoblasts migrating from the neural crest, and Langerhans cells coming from mesenchyme. Langerhans cells have characteristic granules. At 12 weeks, active melanocytes with premelanosomes and melanosomes are common in the basal layer of the epidermis and in the developing hair follicles. By the 5th month, melanocytes have reached about the same number as in adult skin. At that time, they develop dendritic processes and some begin the limited synthesis and transfer of melanin to keratinocytes. All immigrant cells are present in the epidermis with the appearance at 16 weeks of the Merkel cell in the finger tips, nail beds, and glabrous skin. The Merkel cell is the only immigrant cell that forms desmosomes with adjacent keratinocytes, and hemidesmosomes with the basal lamina. Neural crest seems to be the source of Merkel cells; they are possibly modified Schwann cells and are presumed to function as receptors for certain touch stimuli.

References

Breathnach, A. S. Embryology of human skin. J. Invest. Dermatol. 57: 133–143, 1971.

Breathnach, A. S. Development and differentiation of dermal cells in man. J. Invest. Dermatol. 71: 2–8, 1978.

Breathnach, A. S., and L. M. Wyllie. Fine structure of cells forming the surface layer of the epidermis in human fetuses at fourteen and twelve weeks. 45: 179–189, 1965.

Hashimoto, K., B. G. Gross, R. J. DiBella, and W. F. Lever. The ultrastructure of the skin of human embryos. J. Invest. Dermatol. 47: 317–335, 1966.

Holbrook, K. A. Human epidermal embryogenesis. Int. J. Dermatol. 18: 329–356, 1979.

Holbrook, K. A. A histological comparison of infant and adult skin. *In: Neonatal Skin.* H. I. Maibach and E. K. Boisits, eds., Marcel Dekker, Inc., New York and Basel, 1982, p. 3–29.

Holbrook, K. A., and G. F. Odland. Structure of the human fetal hair canal and initial hair eruption. J. Invest. Dermatol. 71: 385–390, 1978.

Holbrook, K. A., and L. T. Smith. Utrastructural aspects of human skin during the embryonic, fetal, premature, neonatal, and adult periods of life. *IN: Morphogenesis and Malformation of the Skin.* R. J. Blandau, ed., Birth Defects: Original Article Series 17: 9–38, 1981.

Hoyes, A. D. Electron microscopy of the surface layer (periderm) of human fetal skin. J. Anat. 103: 321–336, 1968.

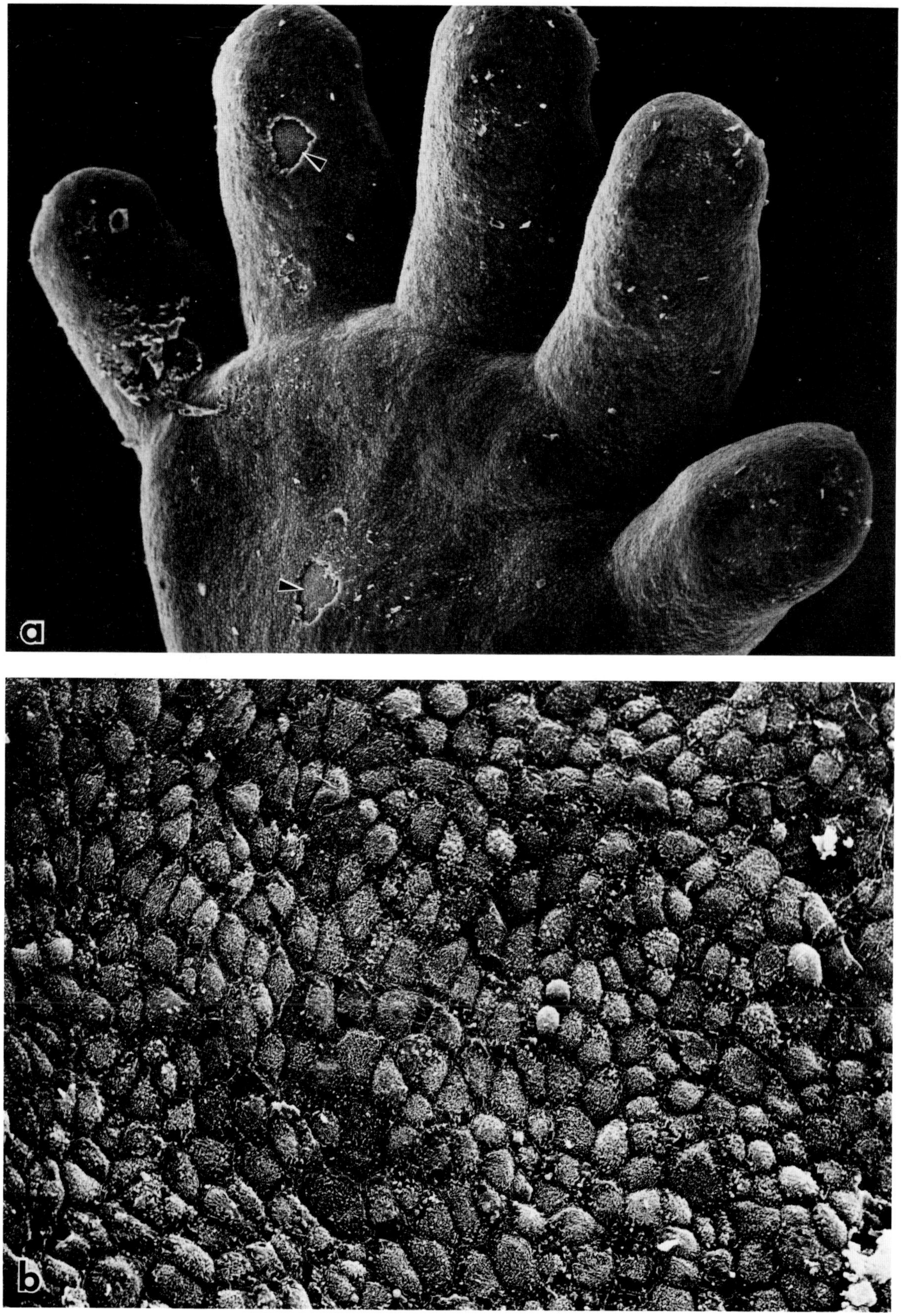

Figure 2–1. Right hand, 6.5 weeks.

a. *The digits are clearly defined and can be numbered one to five with the thumb considered as the first finger. The epidermis consists of two layers, a superficial periderm and a deep basal layer. The basal layer is visible (arrows) where the fragile periderm has been lost from the palm and fourth finger. The flakes of debris on the periderm are from the amniotic fluid. ×70.*

b. *Higher magnification of the periderm of the palm shows outlines of individual cells whose central portions protrude slightly. Microvilli give the exposed surface a "velvety" appearance. The earliest periderm cells are rather flat, squamous cells with tiny microvilli. ×360.*

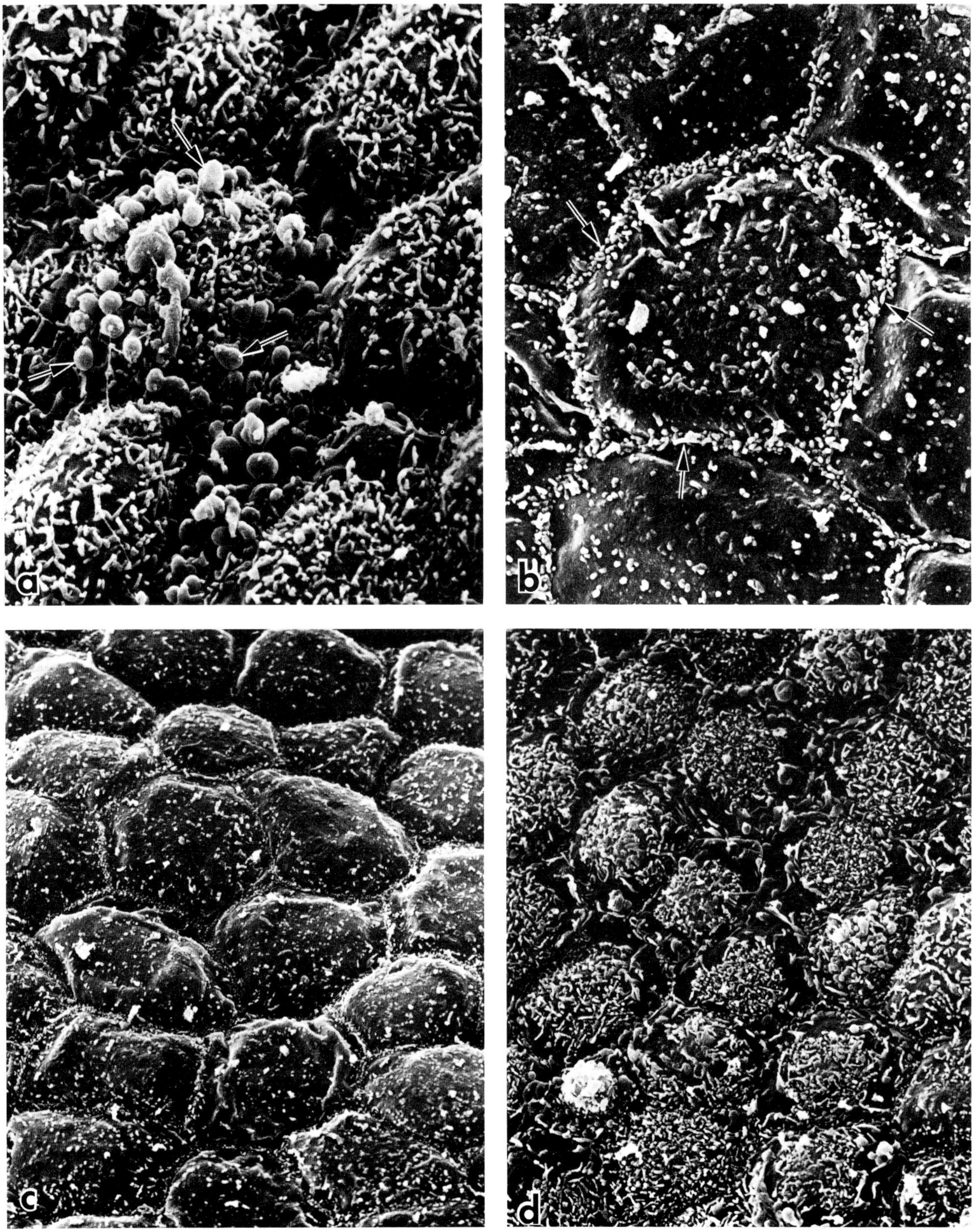

Figure 2–2. Periderm of hand, 6.5 weeks.

a. *Blebs (arrows) and small microvilli suggest that the periderm, as the external layer of the skin, might be involved in the uptake of materials from the amniotic fluid and/or the release of products into the amniotic fluid.* $\times$ *4,630.*

b. *There are fewer microvilli and blebs on the periderm of the fingers than on the thicker epidermis of the palms. Microvilli (arrows) are concentrated at boundaries between adjacent cells.* $\times$ *4,630.*

c. *Lower magnification shows the hexagonal outlines of the periderm cells of the fingers with microvilli in the depressions between individual cells.* $\times$ *1,850.*

d. *This micrograph illustrates the large number of microvilli and blebs on the periderm of the palm. Regional differences in the density of microappendages are found during human skin development.* $\times$ *2,315.*

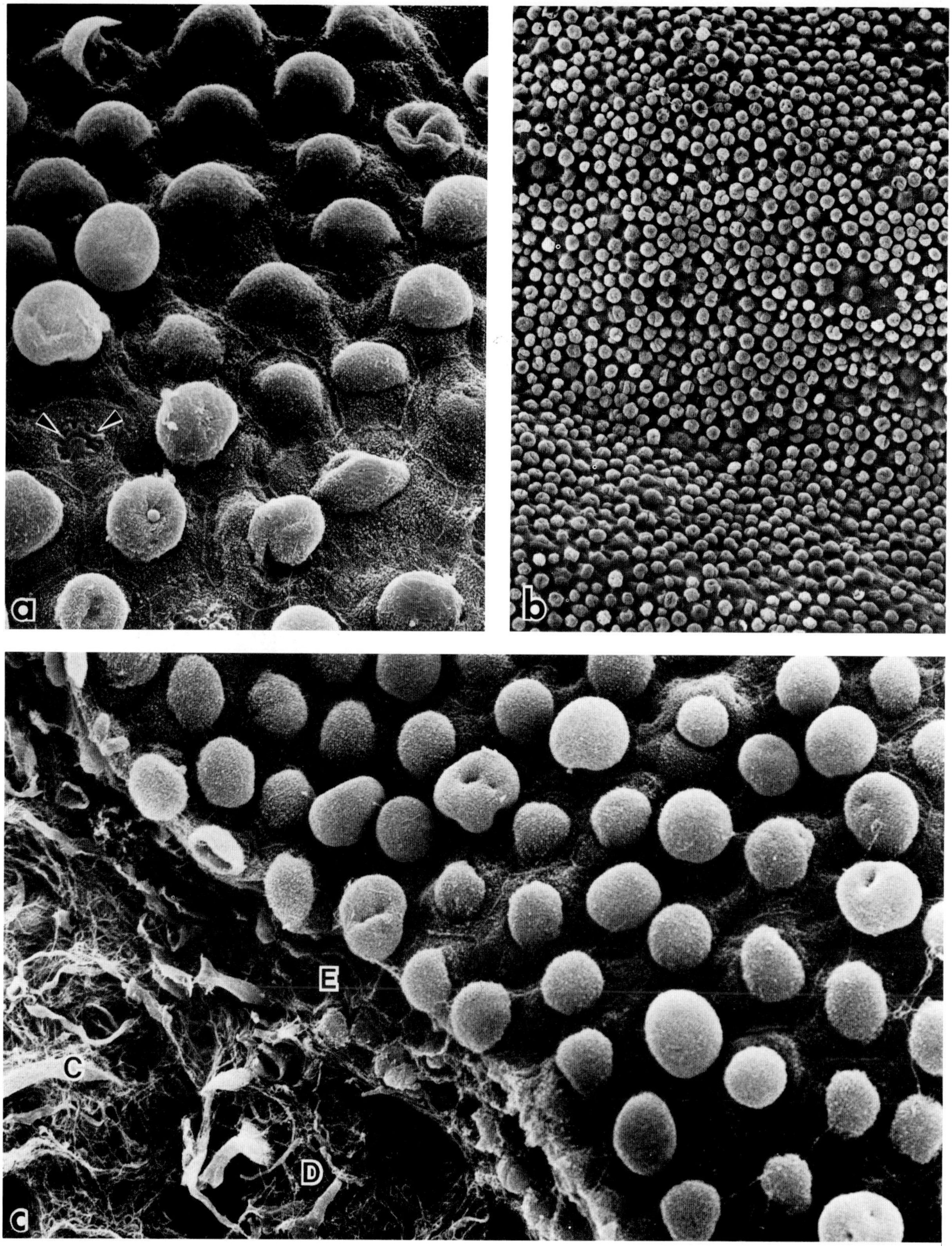

Figure 2–3. Abdominal skin (a) and scalp (b and c), 16.5 weeks.

a. *Abdominal skin with prominent protrusion near center of each periderm cell. Cell boundaries of the polygonal cells are distinct. A porous area (arrows) indicates where a protrusion has detached. LM and TEM observations on fetal skin reveal that glycogen is a major component of the protrusions.* $\times$*935.*

b. *Protrusions of the periderm are especially numerous on the scalp at this stage of development as shown at low magnification in this micrograph. The density of protrusions may be related to the abundance and rapid development of the hairs, sebaceous glands, and sweat glands of the scalp.* $\times$*95.*

c. *Scalp, depicting protrusions of periderm cells, the 3 to 4 layers of epidermal cells (E) beneath the periderm, and the meshwork of connective tissue in the dermis (D). Most connective tissue fibers are young collagenous fibers which are also called reticular fibers. Some collagenous fibers (C) are larger and more mature than others.* $\times$*755.*

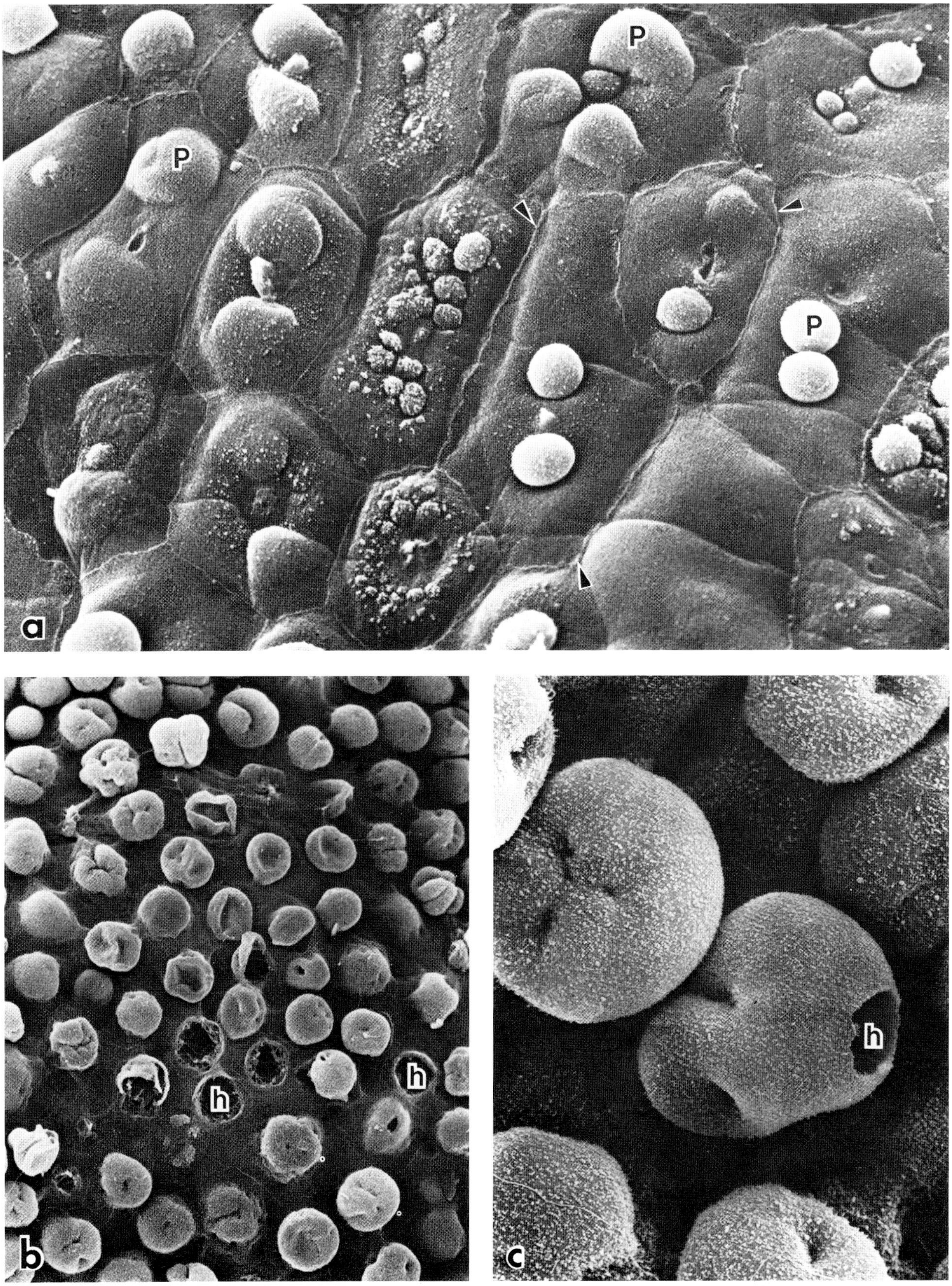

Figure 2–4. Scalp, 16 weeks (a and c); Abdominal skin, 16.5 weeks (b).

a. *Multiple protrusions (P) are present on each of the periderm cells and the cells are separated by distinct boundaries (arrows). As shown in previous micrographs, the periderm is at first flat. The flat stage is followed by a stage in which a cell has a single protrusion, and then by a stage in which a cell has multiple protrusions.* ×*1,325.*

b. *Holes (h) mark sites where protrusions of periderm have been lost.* ×*480.*

c. *The "velvety" appearance and holes (h) associated with protrusions of scalp periderm are illustrated at higher magnification. A protrusion measures about 7 μm at its most expanded portion and often narrows to make a stalk-like connection with the cell surface.* ×*1,915.*

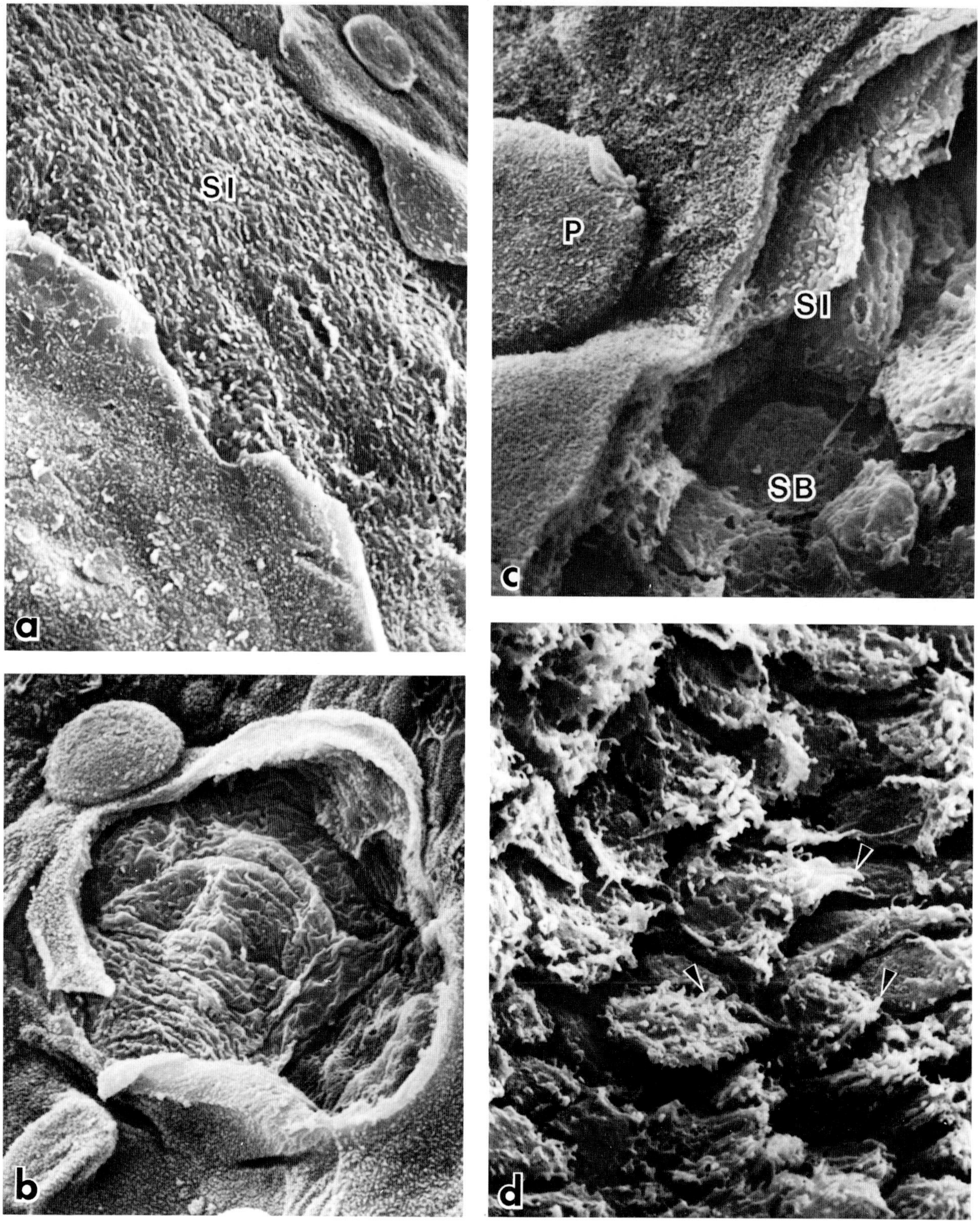

Figure 2–5. Abdominal skin, 14 weeks.

a. *The break in the periderm near center of micrograph has exposed the upper surface of cells in the stratum intermedium (SI).* $\times$ *3,450.*

b. *The break depicted in the lower picture of the first column measures about 25 μm in diameter and typifies a common type of defect in the periderm. The flat portion of the periderm cell at the site of the break measures only 1.2 μm in thickness.* $\times$ *2,760.*

c. *The layers of the epidermis are shown in a terraced-like fashion. Observe the periderm protrusions (P), the stratum basale (SB) with its single layer of basal cells, and the stratum intermedium (SI) which varies from 2 to 3 cells in thickness.* $\times$ *3,220.*

d. *The periderm and stratum intermedium have been removed to expose the apices of cells in the stratum basale. Basal cells have spinous processes (arrows) which are most numerous on their upper surfaces where the cells attach by desmosomes to cells of the intermediate layer.* $\times$ *3,310.*

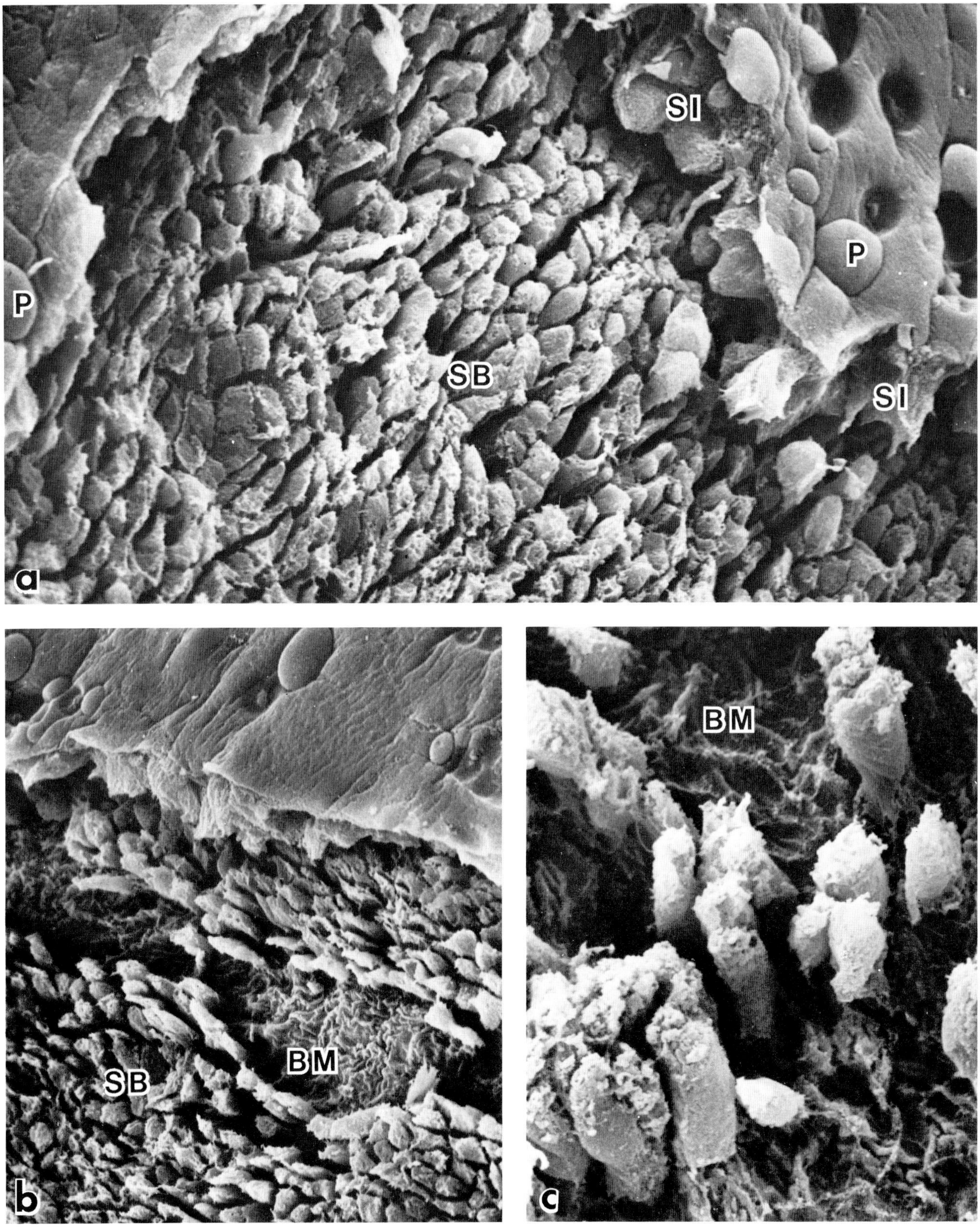

Figure 2–6. Abdominal skin, 14 weeks.

a. *The stratum basale (SB) is revealed beneath the torn periderm with its protrusions (P) and the stratum intermedium (SI). As in adult skin, cells of the stratum basale are mitotically active. They divide and give rise to cells of the intermediate layer, and are the source of all future keratin-producing cells, the keratinocytes. Many melanocytes from the neural crest have entered the basal layer of the epidermis by the 14th week.* × *1,120.*

b. *The stratum basale (SB) and ruffled basement membrane (BM) are shown beneath the periderm and stratum intermedium.* × *830.*

c. *Higher magnification of the basement membrane (BM) and cells of the stratum basale. The latter are columnar cells which attach to the basement membrane. Flocculent material is associated with the spinous processes of the cell apices.* × *1,875.*

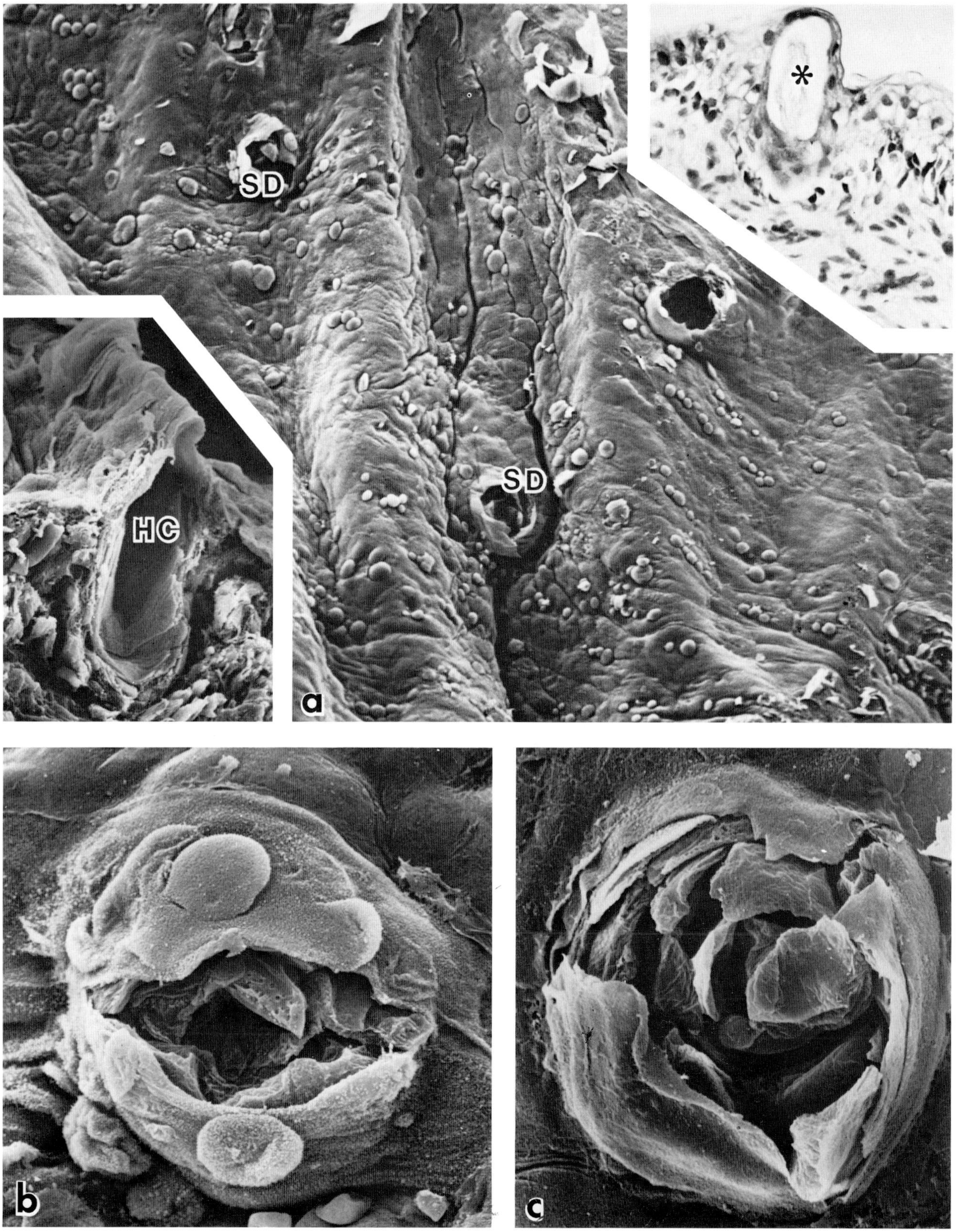

Figure 2–7. Abdominal skin, 14 weeks.

a. *The epidermal ridges are covered by periderm. They are produced by linearly arranged intraepidermal hair canals. Sweat ducts (SD) open between the epidermal ridges.* × 265.

Inset *at lower left shows lumen of hair canal (HC). The lumen is lined by several layers of flattened cells. Cells of the hair canal are the first to keratinize in fetal skin.* × 725.

Inset *at upper right shows another hair canal (*) in an H&E stained paraffin section of 16 weeks old fetal skin.* × 280.

b. *and* c. *Elevated openings of sweat ducts between epidermal ridges.* × 1,410.

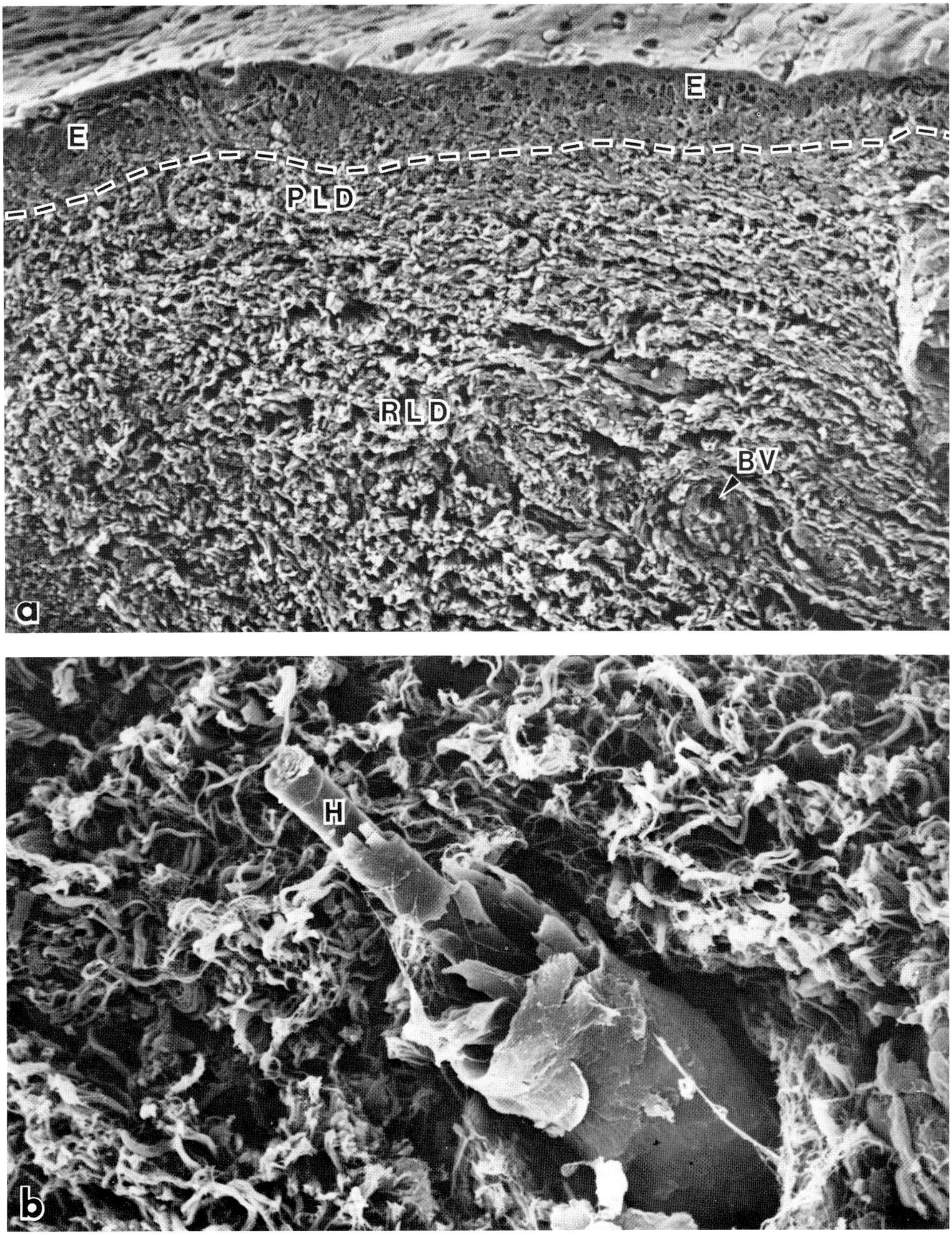

Figure 2–8. Abdominal skin, 14 weeks.
a. *Broken line represents the thin basement membrane area that separates epidermis and dermis. The epidermis (E) varies in thickness from about 8.5 μm to 10.5 μm. The dermis can be divided into a superficial layer and a deep layer. The superficial layer is the future papillary layer of the dermis (PLD), and the deep layer is the future reticular layer of the dermis (RLD). Dermal papillae are not present, and the dermal-epidermal junction is relatively even. Blood vessels (BV) are surrounded by dermal connective tissue. ×300.*

b. *Hair (H) in dermis, showing layers of cells surrounding hair which appear to be flat and keratinized. ×1,065.*

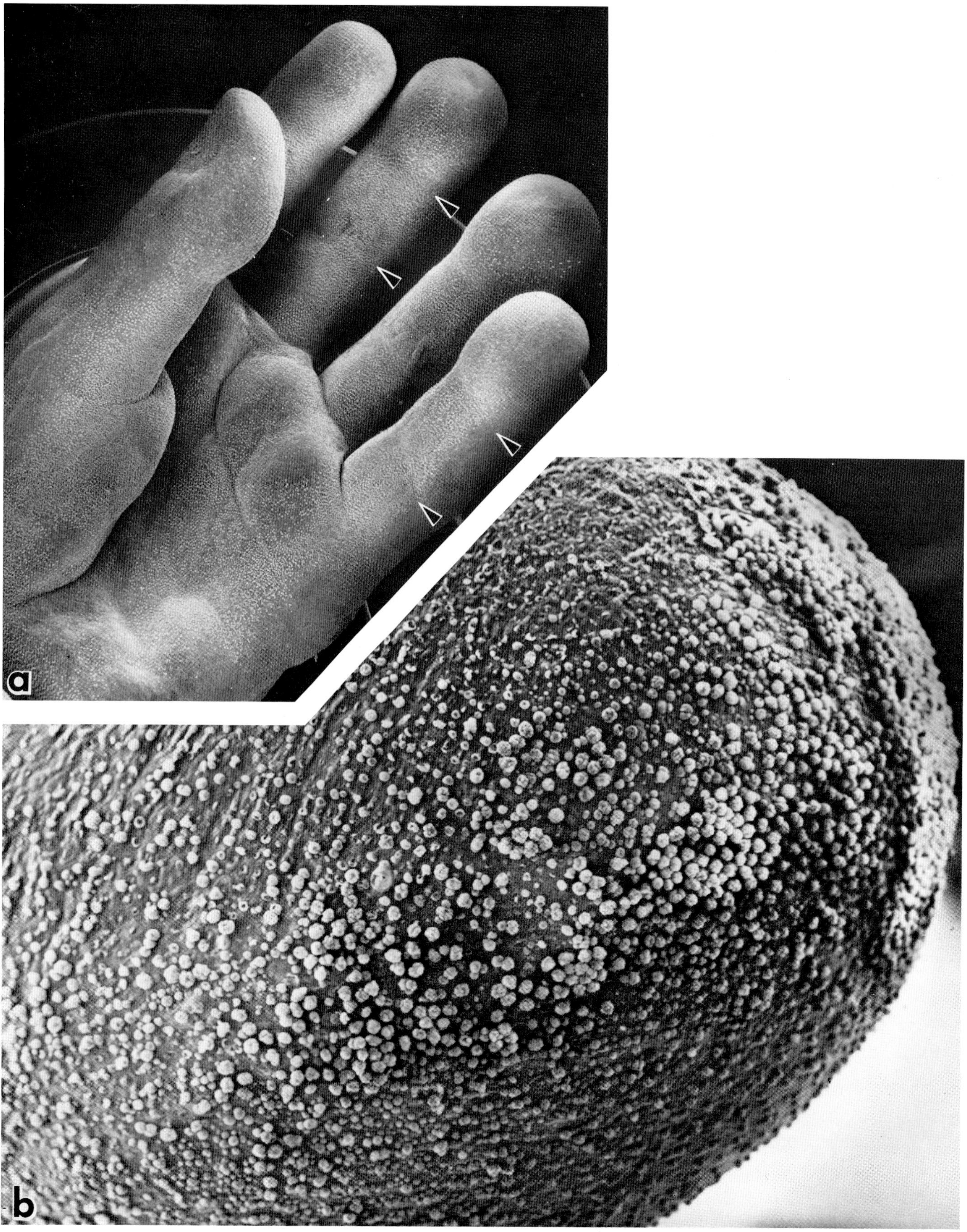

Figure. 2–9. Left hand, 16.5 weeks.

a. *Protrusions of periderm give the surface a stippled appearance. The creases (arrows) that separate the phalanges of the fingers are well defined and two flexure lines are present in the palm. The main creases of the hand appear early in fetal life and are not caused by movements of the digits. The thumb is known as the pollex, the second finger as the index finger, the third as the middle finger, the fourth as the ring finger, and the fifth as the little finger. As in the adult, the third finger projects farther distally than the second or fourth fingers (these two may be equal in length), and all three project farther than the little finger. ×20.*

b. *Periderm protrusions on the ventral surface of the thumb's distal phalanx are shown at higher magnification. ×1,120.*

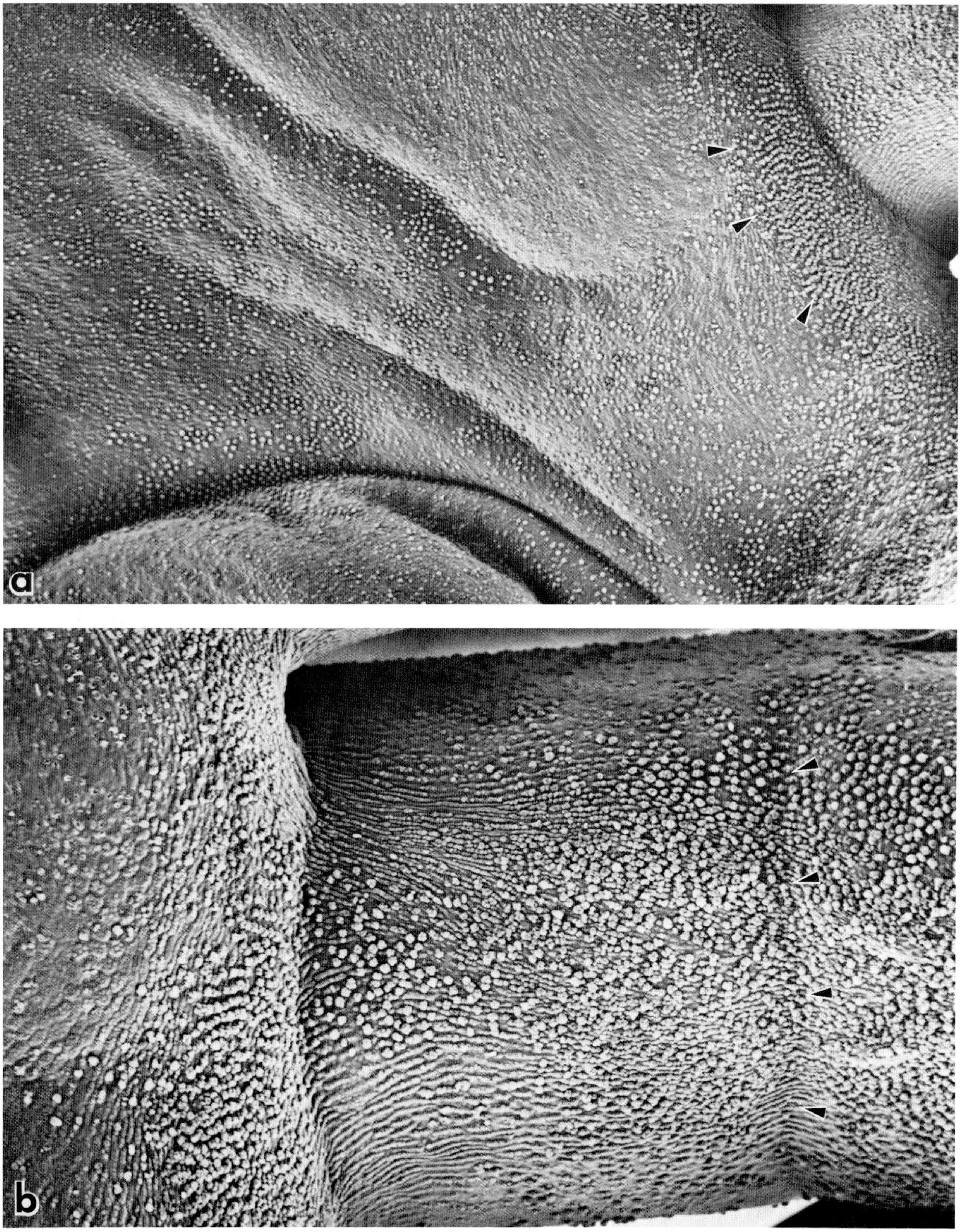

Figure 2–10. Palm of right hand, 16.5 weeks.

a. *Periderm protrusions vary in number in different regions of the palm. They are most numerous at the junction of the hand and fingers (arrows). There are fewer protrusions at other sites, such as the origin of the thumb (lower left) and on the elevated pads of the palm. × 40.*

b. *Part of the ventral surface of the third finger, showing the continuity between hand and finger. Note crease (arrows between proximal and middle phalanges. Small, longitudinal ridges and grooves, the papillary ridges and grooves (arrows), begin at the junction of finger and hand and course distally as they do on fingers of the adult. × 70.*

The distal phalanx is not shown, but it has complex papillary ridges that form the basis for identification by fingerprints (dermatoglyphics). The pattern of papillary ridges is established by the end of the fourth month and remains constant throughout the remainder of gestation and postnatal life.

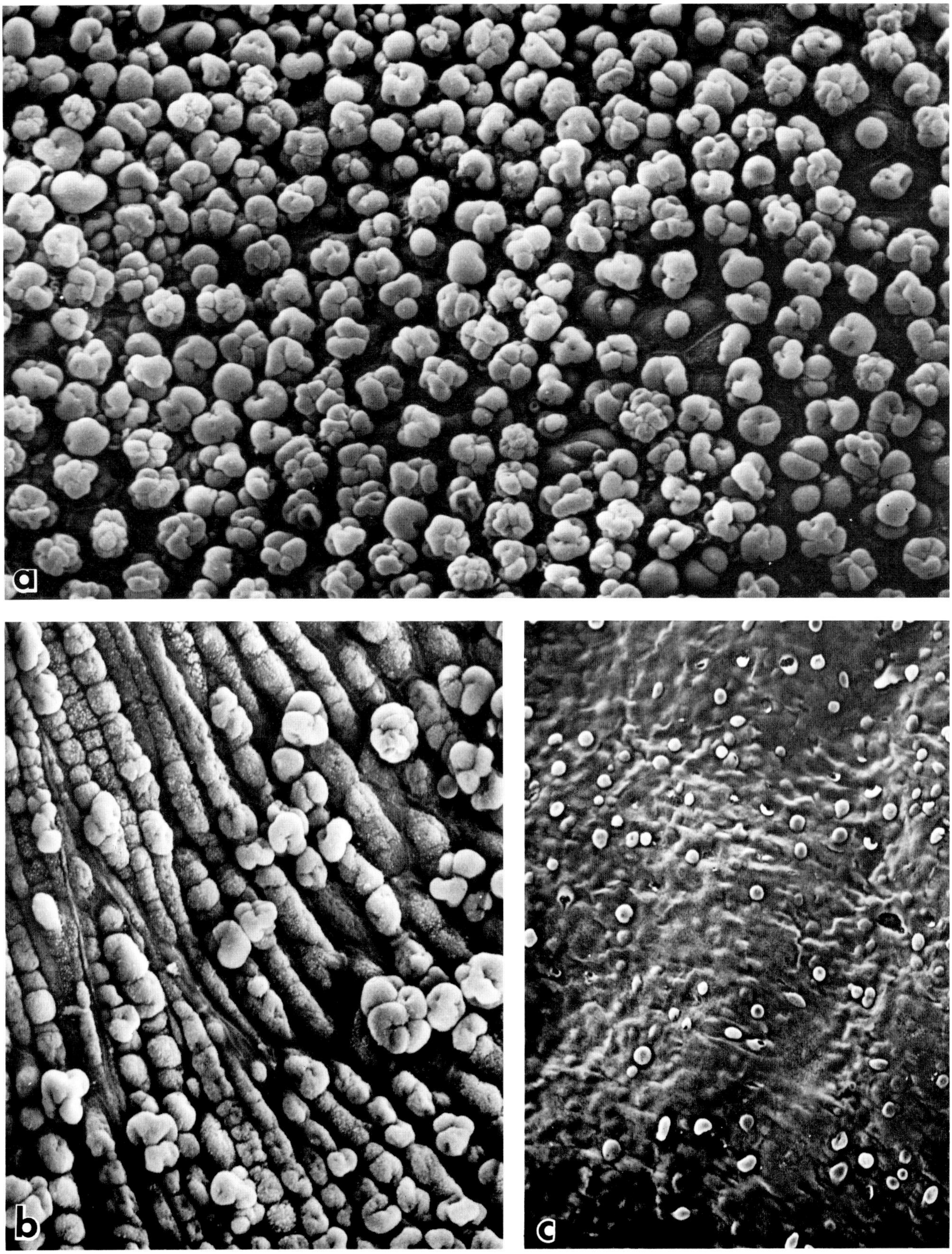

Figure 2–11. Periderm of left hand, 16.5 weeks.

a. *Thenar eminence (ball of thumb) is shown at a developmental stage when periderm protrusions are especially numerous.* ×345.

b. *Observe the longitudinal ridges and grooves of the periderm on the ventral surface of the first (proximal) phalanx of the third finger.* ×465.

c. *Dorsum of hand where periderm protrusions are far fewer in comparison to the number present on the thicker epidermis of the thenar eminence.* ×150.

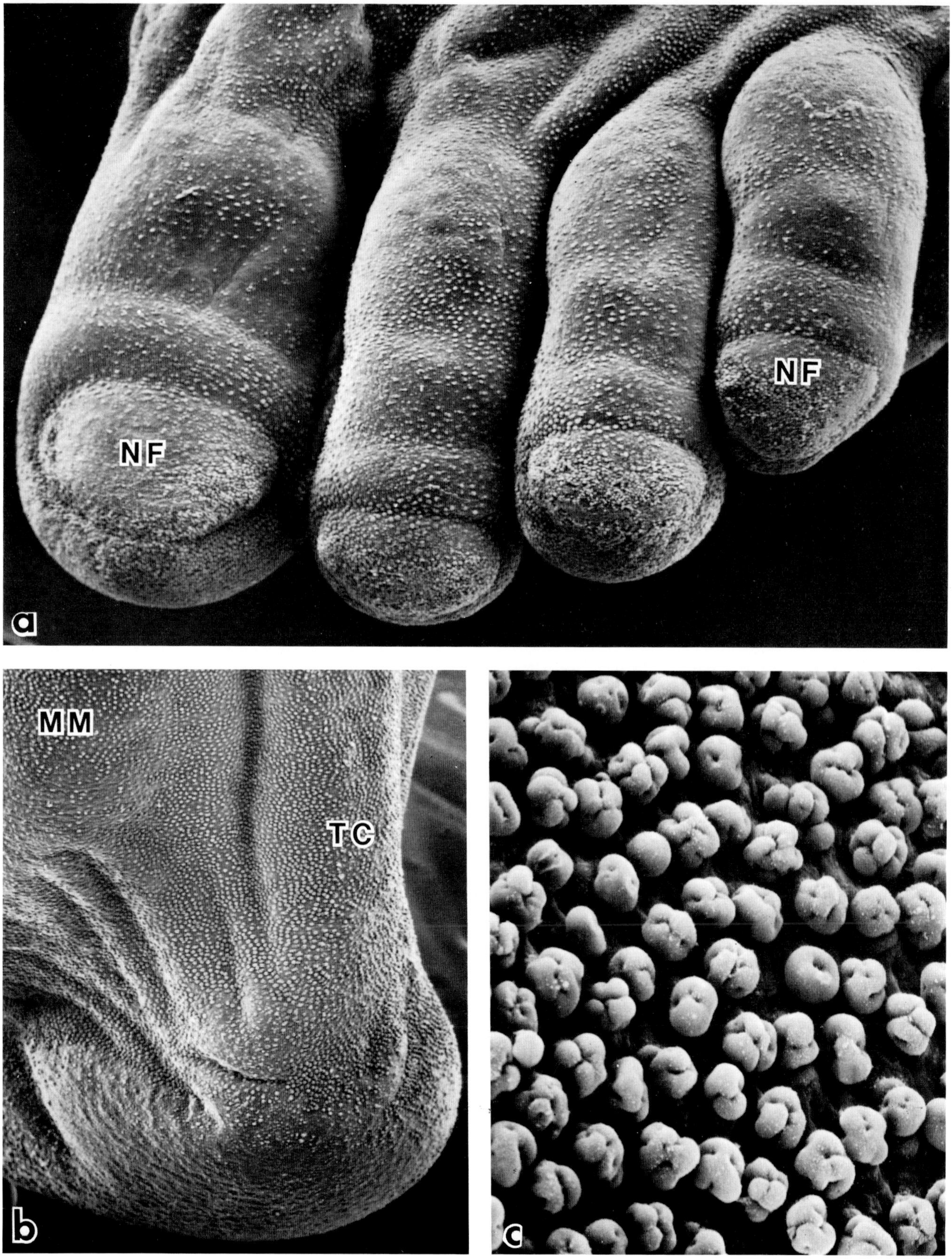

Figure 2–12. Toes and heel of left foot, 16.5 weeks.

a. *Periderm covers the toes which can be numbered one through five, beginning with the big toe or hallux. Part of the fifth (little) toe is hidden beneath the fourth toe. The nail field (NF) is an ectodermal thickening on each terminal phalanx where a nail will develop.* $\times 35$.

b. *Periderm overlies the bulges of the tendo calcaneus (TC), medial malleolus (MM), and heel.* $\times 30$.

c. *Higher magnification of junction of tendo calcaneus and heel, a site where periderm protrusions are abundant.* $\times 480$.

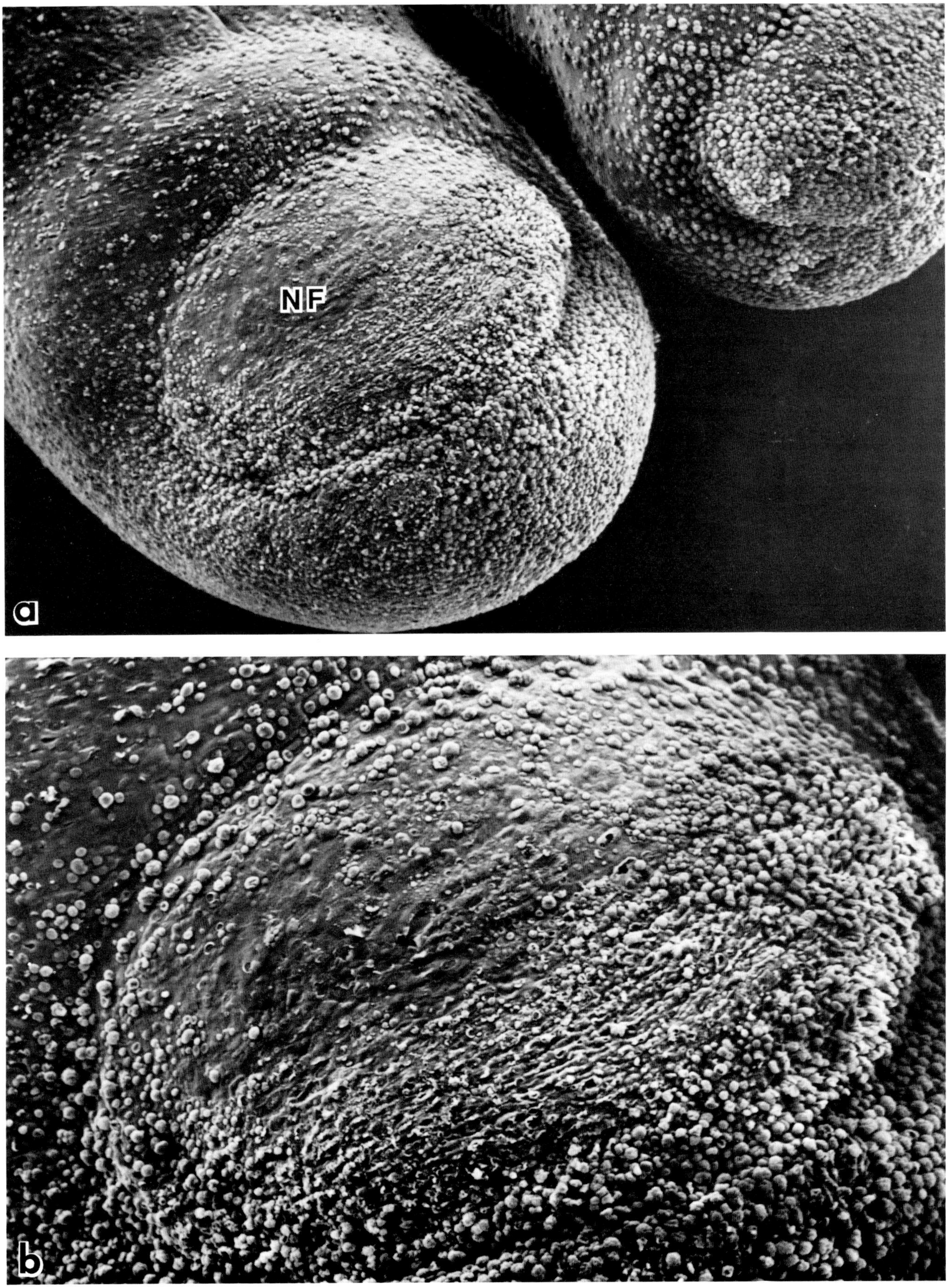

Figure 2–13. Big toe, 16.5 weeks.

a. *The nail field (NF) or site of the future nail does not extend to the tip of the toe. ×70.*

b. *The ectodermal thickening forming the nail field is viewed at higher magnification to show that the periderm protrusions are numerous along the margins of the field and sparse in its center. ×140.*

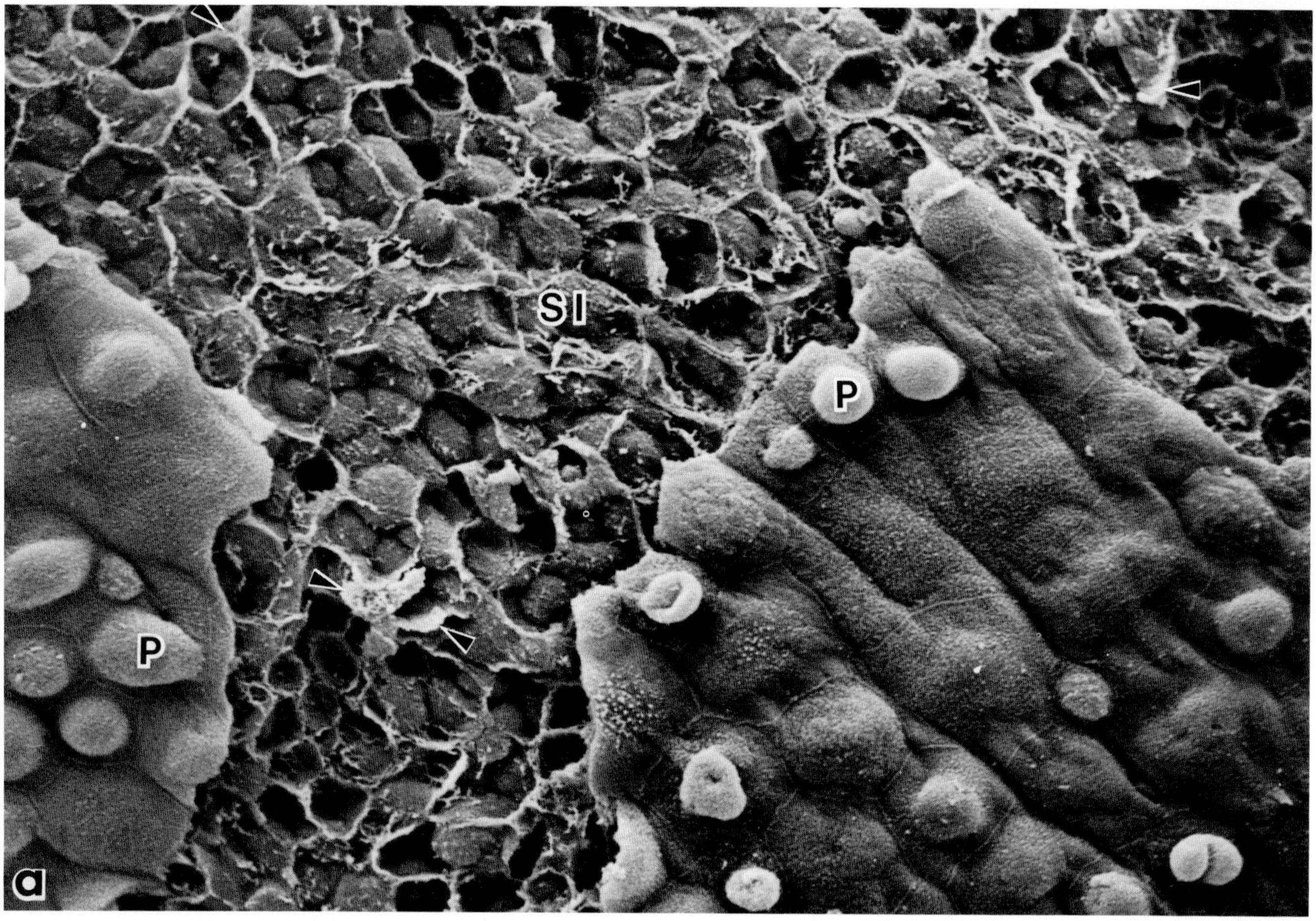

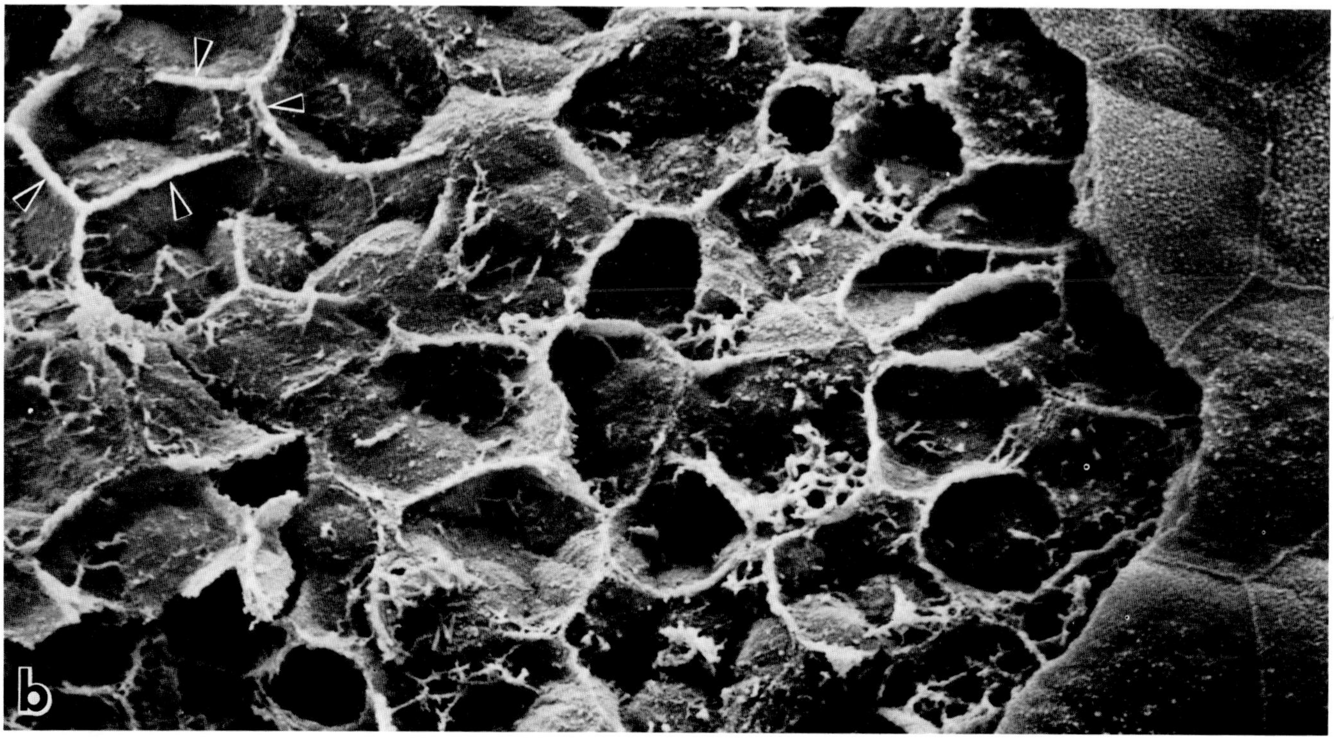

Figure 2–14. Skin of leg, 16.5 weeks.

a. *Most of the periderm has detached, revealing a broad expanse of the uppermost cells of the stratum intermedium (SI). The material (arrows) that is attached to the cells of the stratum intermedium represents remnants of periderm cells. The periderm in this picture has fewer protrusions (P) in comparison to the number shown in previous micrographs of the periderm of the hands, feet, and scalp at comparable stages of development.* × *1,100.*

b. *Periderm remnants (arrows) at higher magnification show the same hexagonal shape as the intact periderm cells at the right margin of micrograph.* × *2,125.*

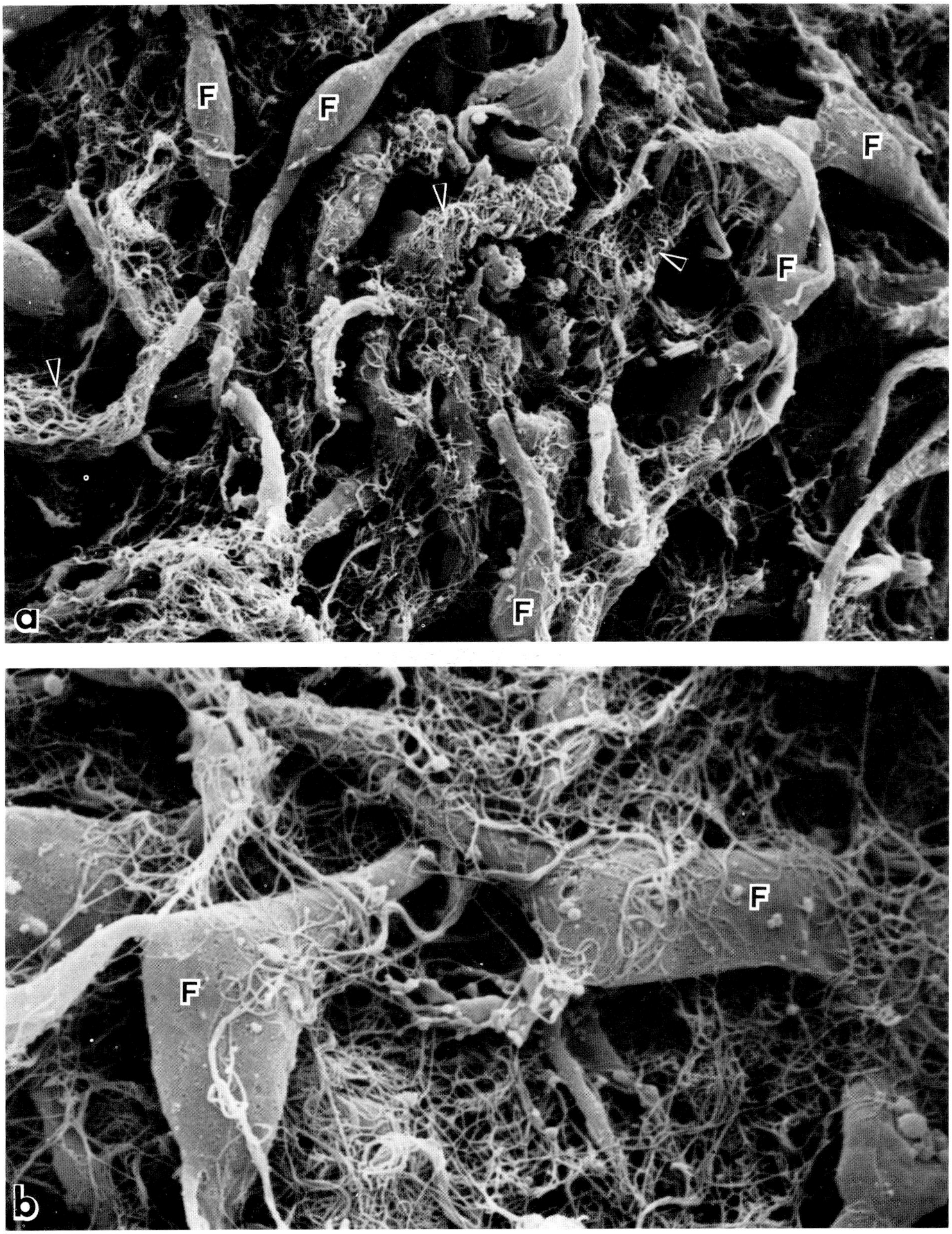

Figure 2–15. Dermis of leg, 16.5 weeks. The epidermis and basement membrane have been removed and the upper dermis is viewed "head on", rather than in profile.

a. *The spindle-shaped cells are active fibroblasts (F) which produce the fine, extracellular connective tissue fibers (arrows). The expanded portion of the fibroblast contains the nucleus. ×2,015.*

b. *At higher magnification, small connective tissue fibers appear to enmesh fibroblasts (F) and their processes. Because these fibers have carbohydrates on their surfaces, they can be stained by the periodic acid-Schiff technique and viewed by light microscopy. Traditionally, small and newly-formed PAS-positive fibers of this type have been called reticular fibers. ×4,000.*

Cells of the dermis can be viewed to best advantage by SEM when the epidermis and basement membrane are removed and one looks into the underlying network of fibers and cells. Such "head on" views, as shown in this figure, are superior to profiles which depict most dermal components in cross-section.

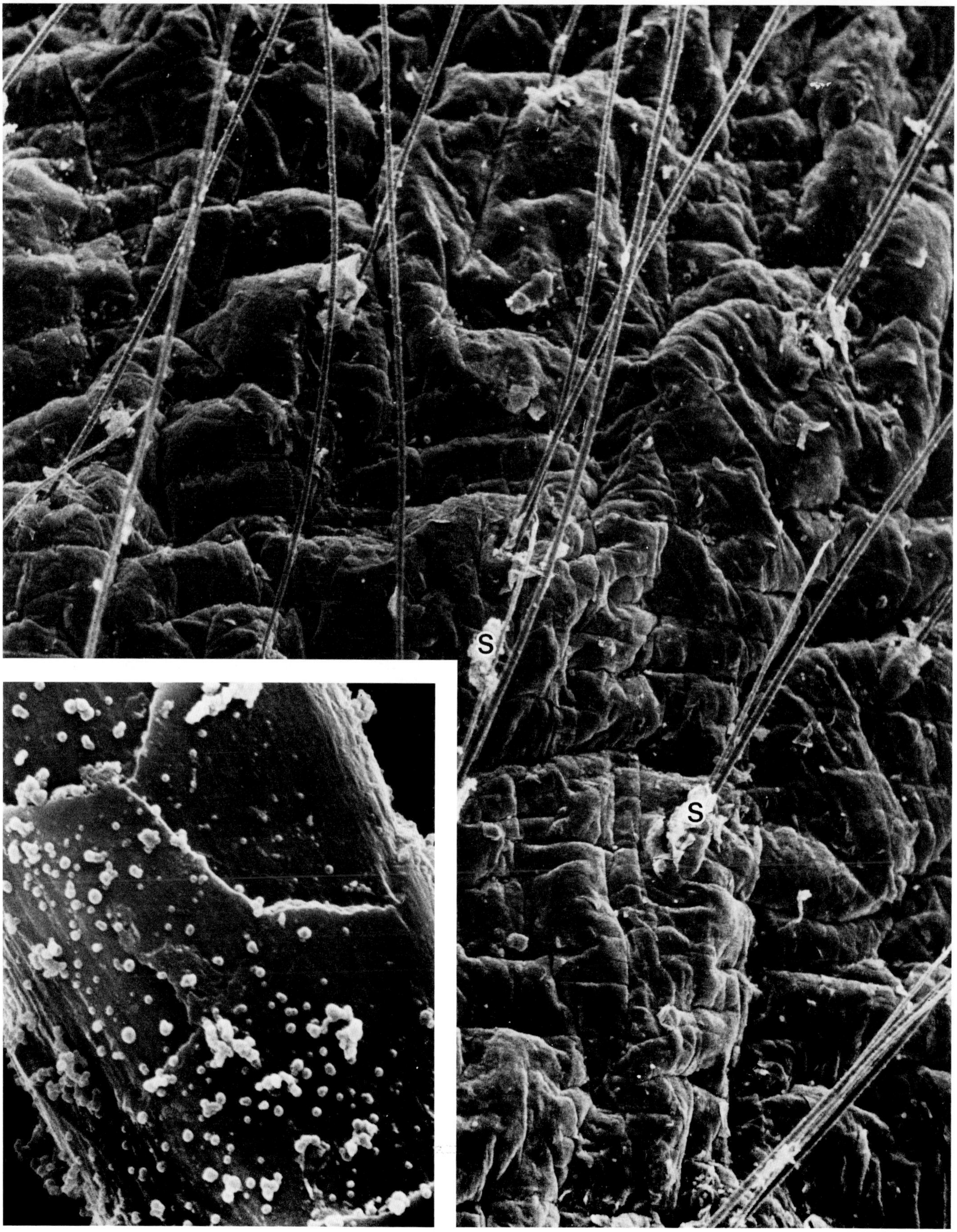

Figure 2–16. Abdominal skin, 24 weeks.

a. *The periderm has been shed and the epidermis is covered with keratinized cells which form the stratum corneum. Shafts of lanugo hairs project from the surface. Sebum (S), as part of the vernix caseosa, is present on the hairs, indicating that the sebaceous glands are functional.* ×*170.*

Inset *hair at higher magnification, depicting well-developed cuticular scales covered with sebum droplets.* ×*9,880.*

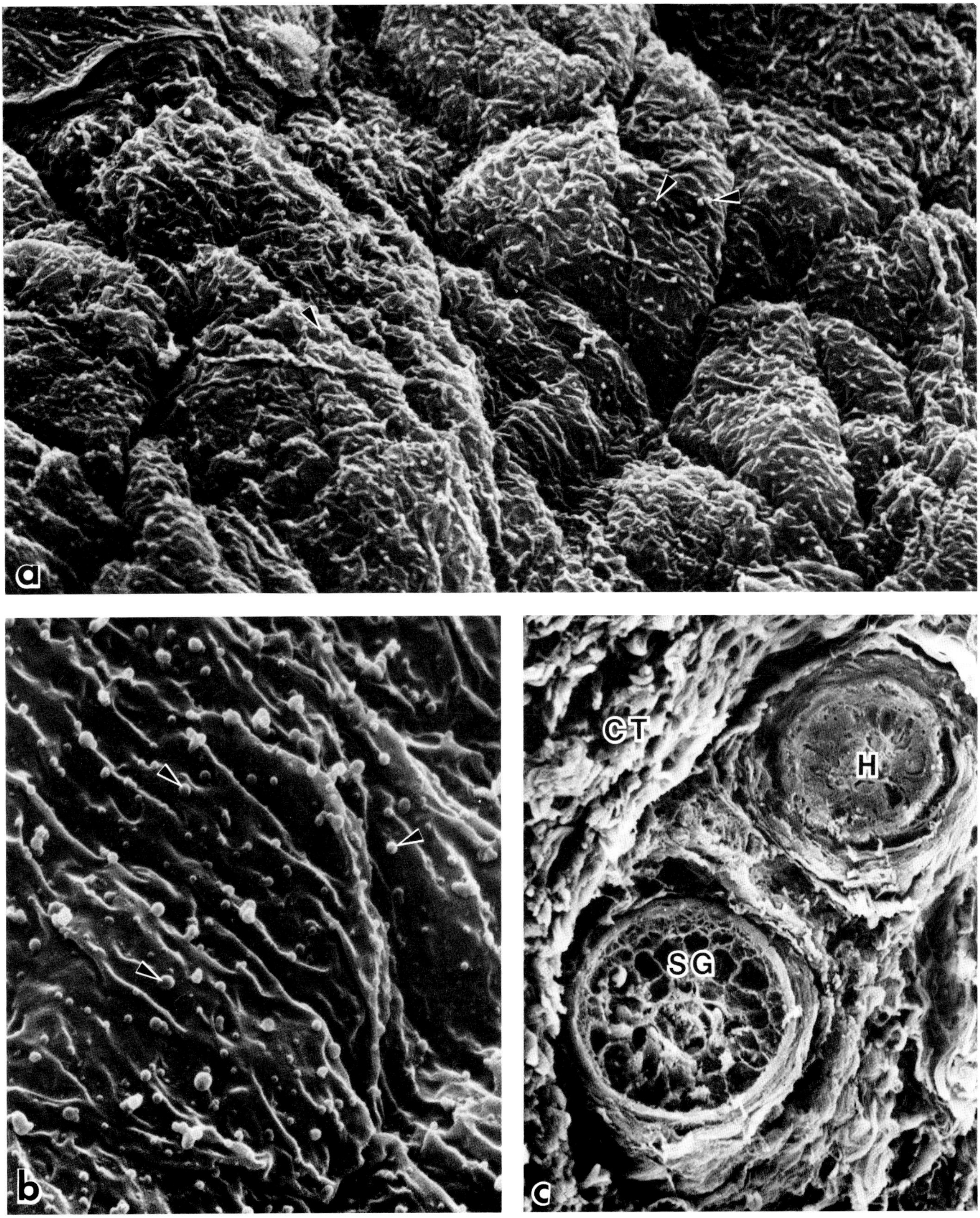

Figure 2–17. Abdominal skin, 24 weeks.

a. *The stratum corneum is thin, ruffled, and incompletely keratinized. Sebum droplets (arrows) are present; lanugo hairs are absent in the area shown. The uneven surface is produced by pressure resulting from growth of the underlying dermis.* ×4,600.

b. *Higher magnification of sebum droplets (arrows) on the ruffled, keratinized cells.* ×12,000.

c. *Connective tissue (CT) of dermis surrounds a small hair (H) and a sebaceous gland (SG). The droplets shown on the skin's surface in* a *and* b *are products of sebaceous glands.* ×830.

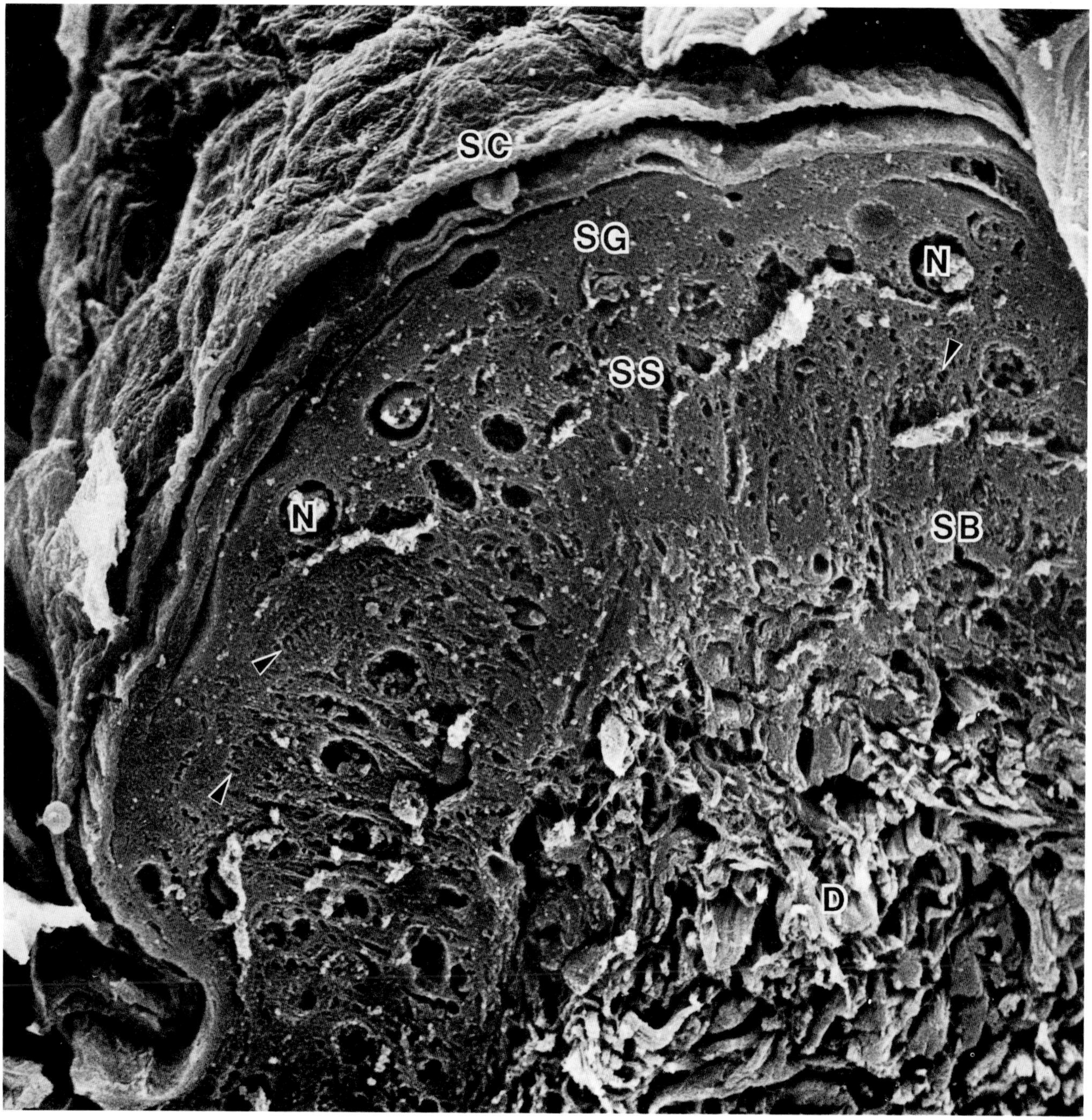

Figure 2–18. Profile of abdominal skin, 28 weeks.

The epidermis has all the layers found in adult skin, including the stratum basale (SB), stratum spinosum (SS), stratum granulosum (SG), and stratum corneum (SC). The epidermis is about 45 μm thick. The thickest layer is the stratum spinosum in which some spinous processes (arrows) are visible even at this low magnification. Four to five layers of flat, keratinized cells comprise the stratum corneum. A few of the uppermost cells are in the process of desquamation. Nucleus (N) of keratinocyte; connective tissue of dermis (D). × 1,840.

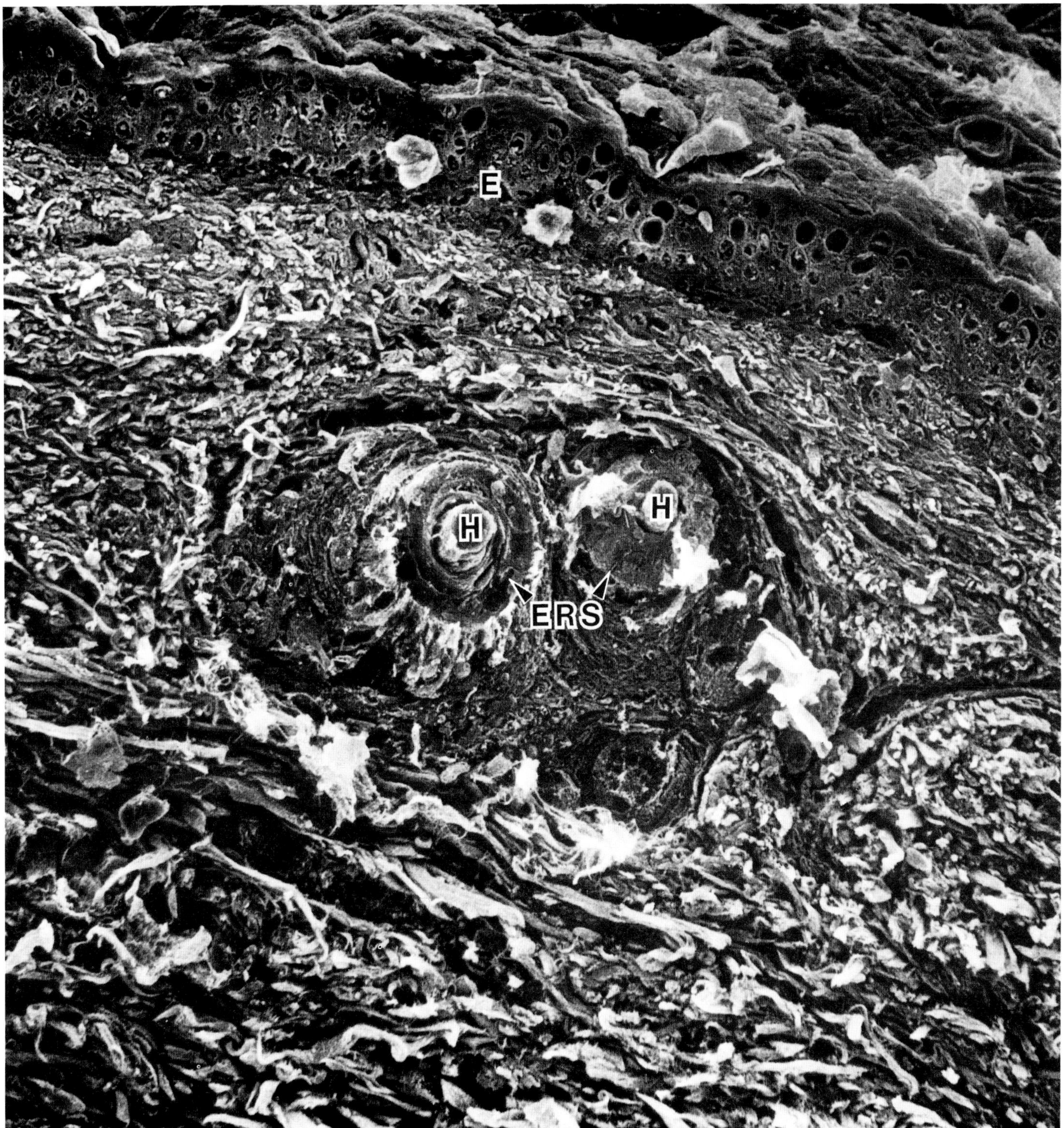

Figure 2–19. Abdominal skin, 30 weeks.

Profile of epidermis (E) and dermis. Each hair (H) in the dermis is surrounded by its own epithelial root sheath (ERS), but both are enclosed by the same connective tissue sheath. ×615.

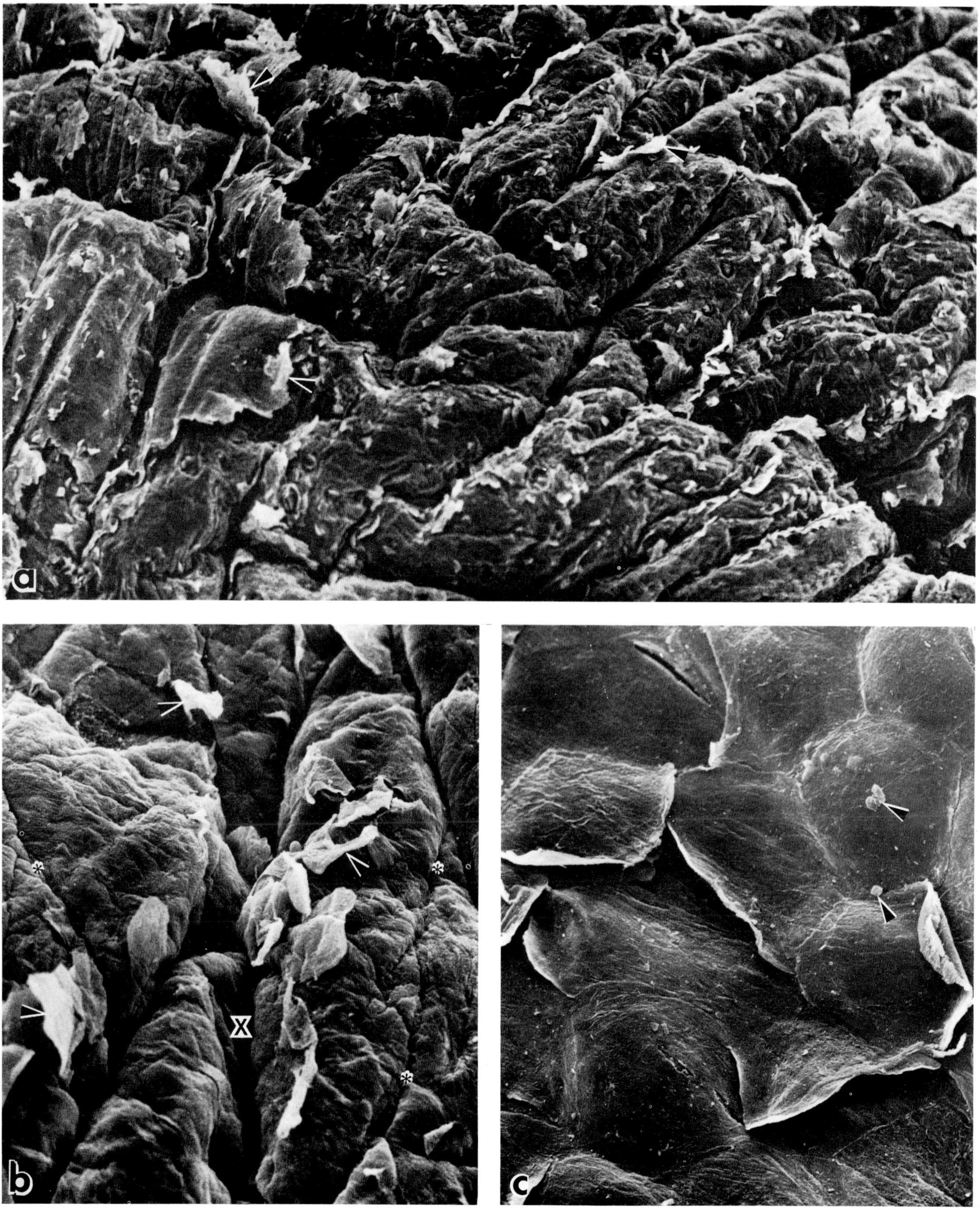
a
b
X
c

Figure 2–20. Abdominal skin, (a) 30 weeks, (b) 32 weeks, and (c) 31 weeks.

a. *The surface is uneven and many of the cornified cells (arrows) are undergoing desquamation. ×105.*

b. *Fetal skin shortly before birth exhibits furrows (X), creases (*), and desquamating cells (arrows). ×720.*

c. *The outer layer of keratinized cells appears smooth, thin, and clean except for a few particles of debris (arrows) on the cells or just beneath their turned-up edges. ×1,200.*

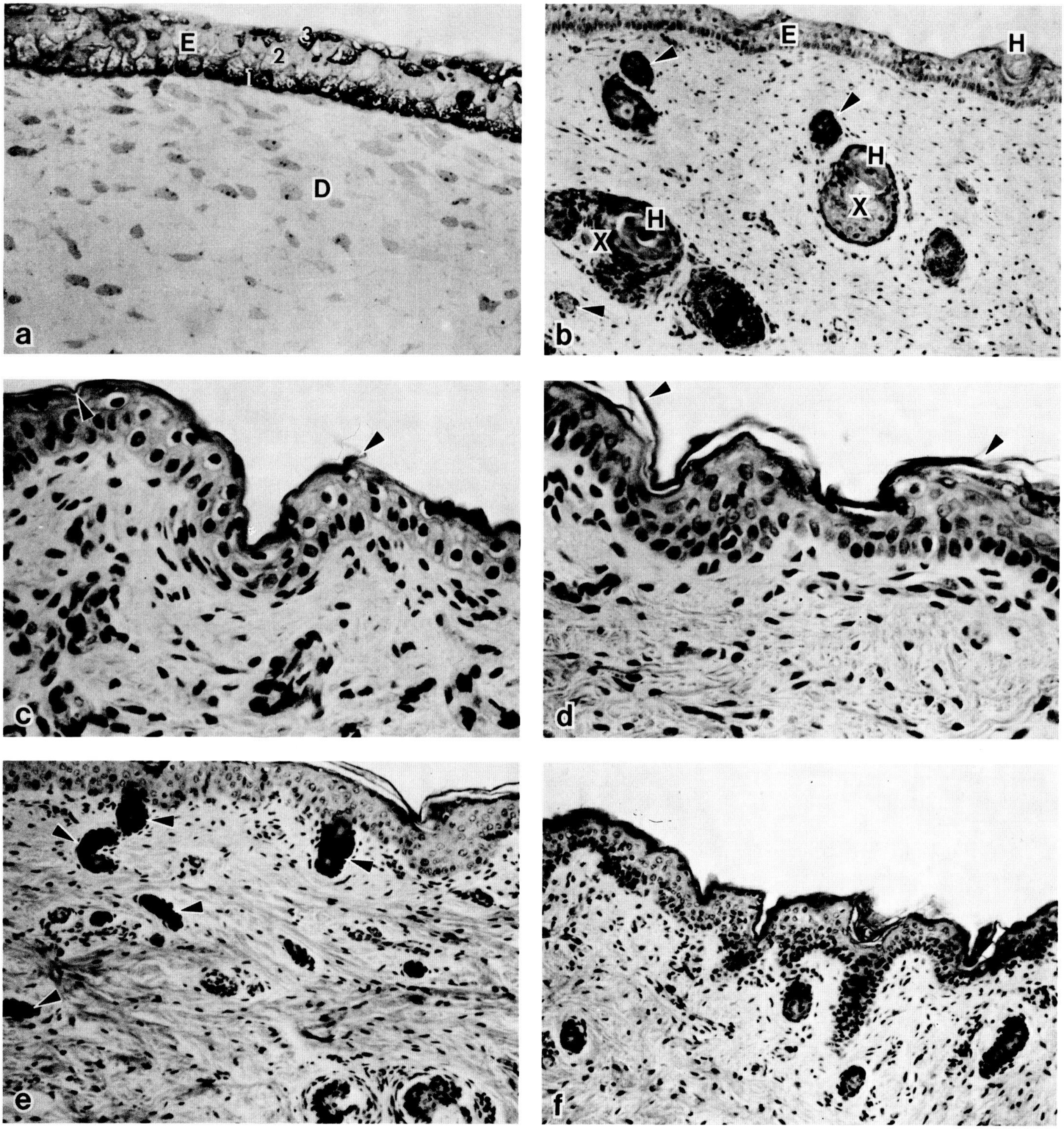
a
E
3
2
1
D
b
E
H
H
X
H
X
c
d
e
f

Figure 2–21. Photomicrographs of fetal skin: (a) 7 weeks, (b) 16 weeks, (c) 24 weeks, (d) 26 weeks, (e) 28 weeks, and (f) 32 weeks.

a. *Plastic section stained with toluidine blue. After 7 weeks of gestation, the epidermis (E) has three layers: basalis (1), intermediate layer (2), and periderm (3). The basal cells and some of the periderm cells are stained dark due to glycogen. Periderm cells lack protrusions and are flat at this stage of development. The dermis (D) consists mostly of widely-spaced mesenchymal cells and blood vessels. ×300.*

b. *Paraffin section stained with H&E. By 16 weeks, the dermis has undergone dramatic changes from the condition at 7 weeks. It now contains pilosebaceous units (X), sweat glands and ducts (arrows), and hairs (H) in various stages of development. The epidermis (E) is the source of the primordia for these structures. ×120.*

c. *Paraffin section stained with H&E. At 24 weeks, the periderm is undergoing degeneration and keratinization is evident in the very thin superficial layer (arrows) of the outermost epidermis. The dermis contains cells and fibers. ×300.*

d. *Paraffin section stained with H&E. By 26 weeks, there is extensive keratinization of the epidermal free surface (arrows) and the dermis has become more fibrous and less cellular due to the increase in connective tissue fibers. ×300.*

e. *Paraffin section stained with H&E. The skin at 28 weeks* in utero *shows a keratinized layer at the free surface, and a richly fibrous and cellular dermis with numerous ducts of eccrine sweat glands (arrows). ×120.*

f. *Paraffin section stained with H&E. At 32 weeks, nearly all features of adult skin are present, including rete ridges, dermal papillae, and patent sweat ducts. ×120.*

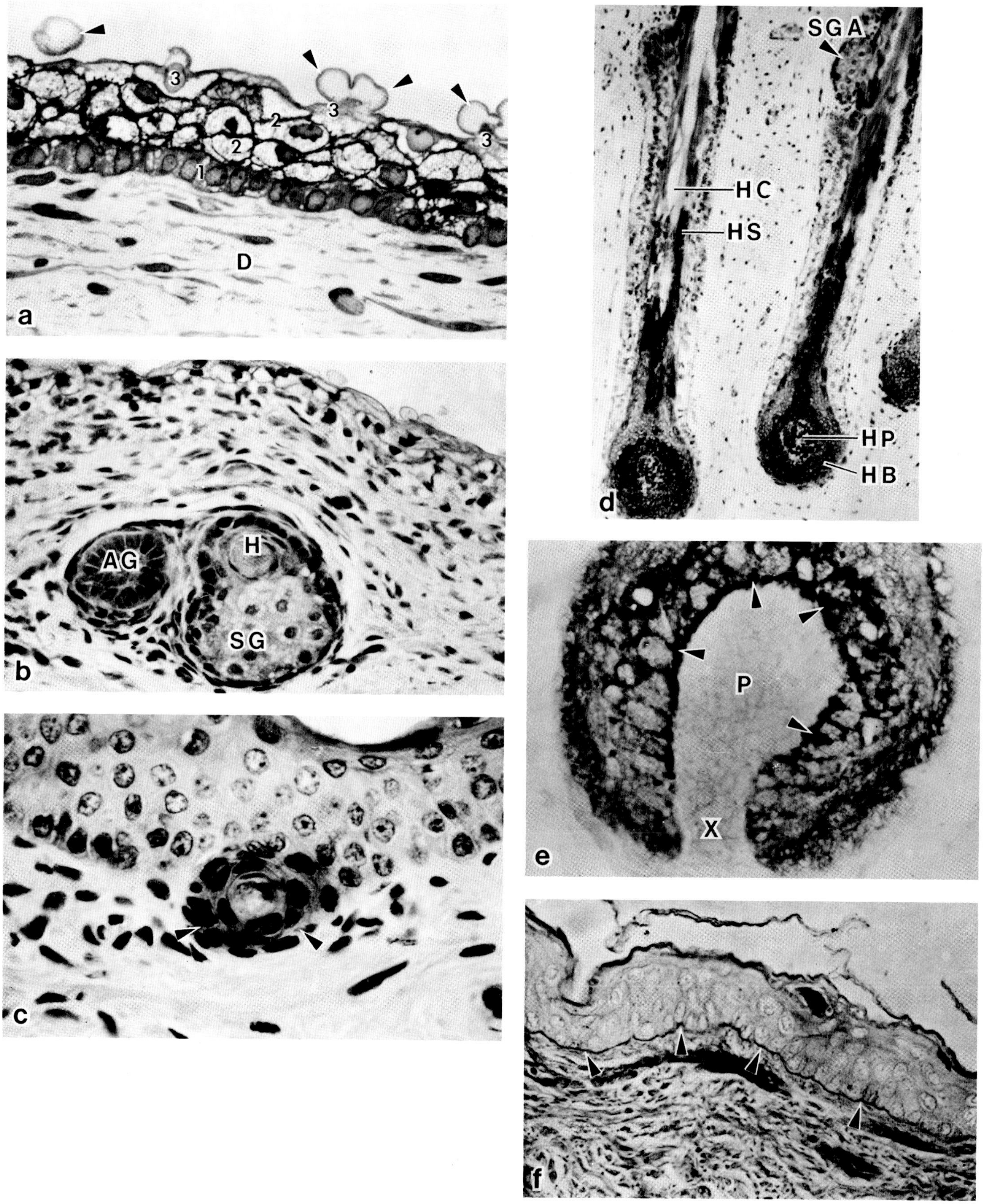

3
2
2
3
3
1
D
a
AG
H
SG
b
c
SGA
HC
HS
HP
HB
d
P
X
e
f

Figure 2–22. Photomicrographs of fetal skin: (a) 16 weeks, (b) 16 weeks, (c) 28 weeks, (d) 16 weeks, (e) 16 weeks, and (f) 28 weeks.

a. *Plastic section stained with toluidine blue. In the epidermis at 16 weeks, the basal cell layer (1) is undergoing mitosis, the intermediate cells (2) are large and vacuolated due to the dissolution of their glycogen content, and the periderm cells (3) have bifid protrusions (arrows). Fibroblasts and collagen fibrils are present in the dermis (D).* $\times 480$.

b. *Paraffin section stained with H&E. Cross section of a developing pilosebaceous unit. The light, foamy cells of the sebaceous gland (SG) contain lipid droplets. Hair (H) and apocrine sweat gland (AG) primordium are shown.* $\times 300$.

c. *Paraffin section stained with H&E. The duct of an eccrine sweat gland (arrows) is shown in a 28 week fetus in the same location where the eccrine gland arises from the epidermal cells.* $\times 480$.

d. *Paraffin section stained with H&E. Longitudinal section through two developing hair follicles at 16 weeks of gestation. The bulges on the left of each follicle represent a sebaceous gland "anlage" (SGA). Note the hair canal (HC), hair shaft (HS), hair bulb (HB), and hair papilla (HP). The skin throughout gestation contains follicles and hairs in different stages of development. Thus, a follicle with a mature appearance may occur adjacent to a hair germ that is developing in the epidermis.*

e. *Paraffin section stained with PAS. At 16 weeks, cells (arrows) of the hair bulb that lie adjacent to the papilla contain glycogen and are PAS-positive. The opening (X) permits blood vessels and nerves to reach the papilla (P).* $\times 480$.

f. *Paraffin section stained with PAS. The thin line (arrows) is the PAS-positive basement membrane at 28 weeks gestation. The basement membrane between epidermis and dermis does not form a continuous layer until late in the fetal life although it is present from the onset of skin development.* $\times 300$.

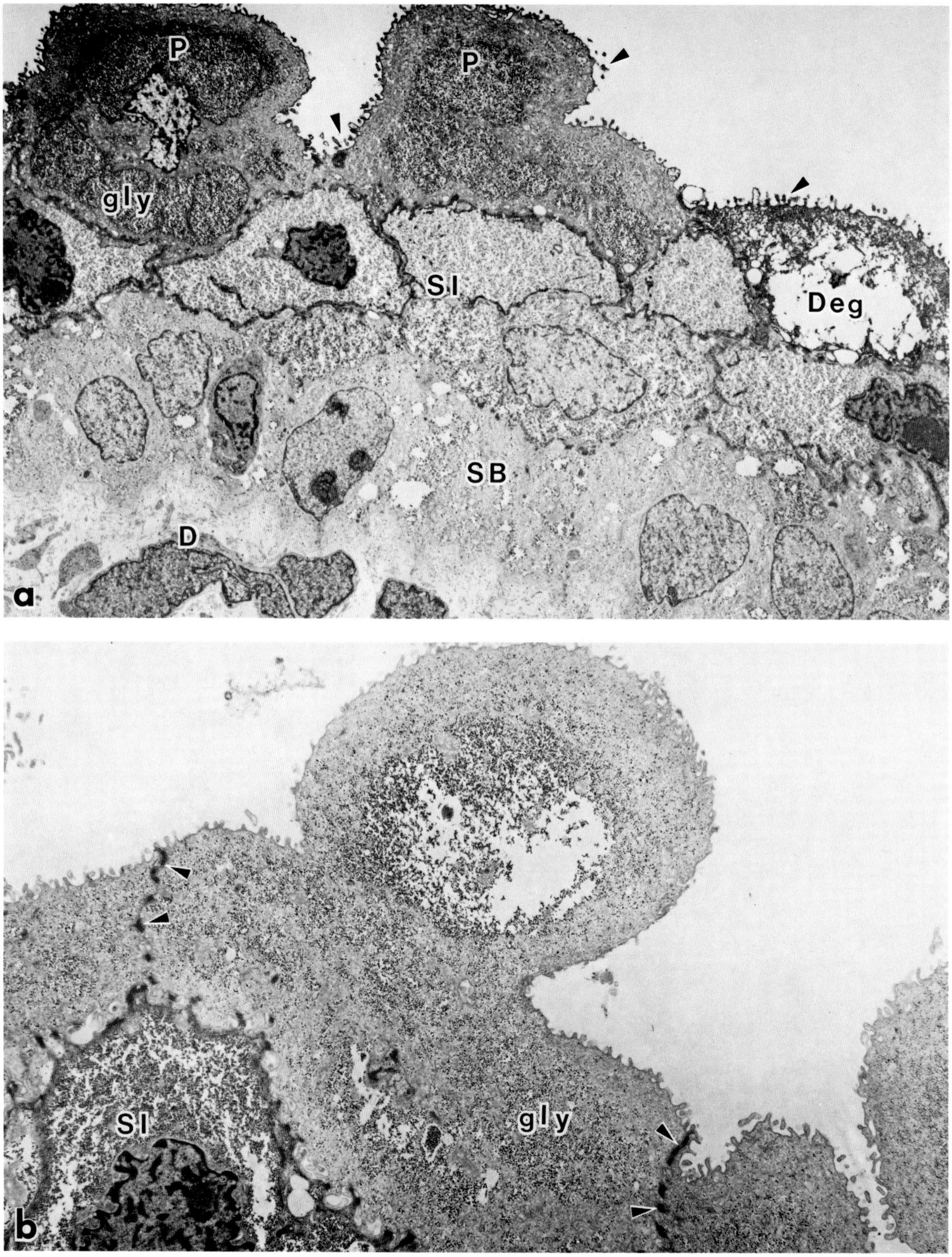

Figure 2–23. TEM, fetal epidermis, 14 weeks. Ruthenium red was added to the fixative to preserve extracellular acid carbohydrates.

a. *The full thickness of the fetal epidermis is shown. The stratum basale (SB) contains less glycogen (gly) than the intermediate layer (SI), or the periderm with its protrusions (P). The periderm cell at upper right is degenerating (Deg). Ruthenium red does not normally penetrate the cell membrane and stain intracellular carbohydrates. The fact that cells of the intermediate layer and periderm are stained indicates that their membranes are porous. Observe the ruthenium red-positive microvilli (arrows) on the periderm cells. Dermis (D). ×3,800.*

b. *The cytoplasm of the periderm cell contains large amounts of dispersed glycogen (gly). Cell apices and their protrusions are lined by short microvilli. Numerous desmosomes (arrows) connect the cells of the periderm. Stratum intermediate (SI). ×6,800.*

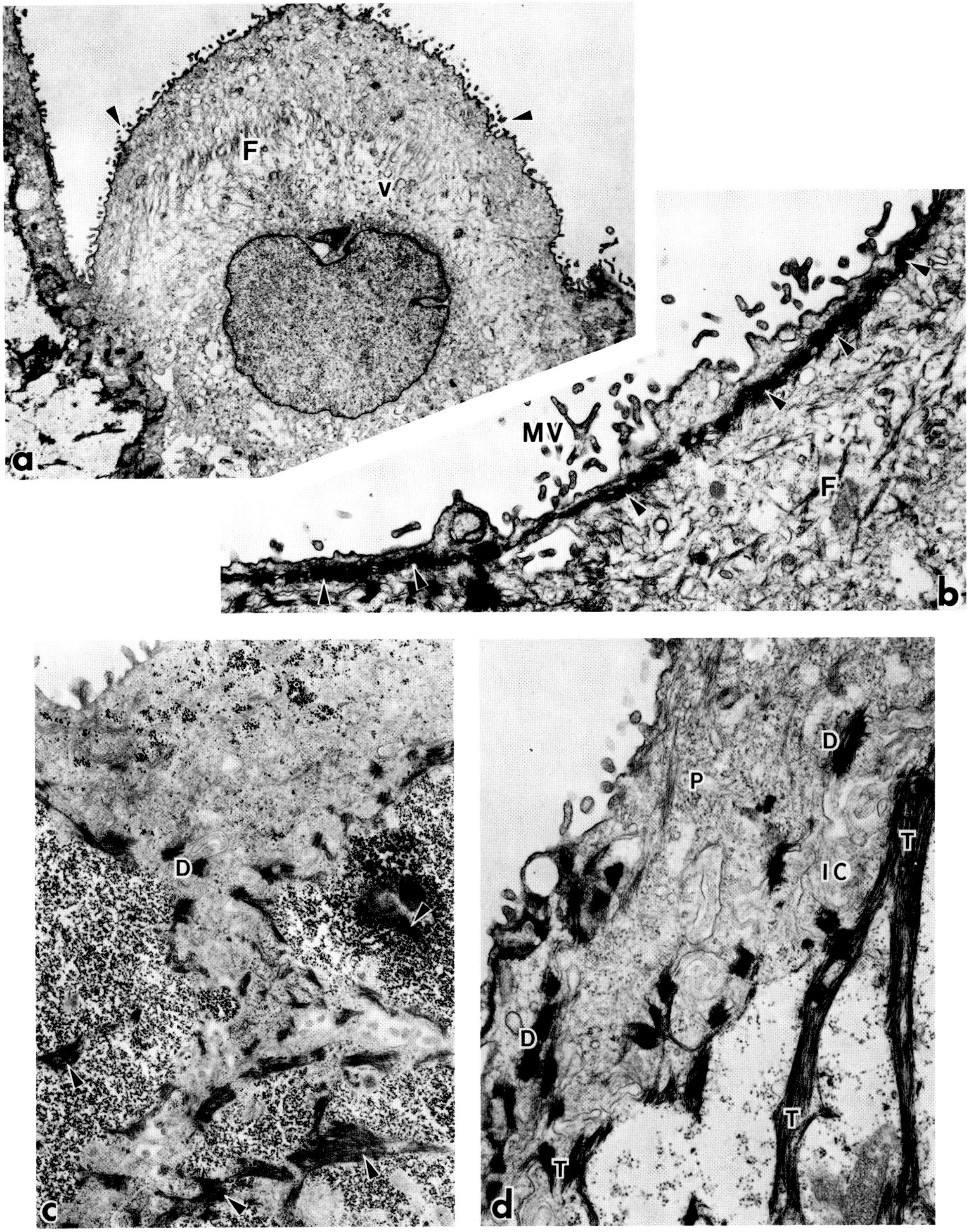

Figure 2–24. TEM, details of periderm at 16.5 weeks (a, b, and d) and 14 weeks (c).

a. *Microvilli (arrows) cover the dome-shaped periderm cell. Filaments (F) and electron lucent vesicles (v) are present in the cytoplasm.* ×4,590.

b. *Numerous desmosomes (arrows) join the thin processes of the two adjacent periderm cells. Microvilli (MV) and fine, dispersed filaments (F) are characteristic of periderm cells.* ×16,380.

c. *At 14 weeks, tonofilaments in the intermediate layer have formed aggregates (arrows). Some aggregates are related to desmosomes (D) and others are in pools of glycogen. Microvilli line the periderm cells.* ×14,850.

d. *Desmosomes (D) demarcate adjacent processes of periderm (P) and intermediate cells (IC). Bundles of tonofilaments (T) are present in the intermediate cell.* ×21,600.

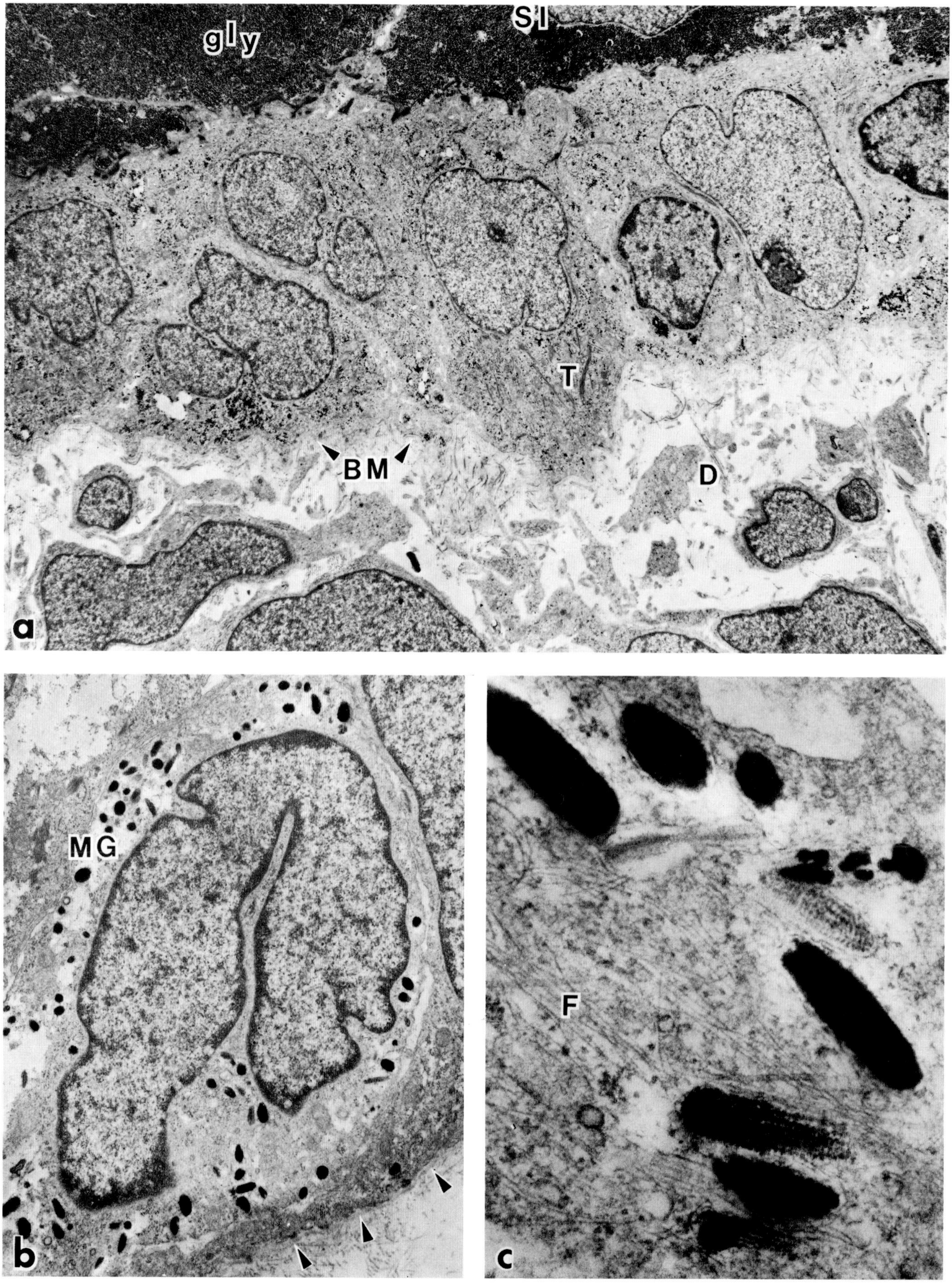
gly
SI
T
BM
D
a
MG
b
F
c

Figure 2–25. TEM, basal layer of epidermis, 15 weeks (a) and 16.5 weeks (b and c).

a. *Glycogen (gly) is sparse in the basal cells and abundant in cells of the intermediate layer (SI). The basal cell in the center of the micrograph has distinct strands of tonofilaments (T). The basal cell layer is the first part of the fetal epidermis to closely resemble the corresponding layer of adult skin. A thin basement membrane (BM) is visible. Fibroblasts and collagen fibrils are present in the dermis (D) at the dermal-epidermal junction. ×5,500.*

b. *Melanocyte in basal layer of epidermis. Melanin granules (MG) are present in the cytoplasm. Observe the basement membrane (arrows) at the dermal-epidermal junction. ×6,750.*

Melanocytes arise from the neural crest and migrate to the skin in the first trimester. Their cell bodies are located in the basal layer and their processes extend between the cells to other layers of the epidermis.

c. *Melanin granules and filaments (F) in melanocyte. ×68,000.*

Melanocytes produce the skin pigment, melanin. The enzyme tyrosinase, which is necessary for melanin synthesis, is formed as protyrosinase by the RER and packaged into vesicles by the Golgi apparatus. The vesicles fuse with other vesicles and become premelanosomes when the enzyme they contain is activated to tyrosinase and melanin synthesis begins. Premelanosomes mature through stages to become melanosomes. At first, premelanosomes are unpigmented and unlaminated. Next, they become laminated, ellipsoidal, and lightly pigmented. The lamellae have a periodicity of approximately 100 Å. Finally, the periodicity is obscured by melanin accumulation. When melanin synthesis ceases, the structure is known as a melanosome which no longer has demonstrable tyrosinase activity and there is no recognizable periodicity. Thus, a melanosome is a membrane-bound granule of melanin pigment that has completed the synthesis of melanin. The terms melanosome, premelanosome, melanin granule, and pigment granule are frequently used interchangeably. The term melanosome complex is used to designate two or more of the aforementioned structures lying close together within the cell's cytoplasm.

Figure 2–26. Diagramatic representation of the development of a hair follicle and sebaceous gland in the fetus. Redrawn from Addison, W.H.F., editor: Piersol's Normal Histology, 15th edition, 1932. J. B. Lippincott, Philadelphia, PA.

Hair development begins early in the third month of fetal life when the basal epidermis thickens to form hair germs. Mesenchyme aggregates about the epidermal thickenings. Hair germs first appear in the skin of the future eyebrows, chin, and upper lip. They develop somewhat later in other sites, and fail to develop in the palms and soles. A hair germ grows slantingly downward through the dermis to reach the subcutaneous connective tissue where its end expands and becomes the "cap-like" hair bulb. Connective tissue invaginates the bulb to form the hair papilla. The hair germ also pushes upward to the free surface to form the hair canal. Two or three thickenings develop on a hair germ. The uppermost thickening is inconstant. When present, it is the bud for the apocrine sweat gland. The second and third thickenings are constant and they are for the sebaceous gland and for the attachment of the arrector pili muscle, respectively.

Fetal skin during the fifth and sixth months is covered with the first generation of hairs, the very delicate lanugo hairs, which are usually shed before birth except those of the eyebrows, eyelids, and scalp. Within a few months after birth, any remaining lanugo hairs are also shed and replaced with coarser hairs. Small hairs called vellus hairs (the downy coat or fleece) emerge from the thin skin covering the remainder of the body. No hair follicles are formed after birth. Large, coarse hairs of the scalp and eyebrows and those that develop with the onset of puberty in the axilla, pubic area, and face of males are called terminal hairs.

Hair is not very important in keeping the human body warm. Hair follicles, however, are important in repairing the epidermis when injury occurs from burns, abrasions, etc. Follicles, along with eccrine sweat glands, also make it possible to perform split-skin grafts.

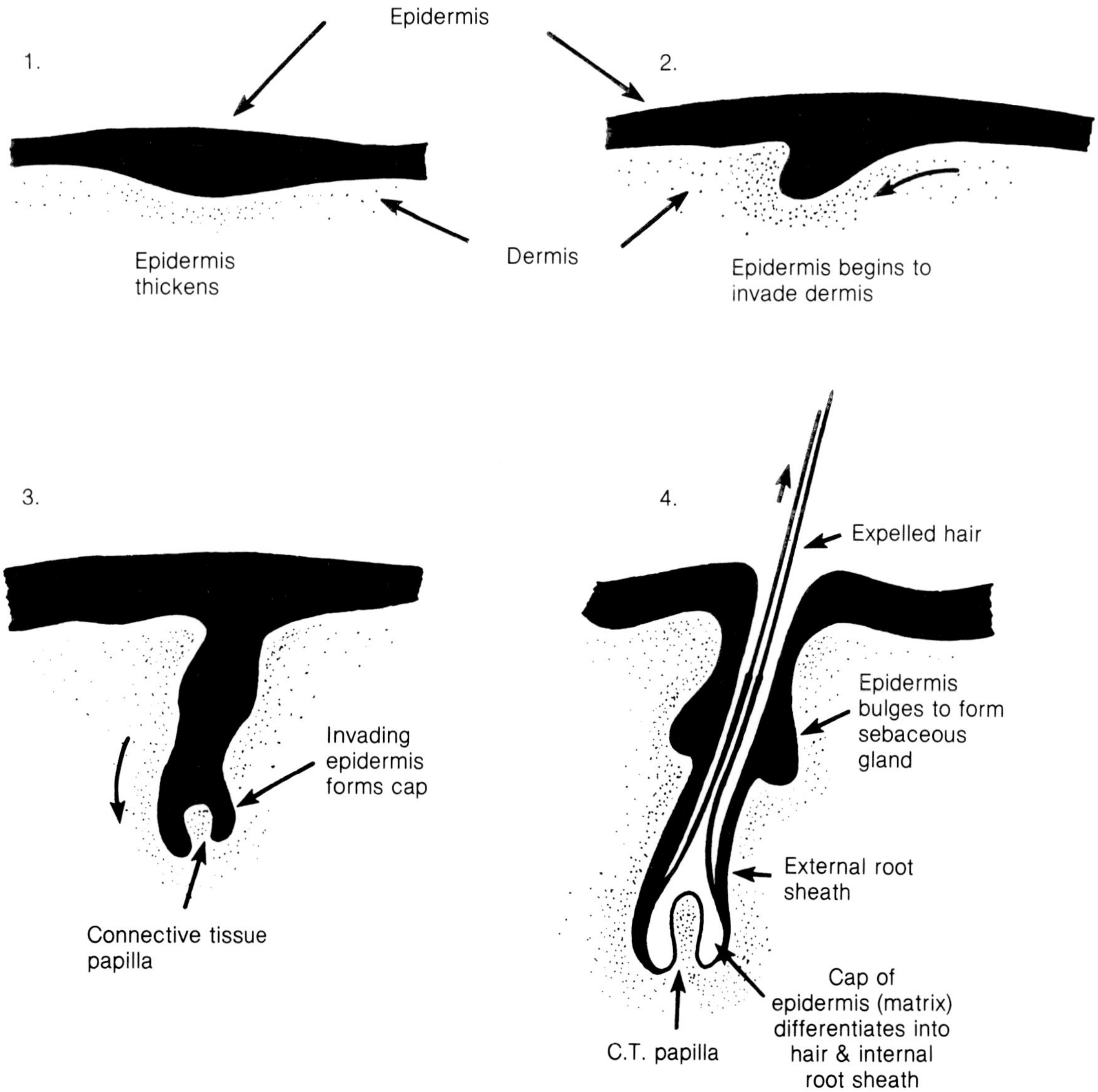

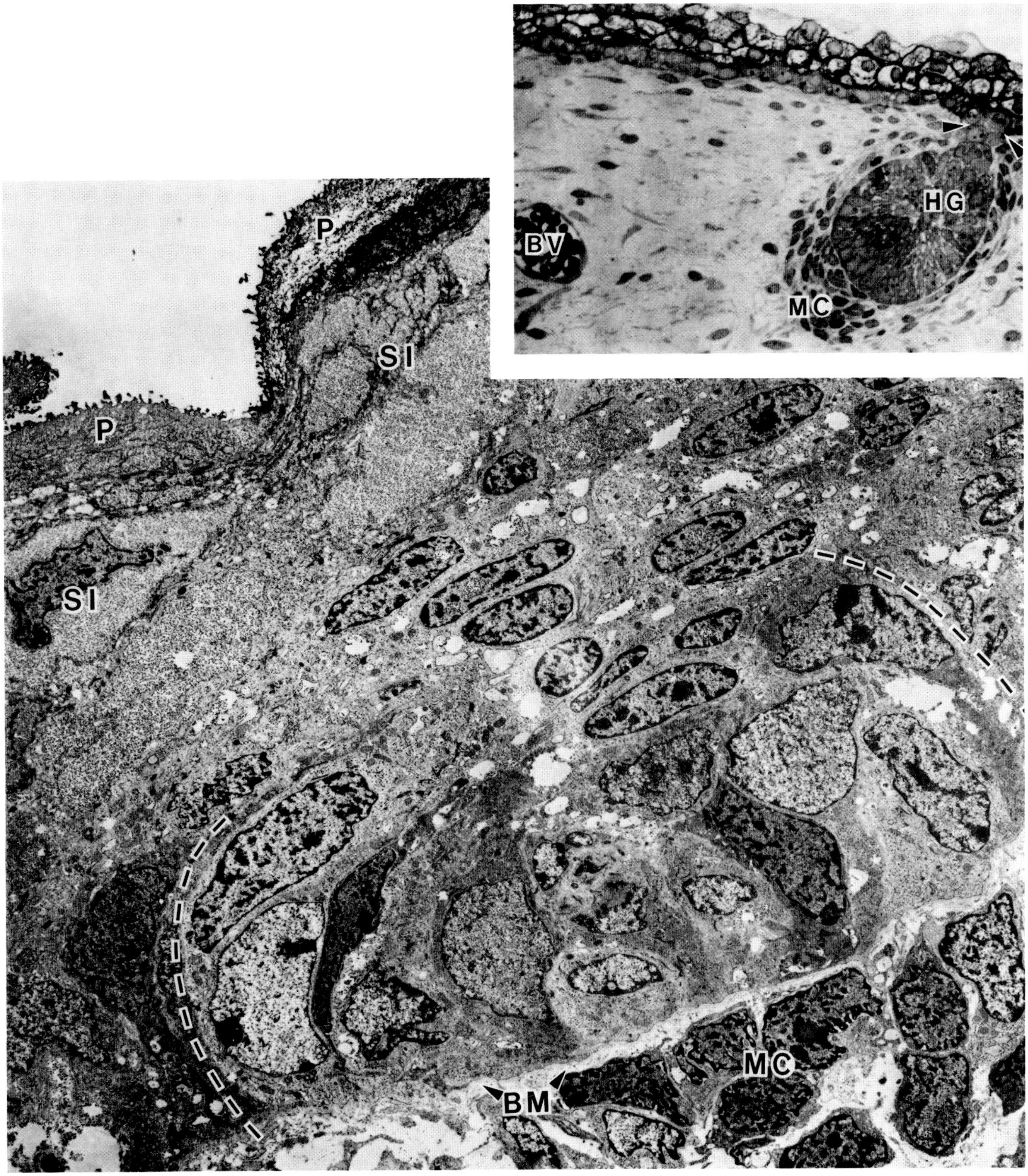

Figure 2–27. Hair germ, 15 weeks and 16 weeks (inset).

TEM, early stage in histogenesis of hair follicle. Cells of the hair germ enclosed by the broken line have come from the basal cells of the epidermis. Through mitotic division and differentiation, the basal cells have become a cell cluster in close association with the aggregate of mesenchymal cells (MC) in the dermis, but they remain separated from the latter by a basement membrane (BM). Stratum intermediate (SI). Periderm (P). $\times$ *4,750.*

Inset, *is a photomicrograph of a plastic section stained with toluidine blue. The ectodermal component of the hair germ (HG) is attached to the epidermis (arrows) at its upper end and is adjacent to the aggregate of mesenchymal cells (MC) at its lower end. Blood vessel (BV).* $\times$ *300.*

In hair development, there is no epidermal invagination of the dermis as traditionally described. Instead, there is ectodermal-mesodermal interaction with the formation of a biological unit that grows inward and outward by its own mitotic activity.

The hair germ eventually gives rise to the hair follicle, apocrine sweat gland, and sebaceous gland. It will serve as the site of attachment for the arrector pili muscle which develops in the mesenchyme just outside the follicle.

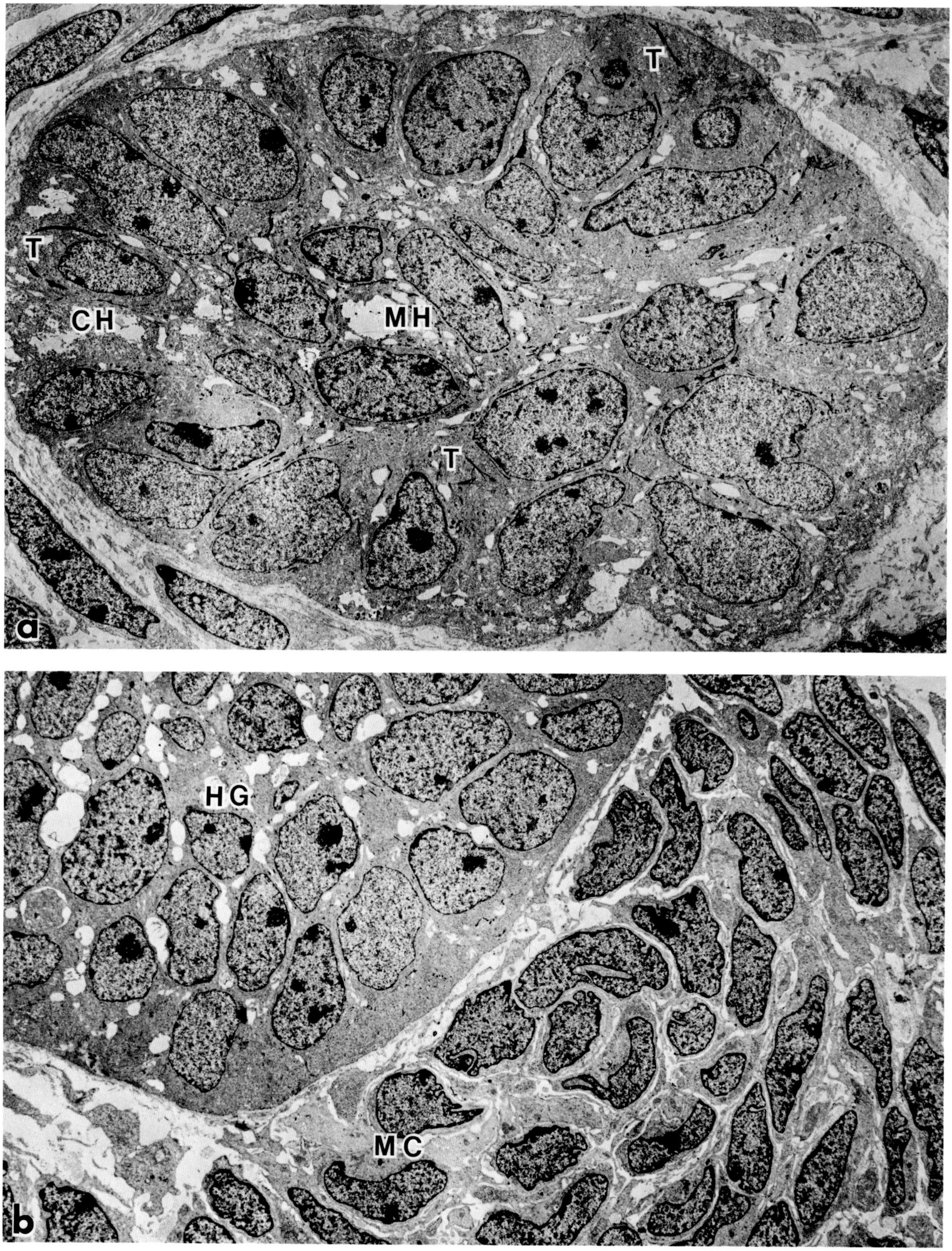

Figure 2–28. Hair germ in dermis, 16.5 weeks.

a. *This cross-section through the midportion of a drop-shaped hair germ shows centrally located cells that will form the medulla of the hair (MH), and peripherally located cells that are destined to give rise to the cortex of the hair (CH). Bundles of tonofilaments (T) are present in the cytoplasm of the future cortical cells. ×3,070.*

b. *Base of hair germ (HG) at site of a future hair bulb. Mesenchymal cells (MC) and ectodermal cells are contiguous but not continuous. The mesenchymal cells are precursors of the fibrous root sheath and hair papilla. ×3,070.*

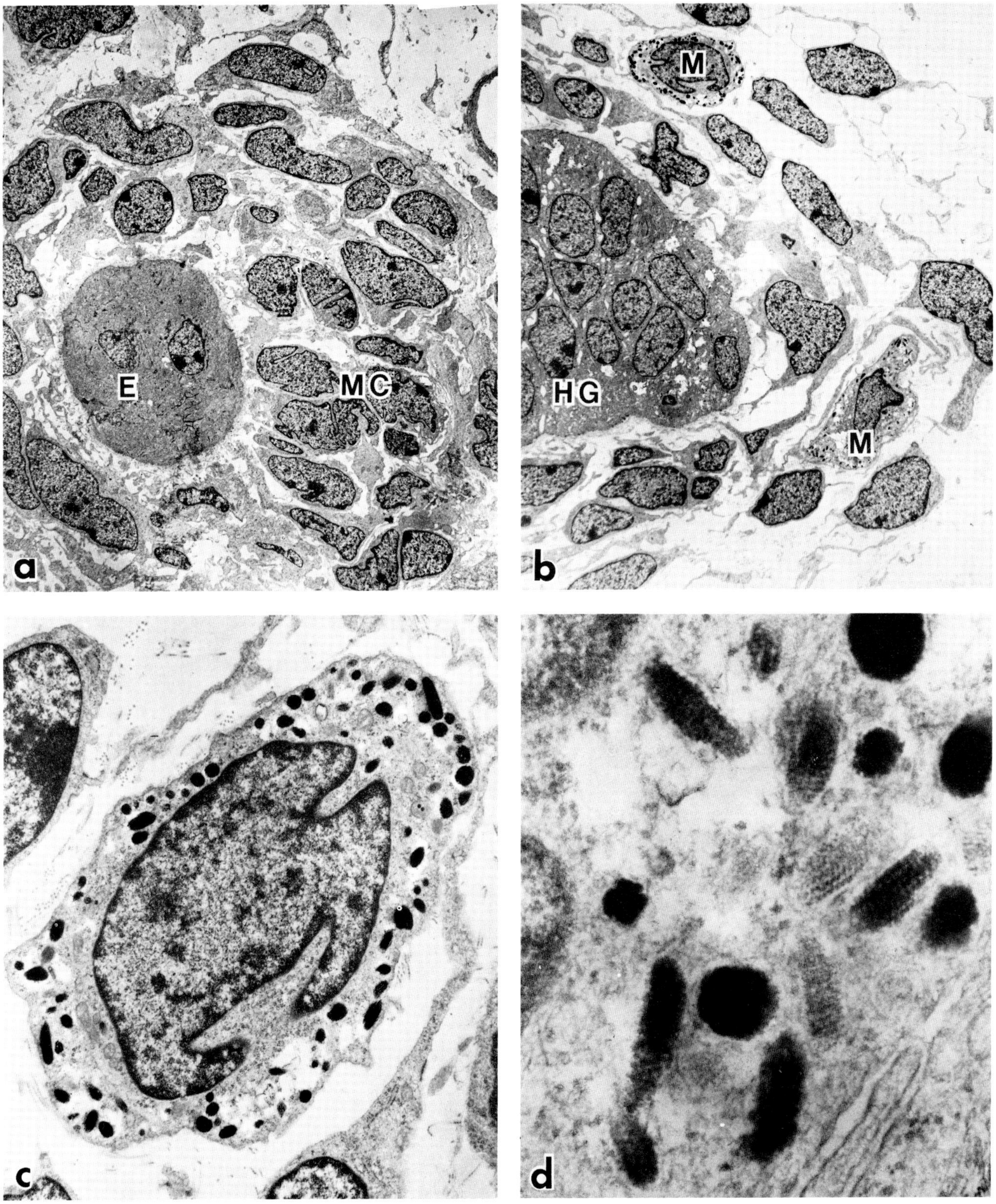

Figure 2–29. TEM, components of fetal dermis, 16.5 weeks.

a. *Ectodermal (E) and mesenchymal (MC) components of eccrine germ. Eccrine sweat glands develop by the same types of ectodermal-mesodermal interactions that were described for the histogenesis of hairs. The epithelial cord acquires a lumen in the seventh or eighth month of fetal life. Eccrine glands, in contrast to apocrine glands, arise independently of hair follicles. ×2,150.*

b. *Two melanocytes (M) are among the mesenchymal cells that surround the closely-packed epithelial cells of the hair germ (HG). ×2,140.*

c. *Higher magnification of a melanocyte in* b *shows the numerous melanin granules in the cytoplasm. ×12,965.*

d. *Melanin granules in different developmental stages. The granules measure 0.3 μm × 0.7 μm and have a complex internal structure with a periodicity of about 100 Å that becomes obscured as melanin accumulates in the granule. ×85,500.*

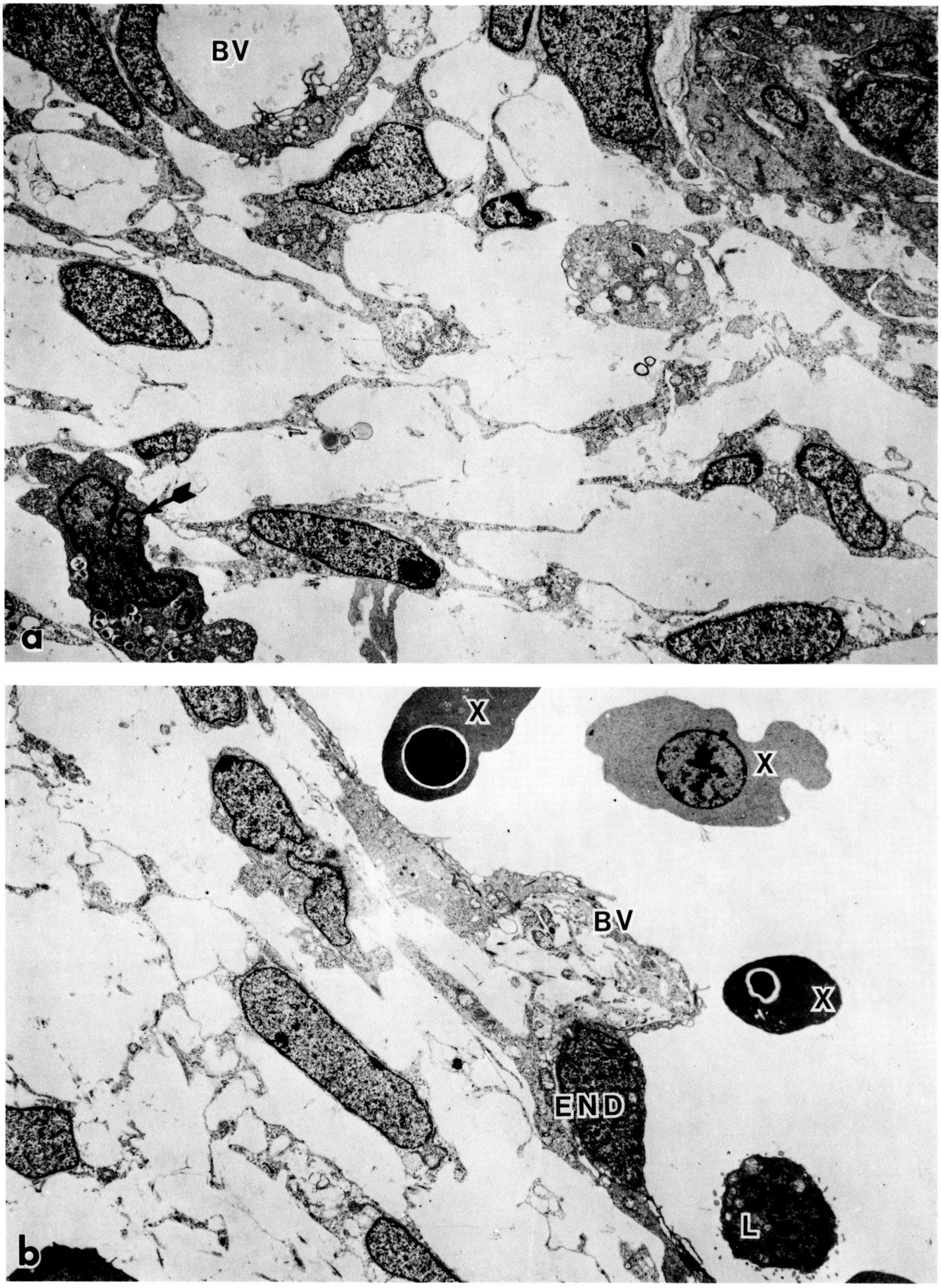

Figure 2–30. TEM, components of fetal dermis, 6.5 weeks.

a. *The fetal dermis consists of a loose network of cell bodies of mesenchymal cells and their processes. The future papillary region is the most cellular. No collagen is present. Once collagen synthesis begins, the dermis will become progressively more fibrous and less cellular. A mast cell (arrow) is present at the lower left, and a developing capillary (BV) is shown in the upper left of the micrograph. ×3,850.*

b. *One wall and lumen of a developing venule (BV) is shown. Three immature red blood cells (X) and a leukocyte (L) are present in the lumen near the endothelium (END). ×3,040.*

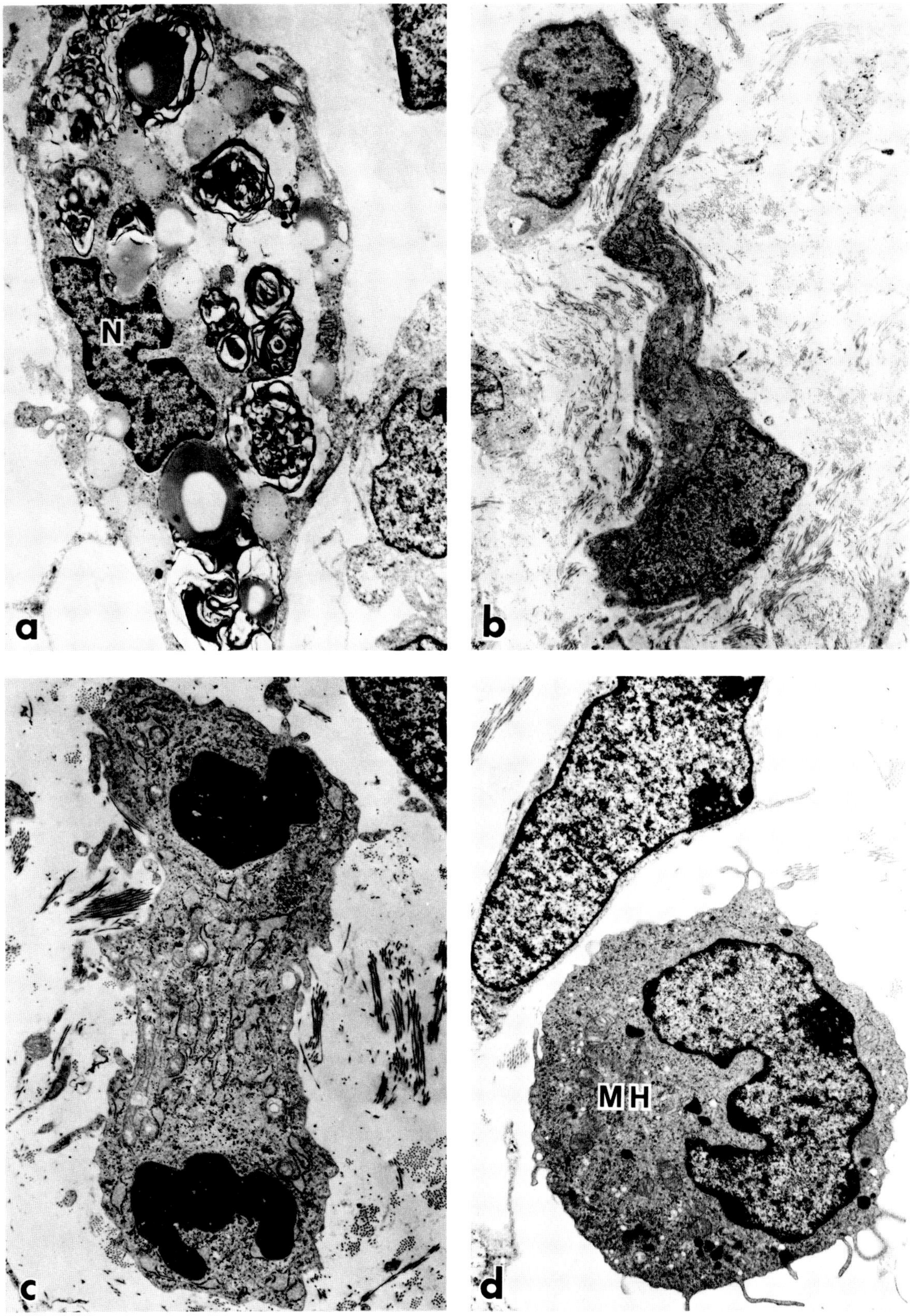

Figure 2–31. TEM, cells of fetal dermis, 6.5 weeks (a), 15 weeks (b and c), and 16.5 weeks (d).

a. *Degenerating phagocytic mesenchymal cell whose cytoplasm surrounding the nucleus (N) is filled with lamellar bodies, lipid droplets, and vacuoles.* $\times 6,210$.

b. *Fibroblast with a long cytoplasmic process rich in RER and surrounded by amorphous ground substance and newly formed collagenous fibrils.* $\times 4,700$.

c. *Fibroblast in telophase of mitosis. Mitotic figures are abundant in the fetal dermis.* $\times 6,210$.

d. *Mesenchymal histiocyte (MH) with indented nucleus and small, electron dense, lysosomal granules. If the uptake of debris had continued, the cell would have come to resemble the one shown in* a. $\times 7,865$.

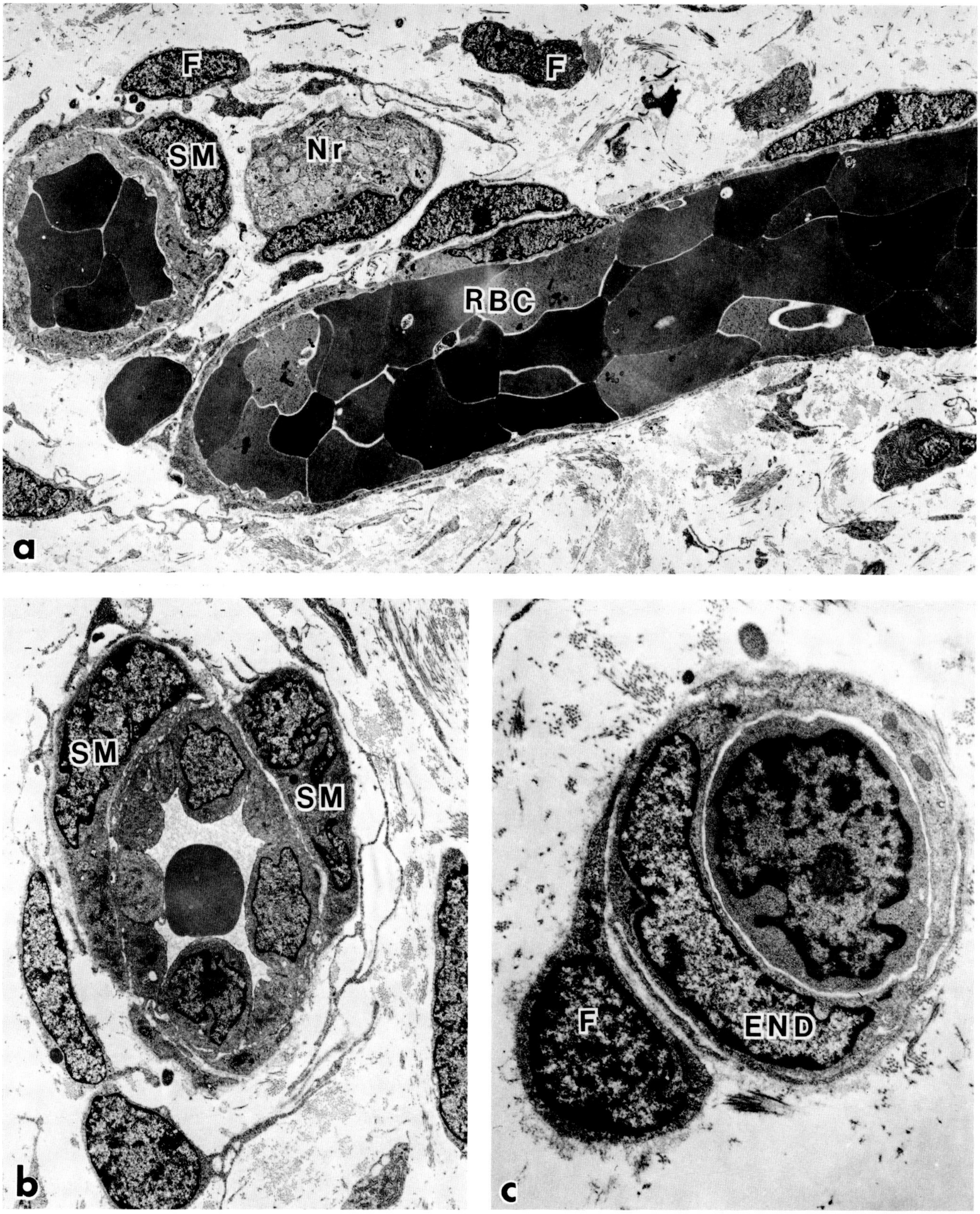

Figure 2–32. TEM, blood vessels in fetal dermis, 15 weeks (a and b) and 14 weeks (c).

a. *Two blood vessels are shown. The thin-walled venule in longitudinal section is filled with red blood cells (RBC). The small arteriole in cross section (upper left) is associated with one layer of developing smooth muscle cells (SM) and lies adjacent to an unmyelinated nerve (Nr) with the nucleus of a Schwann cell at its lower border. The nerve and two blood vessels comprise a neurovascular bundle surrounded by fibroblasts (F) and connective tissue fibers. ×3,200.*

b. *Arteriole in cross section with its single layer of smooth muscle cells (SM). ×5,100.*

c. *Capillary whose lumen is almost filled with a lymphocyte. A fibroblast (F) is adjacent to the elongated nucleus of the endothelial cell (END). ×13,650.*

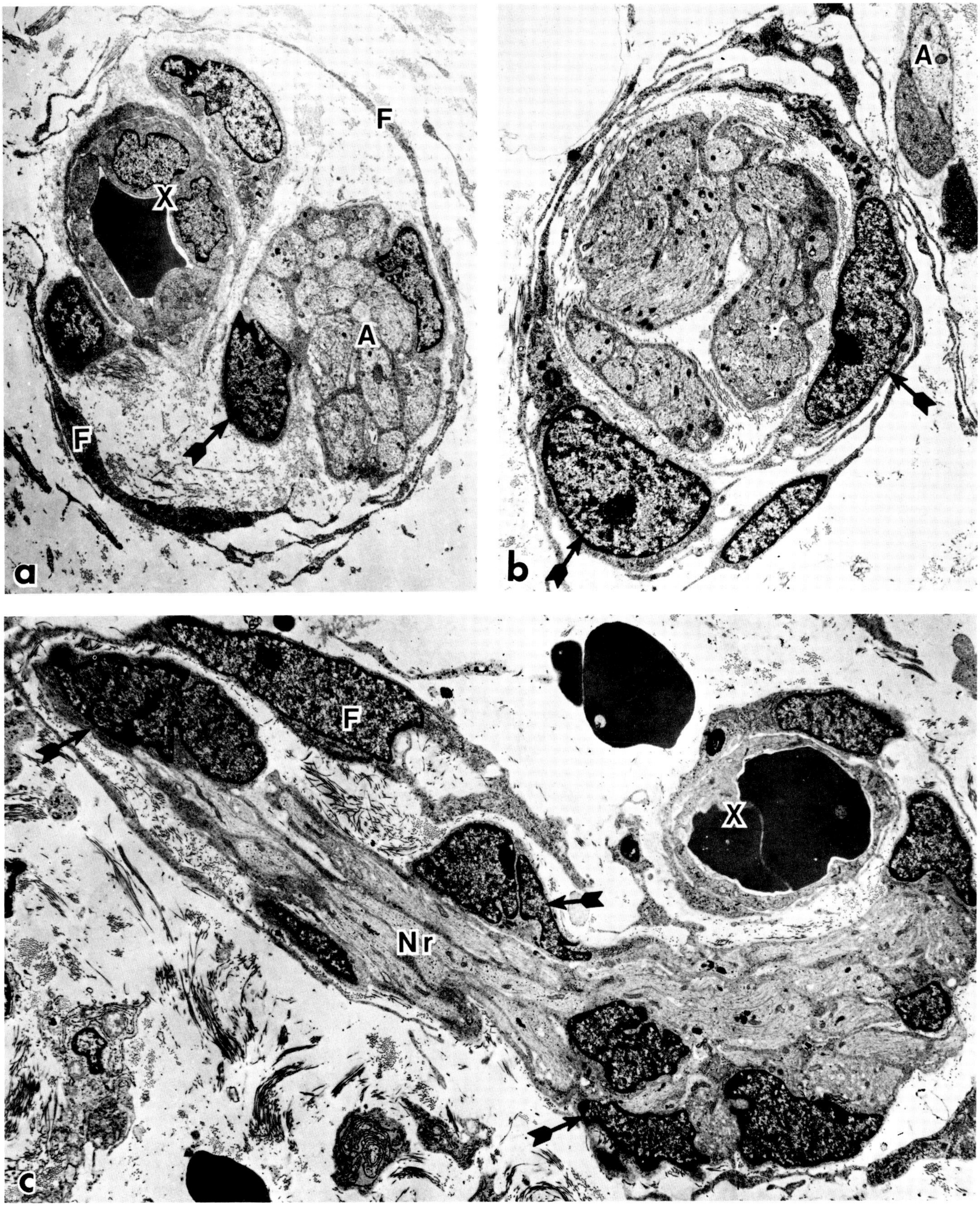

Figure 2–33. TEM, nerves in fetal dermis, 15 weeks (a), 14 weeks (b), and 16 weeks (c).

a. *Neurovascular bundle in cross section. Capillary (X), axons (A), Schwann cell nucleus (arrow), and processes of fibroblasts (F).* ×*5,100.*

b. *Unmyelinated axons of nerve surrounded by two Schwann cells (arrows). A single axon (A) is shown at upper right.* ×*6,1200.*

c. *Longitudinal section through an unmyelinated nerve (Nr) with Schwann cells (arrows) and an adjacent capillary (X). Fibroblast (F).* ×*4,840.*

ADULT SKIN 3

Adult skin is a large, dynamic, and vitally important organ that is highly complex, both structurally and functionally. The skin changes continuously from the time it appears in the embryo until the death of the individual. Adult skin is composed of two anatomically distinct layers, the epidermis and dermis, which arise from ectoderm and mesoderm, respectively. The fatty subcutaneous tissue, the hypodermis, is sometimes considered the skin's third layer.

Skin is also called integument and cutis. Corium is another term for the dermis. The skin appendages are hairs, nails, sweat glands, and sebaceous glands. The integumentary system comprises the skin and its appendages. Appendages arise from the epidermis and project into the dermis sometimes as far as or even into the subcutaneous tissue.

Skin is classified as thick skin and thin skin based on the thickness of the epidermis. Thick skin, also called glabrous skin, is found on the palms and soles. It lacks hairs and sebaceous glands. Thin skin contains hairs and is present over the remainder of the body. Regional differences are well established.

The epidermis contains strata of cells, the keratinocytes, which pass through different phases of their life cycle as they migrate from the lower epidermis to the free surface. Mitotic activity takes place in the stratum basale, differentiation (keratinization) is characteristic of the strata spinosum and granulosum, and exfoliation occurs in the stratum corneum. There is a delicate balance between the mitotic rate and loss of cells at the free surface.

Upon leaving the basal layer of the epidermis, keratinocytes enter the stratum spinosum as polyhedral cells which increase in size and become active in the synthesis of keratins. In the stratum granulosum, cells flatten, cease synthetic activity, and enter a degenerative phase where nuclei and cytoplasmic organelles are eliminated and keratins remain as the chief proteins. Cells of the stratum corneum are cellular skeletons with no metabolic activity. The passage of a cell from the stratum basale to the stratum corneum normally requires about four weeks.

Epidermal cells that are either keratinized or destined to keratinize are called keratinocytes. The keratinocyte is the major epithelial cell of the skin. Other cells that occur in the epidermis are melanocytes, Langerhans cells, and Merkel cells. They are concerned with the synthesis of pigment, immunological reactions, and sensory reception, respectively.

The dermis is 15 to 40 times thicker than the epidermis, and it is thicker in thin skin than in thick skin. The dermis is thickest on the back and thinnest on the eyelids. The dermis contains connective tissue fibers (collagenous, reticular, and elastic), various types of cells, blood and lymph vessels, nerves, hair follicles, and glands. The fibroblast is the main cell of the dermis. It produces the connective tissue fibers and the ground substance.

The number of each dermal component varies in different parts of the body, but it has been estimated that an average sq. cm. of skin contains 100 eccrine sweat glands, 12 ft. of nerves, hundreds of nerve endings, 10 hair follicles, 15 sebaceous glands, and 3 feet of blood vessels. The numbers of these dermal components are especially awesome if the fact is considered that the average person has approximately 18 sq. ft. or 16,000 sq. cm. of skin.

The skin performs numerous functions which are attributable to its multiple components. The stratum corneum provides protection, acts as a barrier, serves as a reservoir for topical medications, prevents dessication, and keeps microorganisms from invading the body. The most essential function of the stratum corneum is to maintain the body's water content and electrolyte concentration. The cornified cells are almost waterproof, making it possible, e.g., to be exposed to fresh water without swelling or to sea water without shrinking. The stratum corneum serves as a barrier to the penetration of many, but not all, molecules. The permeability of the stratum corneum can be increased by elevating the skin's temperature, increasing its water content, or exposing the skin to lipid solvents. Water loss and percutaneous absorption are increased if the stratum corneum is altered. Death may result from dehydration or toxicity if injury to the stratum corneum is severe and extensive.

Regulation of the body's temperature is the chief function of eccrine sweat glands. Excretion of certain metabolites and nitrogeneous waste products is an ancillary function of eccrine sweat glands.

The skin functions as a major sense organ, receiving stimuli for pain, temperature, touch, pressure, and itch. The skin also manufactures vitamin D when exposed to ultraviolet light.

The skin protects the body from too much ultraviolet light. This function is achieved by melanocytes which produce pigment that shields underlying tissues.

The present study of normal skin by SEM has revealed much new information on the skin's intricate and varied terrain. It has contributed to a better understanding of the skin's complex architecture and the distribution of the cutaneous flora. Bacteria and yeasts occur in pockets of scales where they cannot be easily removed by washing. Sebum and microorganisms are found in follicular orifices where hairs project onto the surface. Sebum from continuously-secreting sebaceous glands serves as fuel for some microorganisms. Sweat from eccrine sweat glands is apparently antimicrobial since sweat pores at the surface are usually free of microorganisms. Secretory cells of axillary apocrine sweat glands release their secretory products predominantly by the microapocrine mode characterized by the detachment of small portions of the cell apices. Scales undergo continuous desquamation at the free surface and the stratum corneum becomes thinner with the aging of the skin.

The micrographs and descriptions which follow are representative of the results obtained from the study of many skin specimens by correlative SEM and TEM. In order to provide a strong scientific basis for interpreting cutaneous structures by SEM, this chapter contains more TEM than any other chapter. The study of normal skin by SEM and TEM is an essential prerequisite for recognizing and characterizing the skin disorders in succeeding chapters.

References

Ackerman, A. B. Structure and function of the skin. Section I. Development, morphology, and physiology. *In: Dermatology,* S. L. Moschella, D. M. Pillsbury, and H. J. Hurley (eds). W. B. Saunders Co., Philadelphia, PA, 1975, Vol. 1, pp. 1–60.

Goldsmith, L. A. (editor) *Biochemistry and Physiology of the Skin.* Oxford University Press, New York, N.Y., 1983, Vol. 1 (pp. 1–684) and Vol. 2 (pp. 685–1323).

Grayson, S., A. D. Johnson-Sinegar, and P. M. Elias. Isolation of lamellar bodies from neonatal mouse epidermis by selective sequential filtration. Science 221: 962–964, 1983.

Hurley, H. J., and W. B. Shelley. *The Human Apocrine Sweat Gland in Health and Disease,* Charles C. Thomas, Springfield, IL, 1960, pp. 6–26.

Montagna, W., and P. F. Parakkal. *The Structure and Function of Skin.* 3rd edition, Academic Press, New York, 1974, pp. 1–433.

Montes, L. F., B. L. Baker, and A. C. Curtis. The cytology of the large axillary sweat glands in man. J. Invest. Dermatol. 35: 273–291, 1960.

Montes, L. F., and W. H. Wilborn. Anatomical location of normal skin flora. Arch. Dermatol. 101: 145–159, 1970.

Wilborn, W. H., and L. F. Montes. Scanning electron microscopy of axillary apocrine sweat glands. Scanning Electron Microscopy, Vol. II, 1978, SEM Inc., Chicago, IL, pp. 245–252.

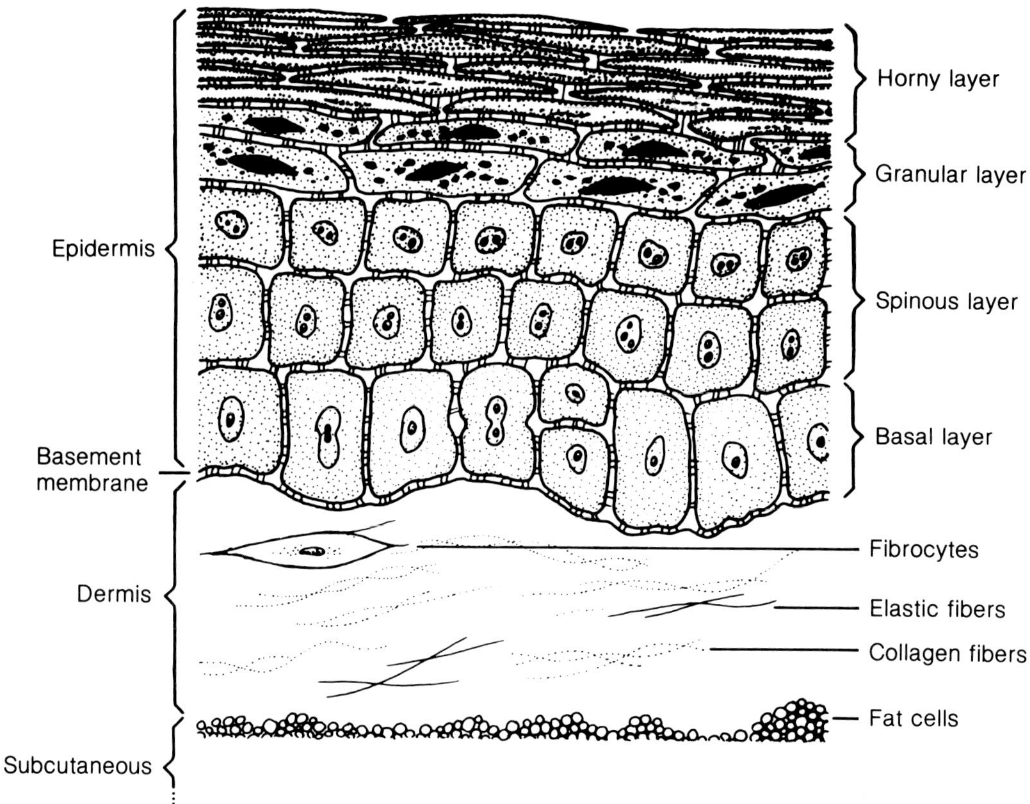

Figure 3–1. The skin has two layers, the epidermis and dermis, separated by a basement membrane. The epidermis is a keratinized, stratified, squamous epithelium composed from top to bottom of the following strata: (1) stratum corneum (horny layer), (2) stratum granulosum, (3) stratum spinosum, and (4) stratum basale (basal layer). The entire epidermis is about 1 mm thick over the palms and soles and about 0.1 mm thick over the remainder of the body. The thickness of the latter approximates the thickness of a sheet of typing paper. In the thick epidermis of the palms and soles, a stratum lucidum is sometimes interposed between the granular and horny layers. The epidermis is derived from ectoderm. It is avascular and must be nourished by diffusion of nutrients from blood vessels in the dermis. Cells of the basal layer divide and are pushed toward the surface of the skin. During this process, the cells keratinize and eventually desquamate at the free surface. The entire process from the time a cell is formed until its desquamation at the free surface requires about four weeks in normal, healthy skin. This compares with four days for actively dividing psoriatic skin.

The dermis or corium is classified as dense irregular connective tissue consisting of cells, fibers, and ground substance. It contains sweat glands, sebaceous glands, hairs, bands of smooth muscle (arrector pili), blood vessels, and nerves. Cells present in the dermis are fibroblasts (fibrocytes), macrophages (histiocytes), mast cells, and all types of cells that are found in peripheral blood (lymphocytes, neutrophils, eosinophils, and monocytes). Connective tissue fibers in the dermis are the collagenous, reticular, and elastic fibers, and all are made by fibroblasts. The dermis is derived from mesoderm. Leather is made from the dermis of animals.

Fat cells are especially abundant in the subcutaneous connective tissue (hypodermis).

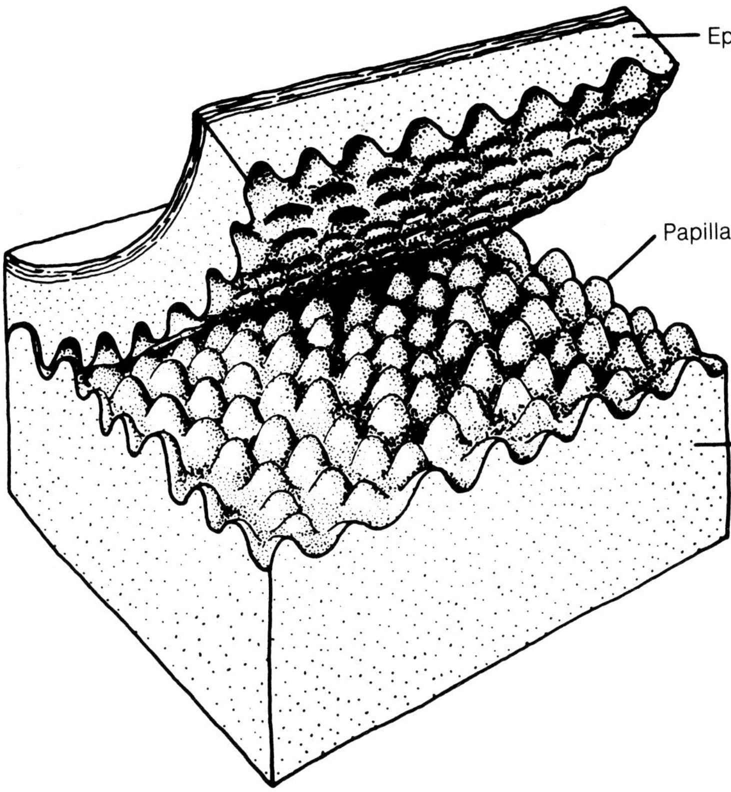

Figure 3–2. In this drawing, the epidermis has been lifted from the dermis (corium) to show the three-dimensional appearance of the dermoepidermal junction. Each dermal papilla fits into a depression of the epidermis. Epidermal ridges (rete ridges) surround each depression and produce the irregular border of the epidermis that is visible in histological sections.

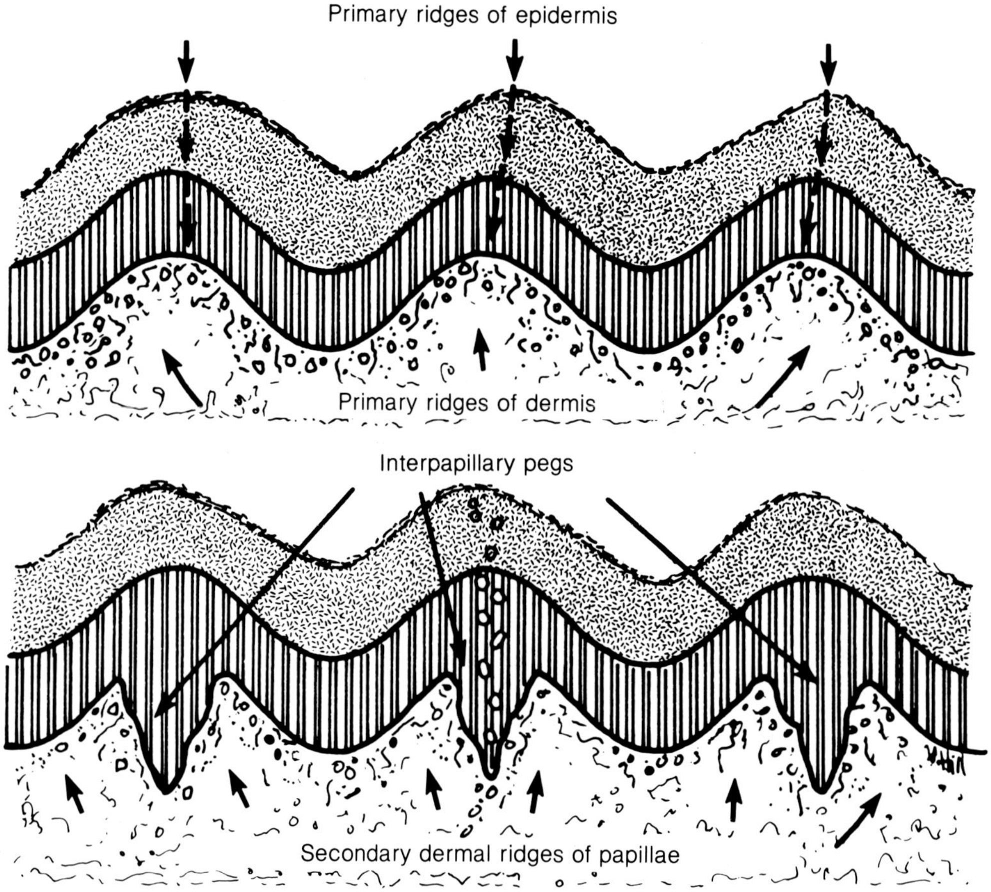

Figure 3–3. In the upper diagram, the primary ridges of epidermis and dermis are depicted. Furrows separate the primary epidermal ridges at the free surface of the skin. The lower diagram shows the interpapillary pegs and secondary dermal ridges or papillae. Ridges and furrows of the skin form during fetal life. Their pattern is determined chiefly by hereditary factors although this can be modified somewhat by disturbances of growth. Since the basic pattern is distinctive for an individual and does not change except to enlarge, it is used as the basis for the science of dermatoglyphics which permits the identification of an individual by fingerprints.

The upper diagram shows that the primary epidermal ridges overlie primary dermal ridges. The lower diagram illustrates that an interpapillary peg of epidermis grows downward from the apex of each primary dermal ridge. An interpapillary peg divides each primary dermal ridge into two secondary ridges or papillae. Ducts of eccrine sweat glands enter interpapillary pegs and open onto primary epidermal ridges.

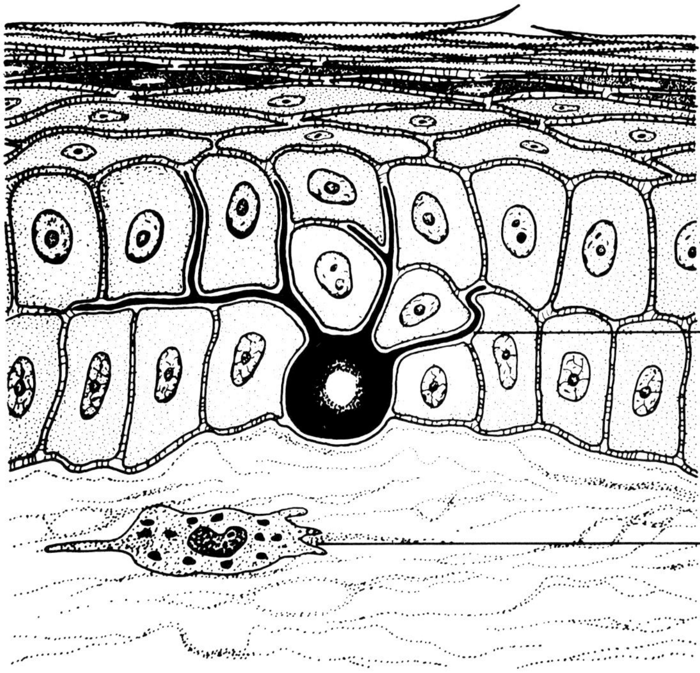

Figure 3–4. Drawing of epidermal melanocyte and its dendritic processes. The processes ramify in the intercellular spaces between the basal and spinous layers and between the keratinocytes of the spinous layer. Melanocytes produce melanin and transfer it to keratinocytes. The cells arise from the neural crest during embryonic development and migrate to the epidermis. The body of the cell in this illustration lies in the stratum basale and its processes extend into the stratum spinosum. It is estimated that there are 100,000 to 200,000 melanocytes/cm^2 of skin surface. Melanocytes are most numerous in the skin of the face, areola, and external genitalia. In other regions, they comprise about 10% of the cells of the basal layer in comparison to 20% to 25% in the aforementioned areas. Melanocytes are also present in hair follicles. One melanocyte supplies about thirty keratinocytes with melanin. Melanocytes use the amino acid tyrosine and the enzyme tyrosinase to synthesize melanin. Dihydroxyphenylalanine (DOPA) is used on unfixed cryostat sections of the skin to demonstrate melanocytes. Although most melanin stays in the epidermis, some is transferred through the basement membrane to the dermis where it is taken up by dermal macrophages (melanophages). Phagocytosis of pigment by macrophages in the dermis is the basis for tattoos.

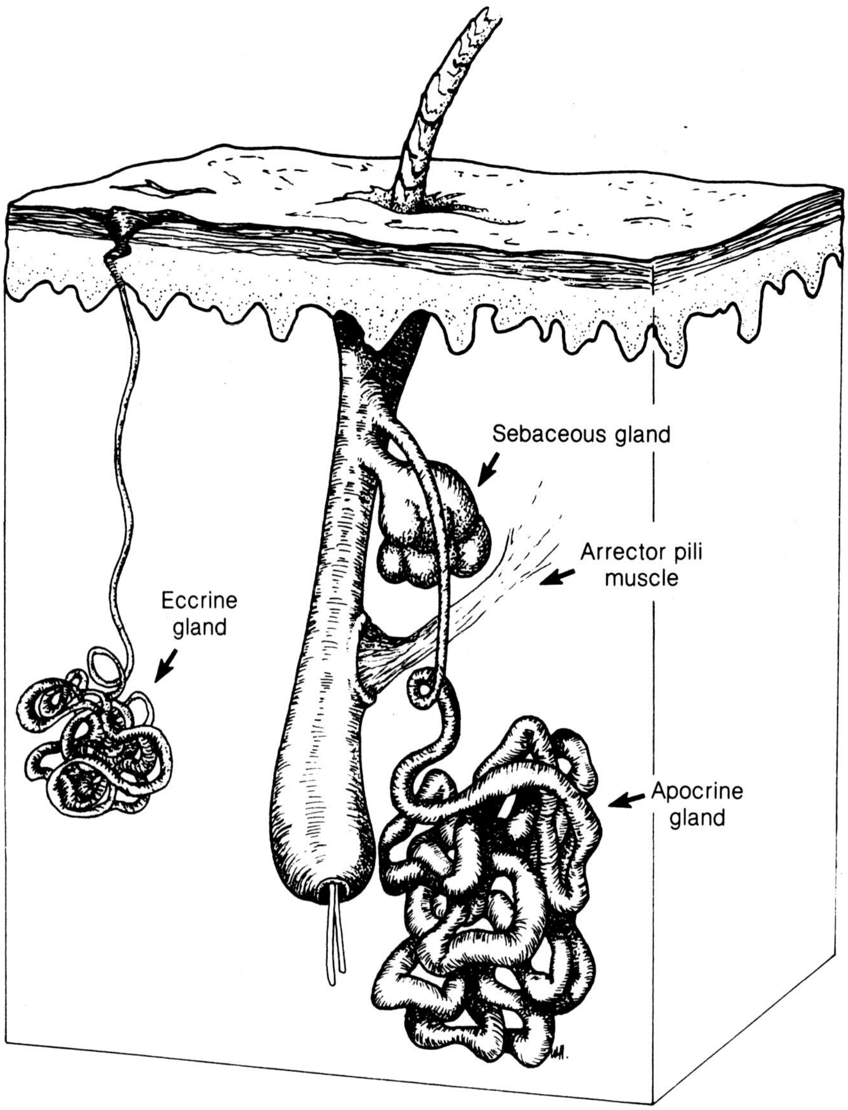

Figure 3–5. Diagramatic illustration of eccrine sweat gland, hair, and structures associated with the hair follicle, including sebaceous gland, arrector pili muscle, and apocrine sweat gland. The duct of an apocrine gland enters the hair follicle above the entrance of the sebaceous duct. The arrector pili muscle is a band of smooth muscle that extends from the papillary layer of the dermis to the connective tissue sheath of the hair follicle. Contraction of this muscle erects the hair and squeezes the sebaceous gland to aid in the release of its oily secretion, sebum. Cold temperatures stimulate arrector pili muscles to contract. Sebum spreads over the skin surface and helps to conserve body heat by slowing evaporation. Fear and certain other emotional states can cause contraction of the arrector pili and make the hair "stand on end." Upon contraction of the muscle, the skin may "dimple in" above the site of muscle attachment, resulting in a "goose pimple."

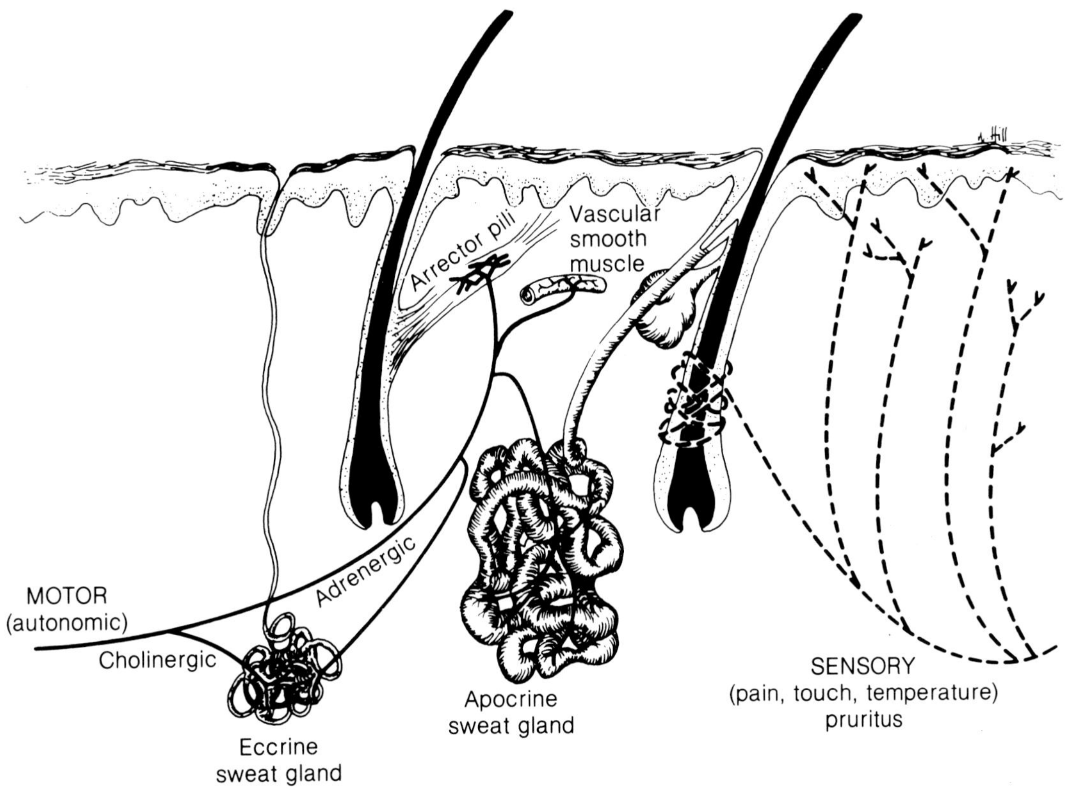

Figure 3–6. The skin contains numerous sensory and motor nerve endings. Sensory nerves for pain, temperature, and itch (pruritus) stimuli terminate as free nerve endings in the dermis, in association with hair follicles, and in the lower epidermis. In addition, there are many types of encapsulated receptors in the skin that serve a variety of sensory modalities (see Figure 3–7). Motor fibers to the skin are supplied by postganglionic fibers of the sympathetic division of the autonomic nervous system. Sympathetic adrenergic fibers innervate vascular smooth muscle, arrector pili muscles, and myoepithelial cells in apocrine sweat glands. Sympathetic cholinergic fibers innervate myoepithelial cells in eccrine sweat glands. Sebaceous glands depend on hormones, instead of nervous stimuli, for functional activity.

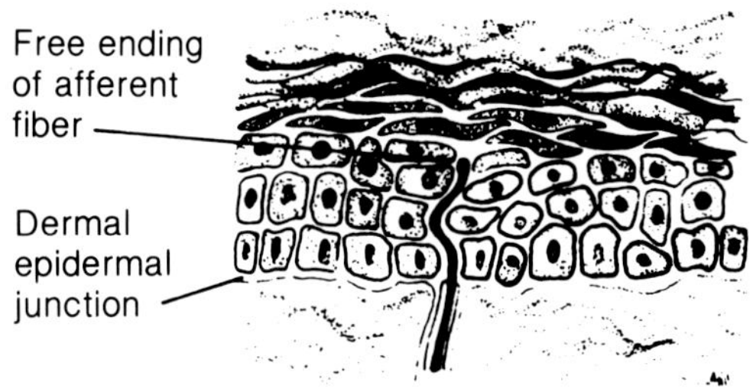

1 FREE EPIDERMAL NERVE ENDINGS

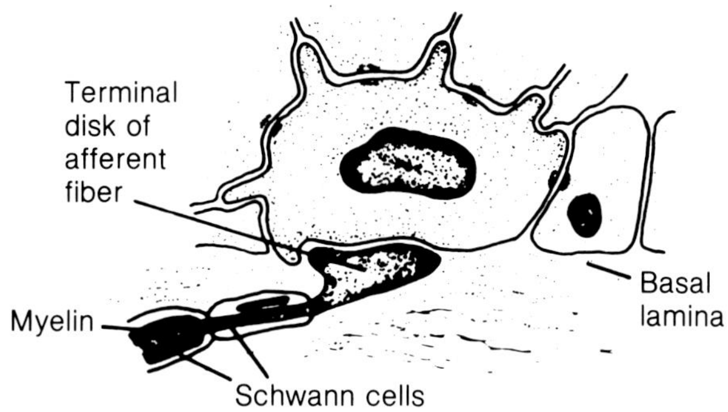

2 MERKEL ENDING

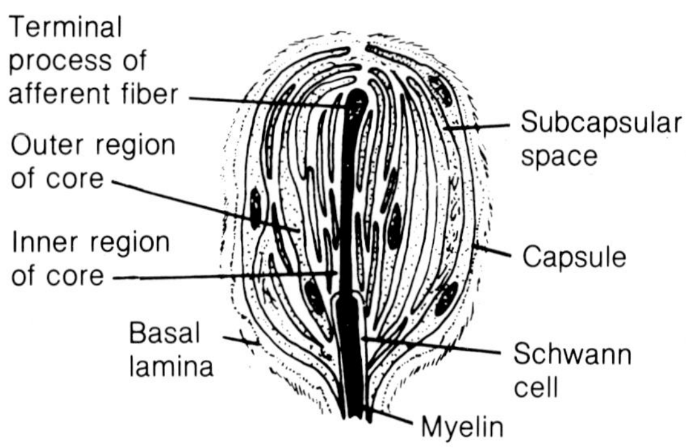

3 PACINIAN CORPUSCLE

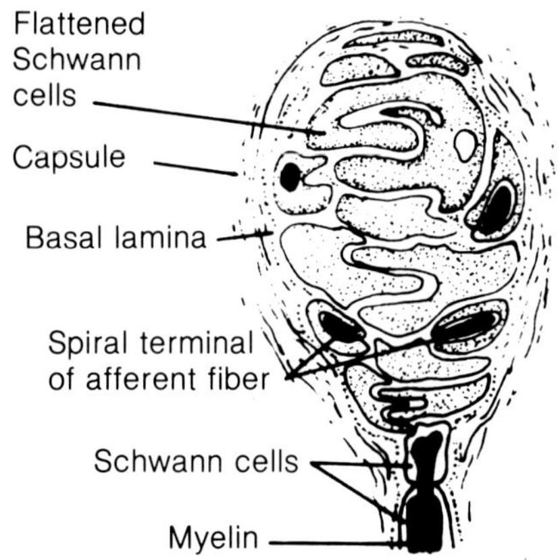

4 MEISSNER'S CORPUSCLE

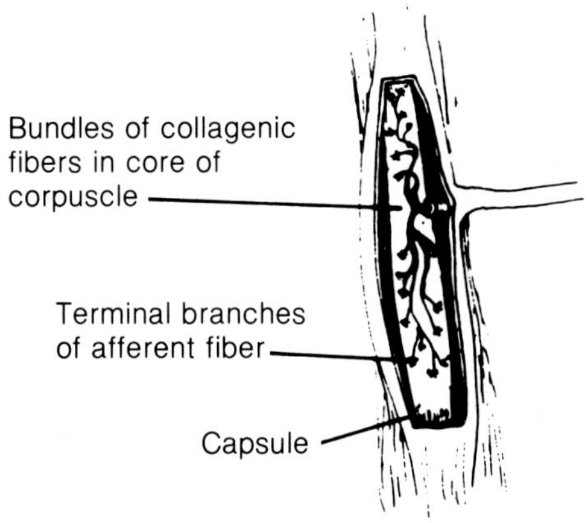

5 RUFFINI CORPUSCLE

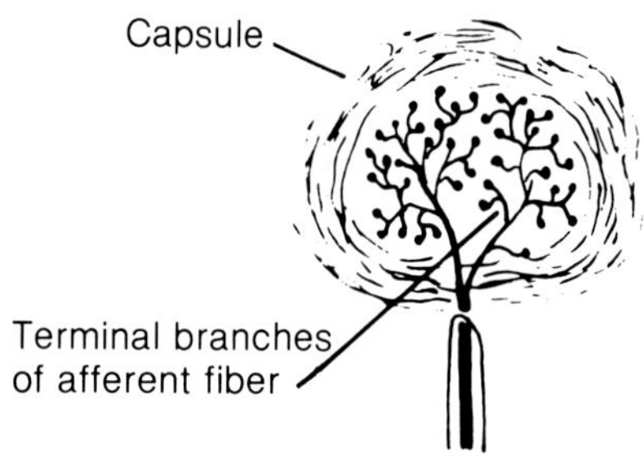

6 KRAUSE END BULB

Figure 3–7. Diagram of the different morphological types of sensory receptors in the skin. Functionally, cutaneous receptors are classified as (1) mechanoreceptors (stimulated by displacement due to pressure or touch), (2) thermoreceptors (respond to changes in temperature), and (3) nocioreceptors (respond to injurious agents capable of eliciting pain). Cutaneous receptors fit into two broad categories: free nerve endings and encapsulated nerve endings.

(1) Free Epidermal Nerve Endings. *These are unmyelinated fibers that register the sensations of pain, temperature, and itching.*

(2) Merkel Endings. *These receptors are found in the stratum basale. They are more numerous in the epidermis of the palms and soles than elsewhere. The nerve fiber to the Merkel endings is myelinated until it penetrates the basal lamina (basement membrane) to enter the epidermis. At that point, the fiber loses its myelin sheath and expands to end about an enlarged, modified epidermal cell called a Merkel cell. These endings serve the sense of touch.*

(3) Pacinian Corpuscle. *These encapsulated pressure receptors are distributed in the deep dermis and hypodermis. They are most abundant in the fingers, external genitalia, and breasts. Pacinian corpuscles are also present at other sites, e.g., joints, mesentery, and urinary bladder. Each is supplied by a myelinated nerve fiber that loses its myelin just inside the capsule. The capsule is composed of numerous lamellae of flattened cells that give sections of the corpuscle the appearance of a sliced onion.*

(4) Meissner's Corpuscle. *These encapsuled receptors for touch are located in the dermal papillae and are most numerous in the fingers, toes, lips, nipples, external genitalia, and eyelids. Each corpuscle is an ovoid connective tissue unit which contains ramifying myelinated and unmyelinated nerve fibers.*

(5) Ruffini Corpuscle. *These spindle-shaped encapsulated mechanoreceptors are found in the deep dermis and subcutaneous connective tissue. The receptors contain afferent branching nerve endings that ramify between bundles of collagenous fibers and sense the tension in them.*

(6) Krause End Bulb. *This type of encapsulated receptor is found mainly in mucocutaneous regions — for example, the dermis of the conjunctiva, lips, tongue, and external genitalia. The afferent nerve fiber enters the poorly formed capsule, branches repeatedly, and forms a network of nonmyelinated endings. Krause end bulbs vary considerably in structure. The precise function is not known, but they are believed to be mechanoreceptors.*

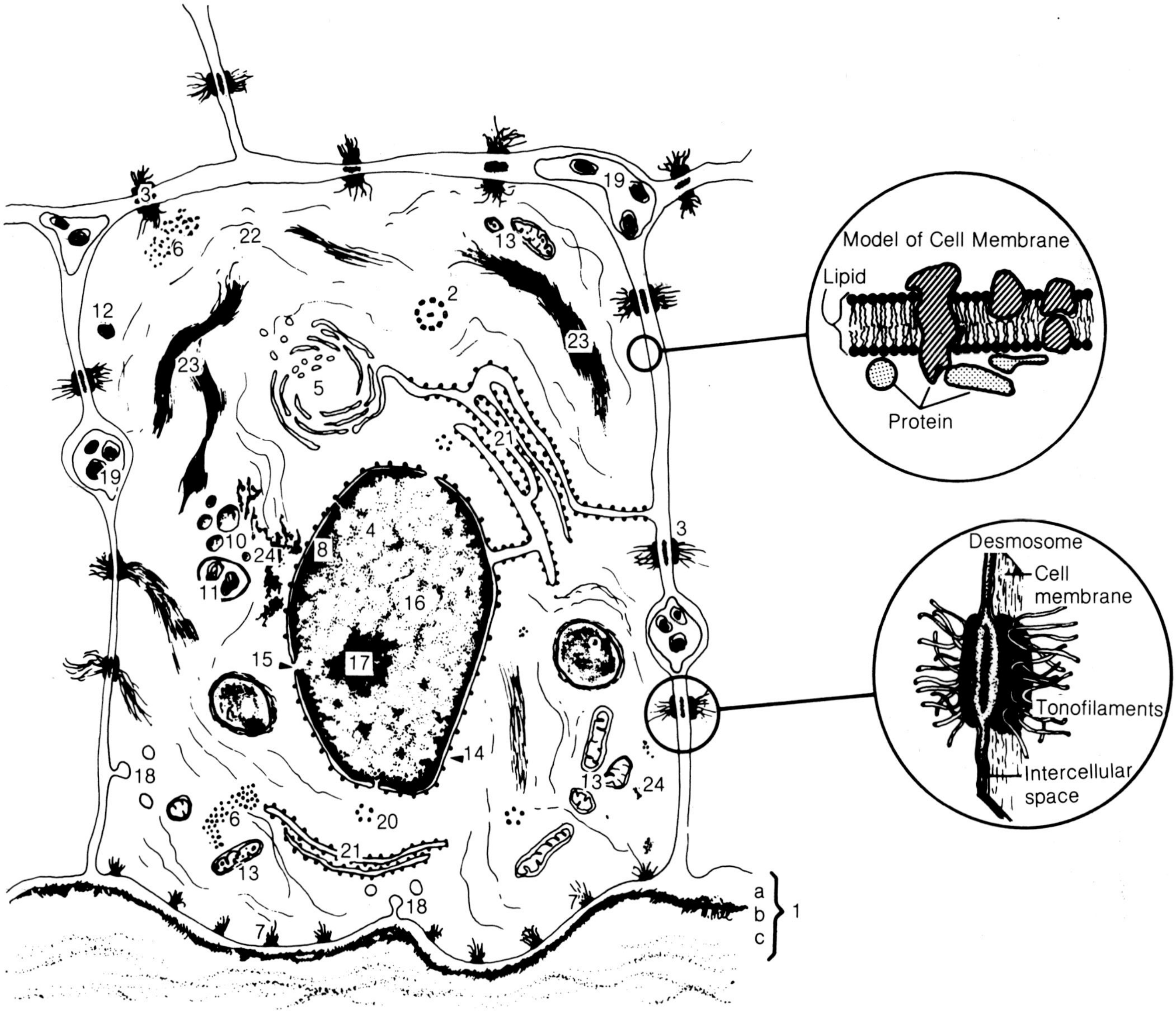

Figure 3–8. Diagram of a typical keratinocyte in the stratum basale as it would appear in an ultrathin section viewed by TEM. Cell components are numbered as follows: (1) Basement membrane, consisting of (a) lamina lucida, (b) basal lamina, and (c) reticular lamina; (2) Centriole; (3) Desmosome; (4) Euchromatin; (5) Golgi apparatus; (6) Glycogen; (7) Hemidesmosome; (8) Heterochromatin; (9) Lipid; (10) Lysosome, primary; (11) Lysosome, secondary; (12) Melanin pigment granule; (13) Mitochondrion; (14) Nuclear envelope, outer membrane; (15) Nuclear pore; (16) Nucleus; (17) Nucleolus; (18) Pinocytotic vesicles; (19) Process of melanocyte; (20) Ribosomes, free; (21) Rough endoplasmic reticulum; (22) Tonofilaments, solitary; (23) Tonofilaments, bundle; and (24) Tonofilaments, cross section.

Top inset. *Model of cell membrane (plasma membrane or plasmalemma). The cell membrane is about 75 Å thick. It is a lipoprotein with the bulk consisting of a phospholipid bilayer. Each lipid molecule has a hydrophilic head (solid circle) and two hydrophobic tails (wavy lines). Protein molecules are present on the inner and outer aspects of the membrane and may extend wholly or partly through the lipid bilayer. The trilaminar cell membrane is called a unit membrane because other membranes of the cell, such as those that surround organelles, have the same basic structure as the cell membrane.*

Bottom inset. *A desmosome (macula adherens) consists of a dense plaque on each adjacent cell membrane, tonofilaments, and the dense material in the intercellular space. The cytoplasmic aspect of each cell membrane is associated with a plaque of electron dense material. Within the cytoplasm, tonofilaments make hairpin loops in or near the dense material of the plaque. The filaments are composed of keratins. They are a major cytoskeletal element within most epithelial cells and differ chemically and in size from the smaller actin filaments of the terminal web and zonula adherens.*

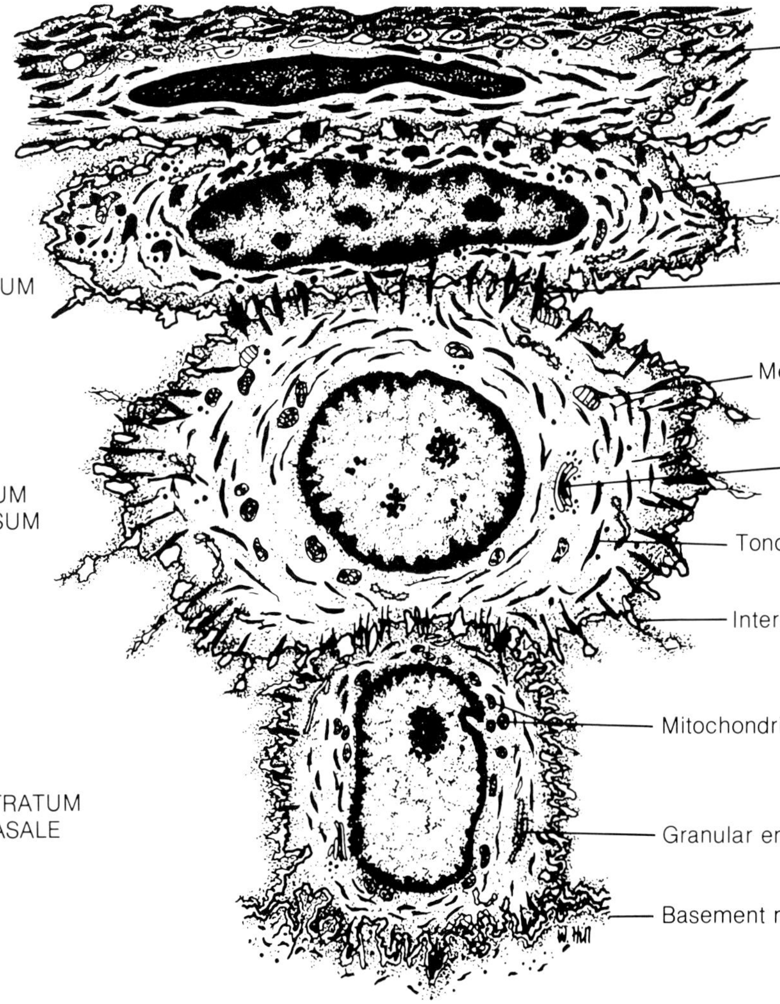

Figure 3–9. Diagram of a cell in each stratum of the skin as it might appear by TEM. The layer of cells on the basement membrane constitutes the stratum basale. This layer is followed by the stratum spinosum, stratum granulosum, and stratum corneum. Through the process of keratinization, cells derived from the vertically oriented columnar basal cells are transformed into horizontally aligned, thin, cornified cells that form a protective barrier over the body's external surface.

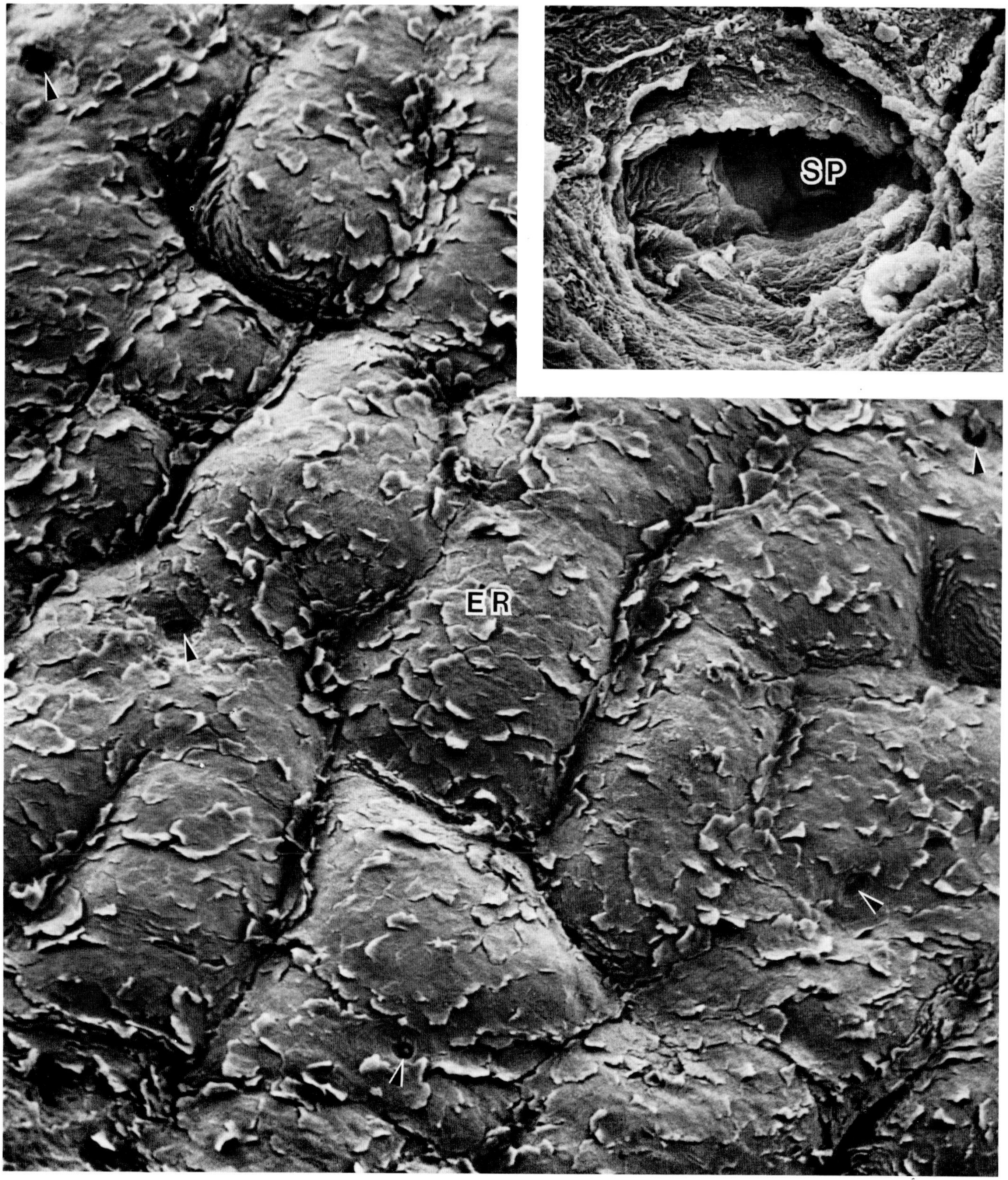

Figure 3–10. Dorsolateral surface of distal phalanx, 3rd finger, right hand. The epidermal ridges (ER) and grooves are responsible for the unevenness of the skin's surface. Sweat ducts, as sweat pores (arrows), open into the ridges. Many cells of the stratum corneum have turned-up edges, and are in the process of desquamation. × 180.

The inset shows a sweat pore (SP) at higher magnification. × 1,660.

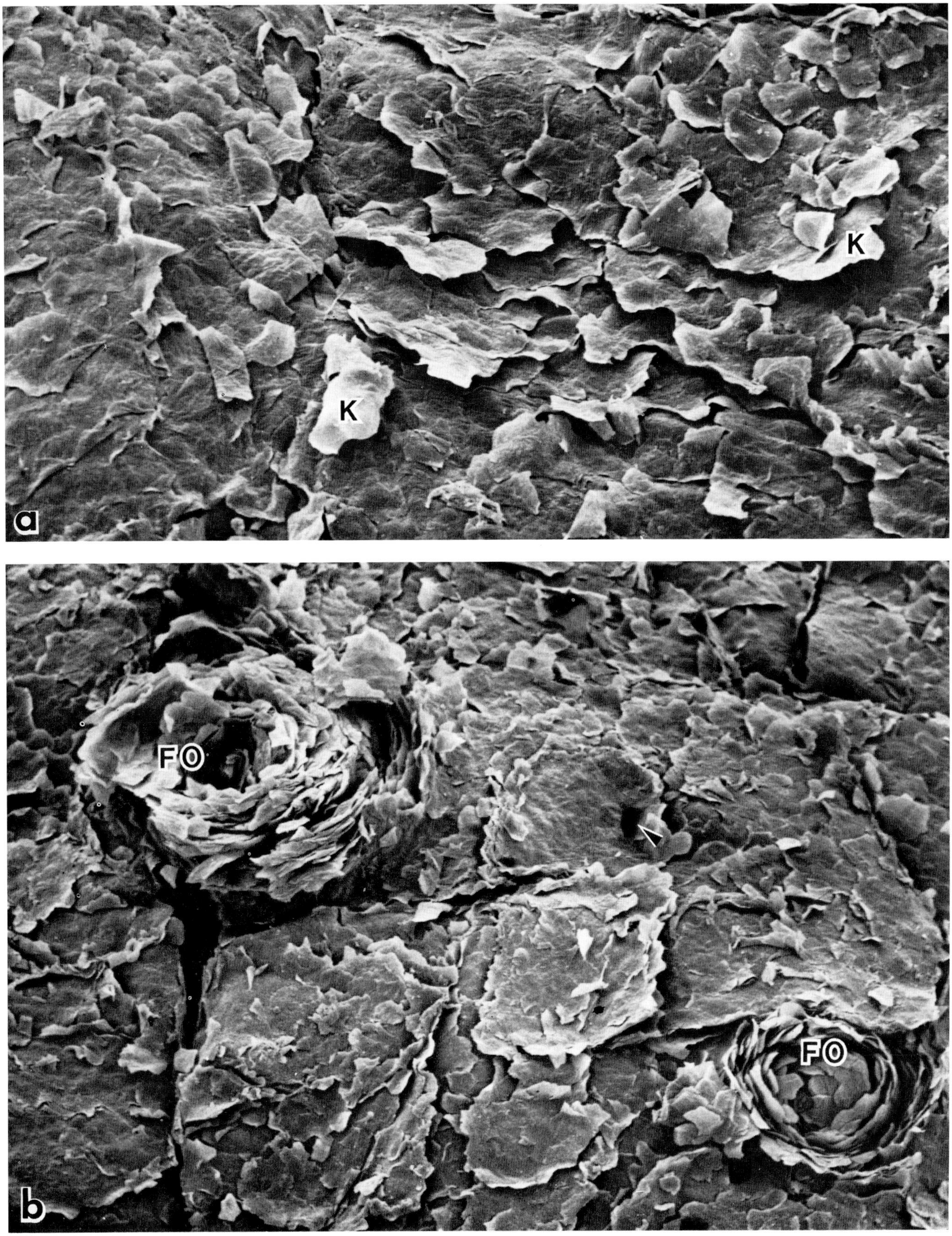

Figure 3–11. a. *Dorsal surface of forearm. The outermost keratinized cells (K) of the stratum corneum are loosely attached. They are shed continuously and comprise the stratum disjunctum. Individual cells of the stratum corneum are called different names, including keratinized cells, scales, squames, and horny cells.* ×290.

b. *Hairs are absent from the two follicular orifices (FO). Hairs are "wiry" and are frequently lost from their follicles during tissue processing. Follicular orifices are slightly elevated because of the increased numbers of keratinized cells present at such openings. Note the sweat pore (arrow).* ×145.

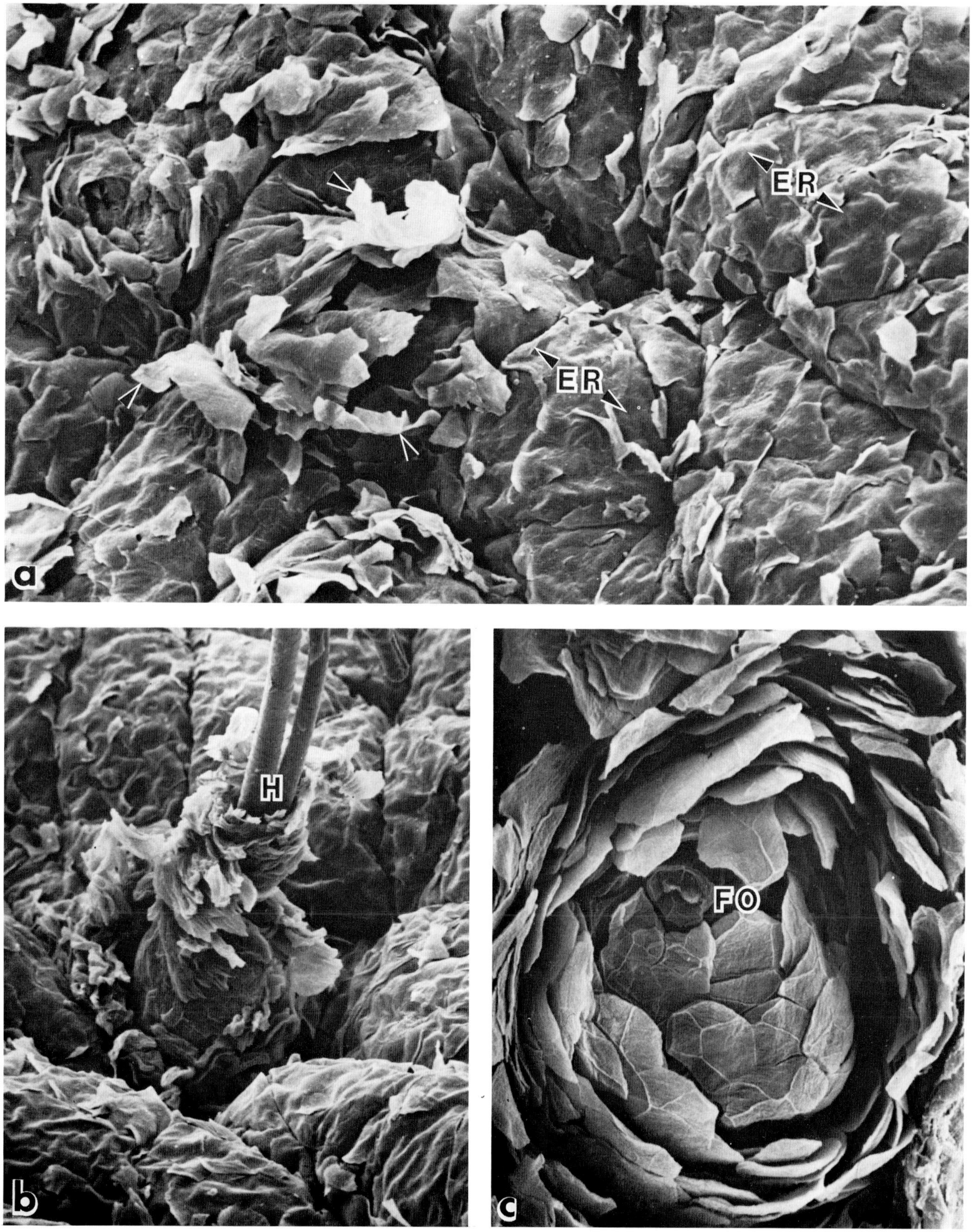

Figure 3–12. a. *Back, showing desquamation of scales (arrows) from epidermal ridges (ER).* ×290.

b. *Back, illustrating two small hairs (H) emerging from the same orifice. Follicles with multiple hairs are most frequent on the face, back, and arms in the order named.* ×240.

c. *Arm, depicting follicular orifice (FO) without hair and plugged with keratin.* ×480.

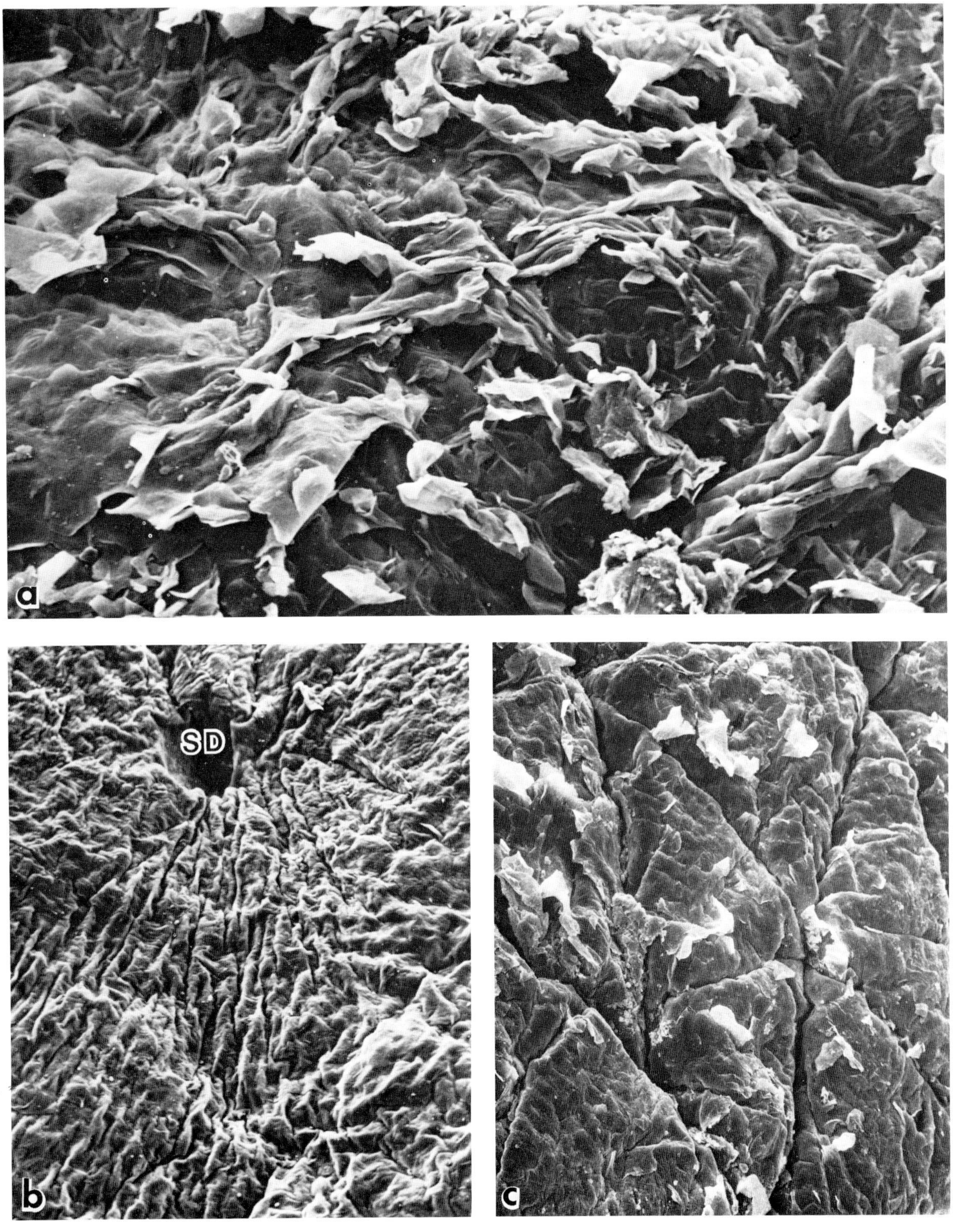

Figure 3–13. The effects of age on the skin and the effects of removing tape from "unprotected" skin and from "protected" skin.

a. *Abdominal skin, 77 year old male. Many scales are loose and in the process of detaching. Exfoliation increases with age as the skin becomes dryer due to atrophy and inactivity of the sebaceous glands. Consequently the epidermis becomes thinner with advancing age.* ×240.

b. *Back, 47 year old male. Adhesive tape was applied directly to unprotected skin and removed after 24 hours. The tape "stripped" the majority of cells from the free surface. The "wrinkles" are a result of the tape. They course in the direction of the sweat duct (SD) opening. The epidermis is removed and bleeding results upon the repeated application of tape.* ×190.

c. *Abdomen, 21 year old male, Adhesive tape was applied over a protective dressing (Skin Prep®, United, Largo, FL). The protected skin was not damaged when the tape was removed after 24 hours, and it was similar to biopsies of control skin taken from the same patient. This protective dressing lessens skin trauma when used with any adhesive that must be applied frequently to the skin.* ×165.

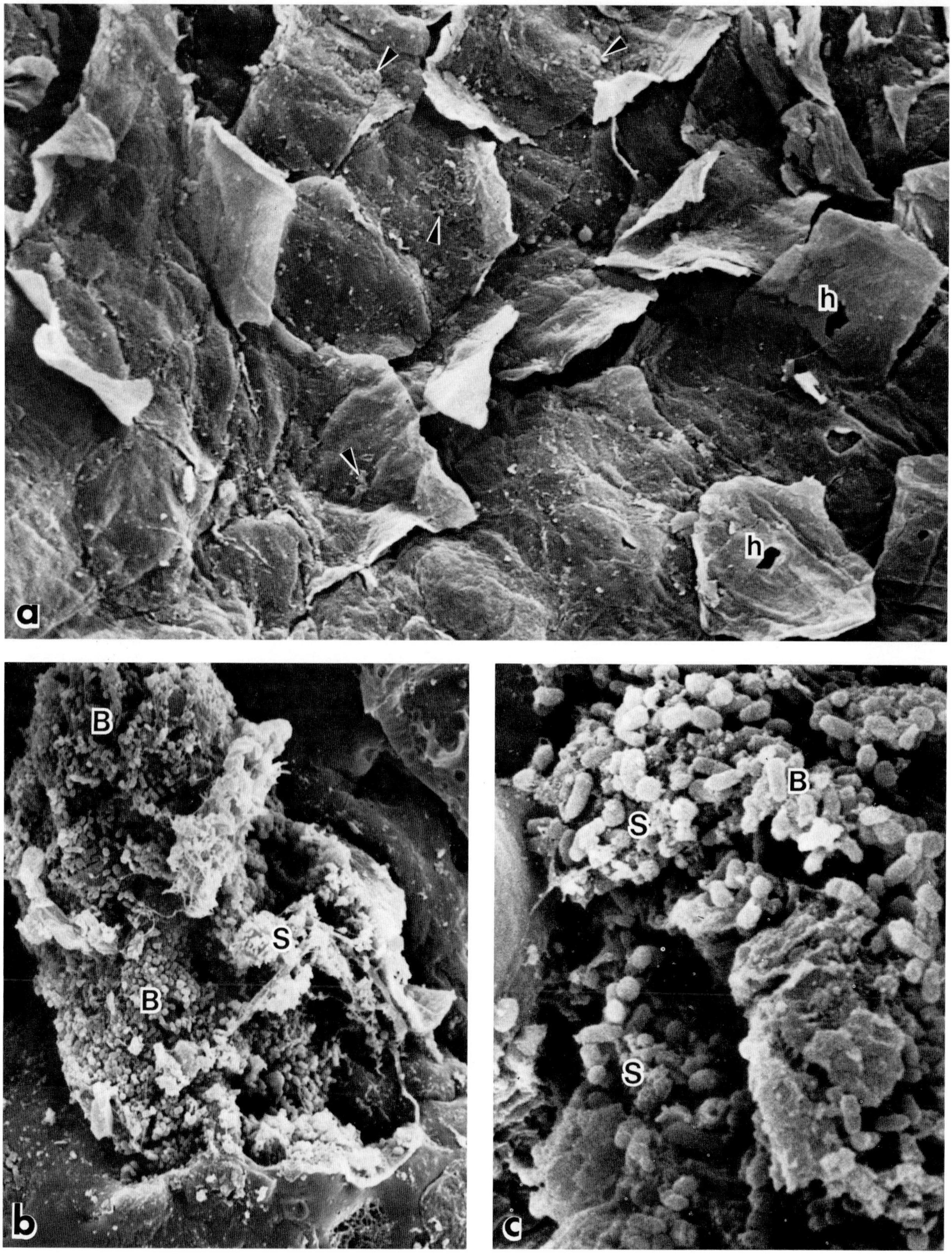

Figure 3–14. Microorganisms on the skin.
a. Microorganisms (arrows), barely visible at this magnification, are widely distributed on the scales shown in this micrograph of the forearm. SEM has been especially valuable for visualizing cutaneous flora. It has been estimated that some areas of normal skin harbor as many as 5,000,000 microorganisms/cm^2. Both bacteria and yeasts are present. Yeasts are larger than bacteria and some species have keratolytic activity. The latter may account for the holes (h) in the scales. The number of microorganisms varies from one individual to another and in different regions of the body of the same person. × 1,060.

b. Microcolony of bacteria mixed with sebum. Most bacteria (B) of the skin are associated with sebum (S) which occurs as single or multiple droplets. × 1,485.

c. Microcolony of bacteria and sebum in skin crease. The close association of bacteria (B) and sebum (S) indicates that sebum is a choice fuel for some cutaneous bacteria. × 6,075.

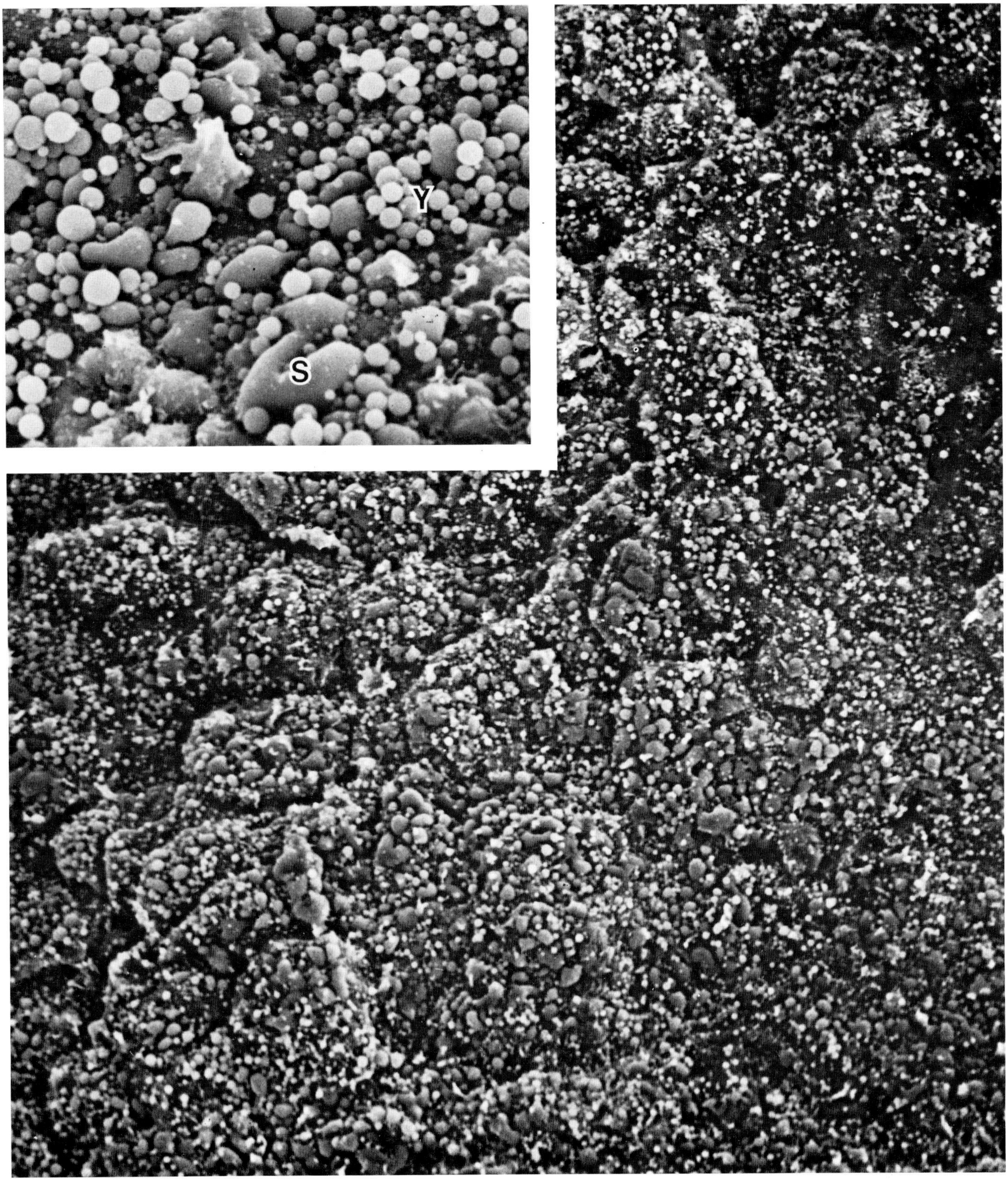

Figure 3–15. Scalp. Hair is absent in the area shown, and the skin is completely covered with sebum and yeast cells (Pityrosporum). ×770.

Inset. *Higher magnification of yeast cells (Y) and sebum (S). The yeasts reproduce by budding. ×2,875.*

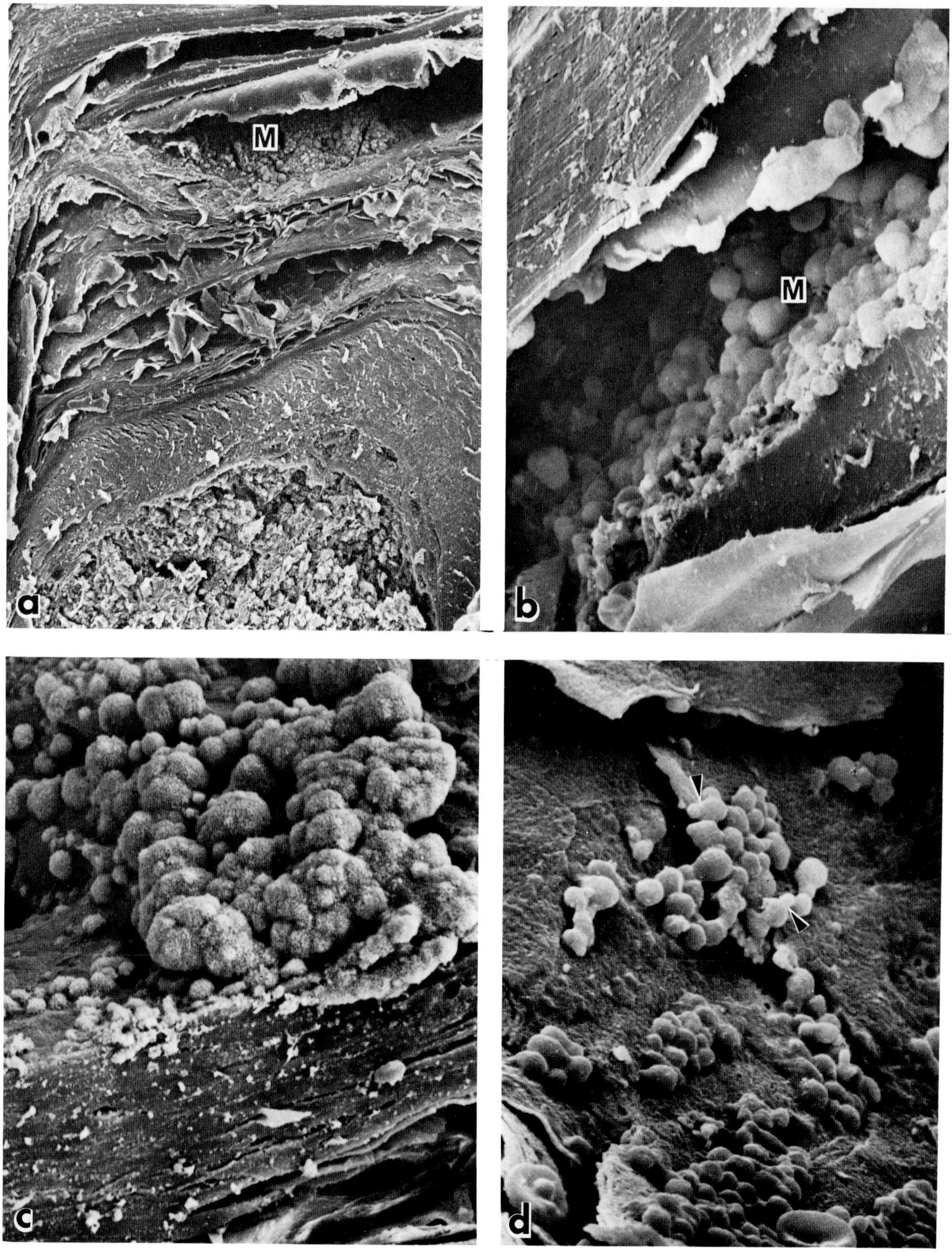

Figure 3–16. Scales in profile reveal microorganisms that are usually hidden from view.

a. *Profile of stratum corneum, depicting microorganism (M) in one of several "pockets" between the scales. ×85.*

b. *Nest of microorganisms (M) between two lamellae of scales. Most of the microorganisms resemble yeasts in size and shape. ×965.*

c. *Microcolony of yeasts covered with a fuzzy coat and located on a shelf of compact scales. ×960.*

d. *Microcolony of yeasts whose smooth surfaces differ from the fuzzy surfaces shown in c. Buds (arrows) occur at sites where yeasts are reproducing. ×1,530.*

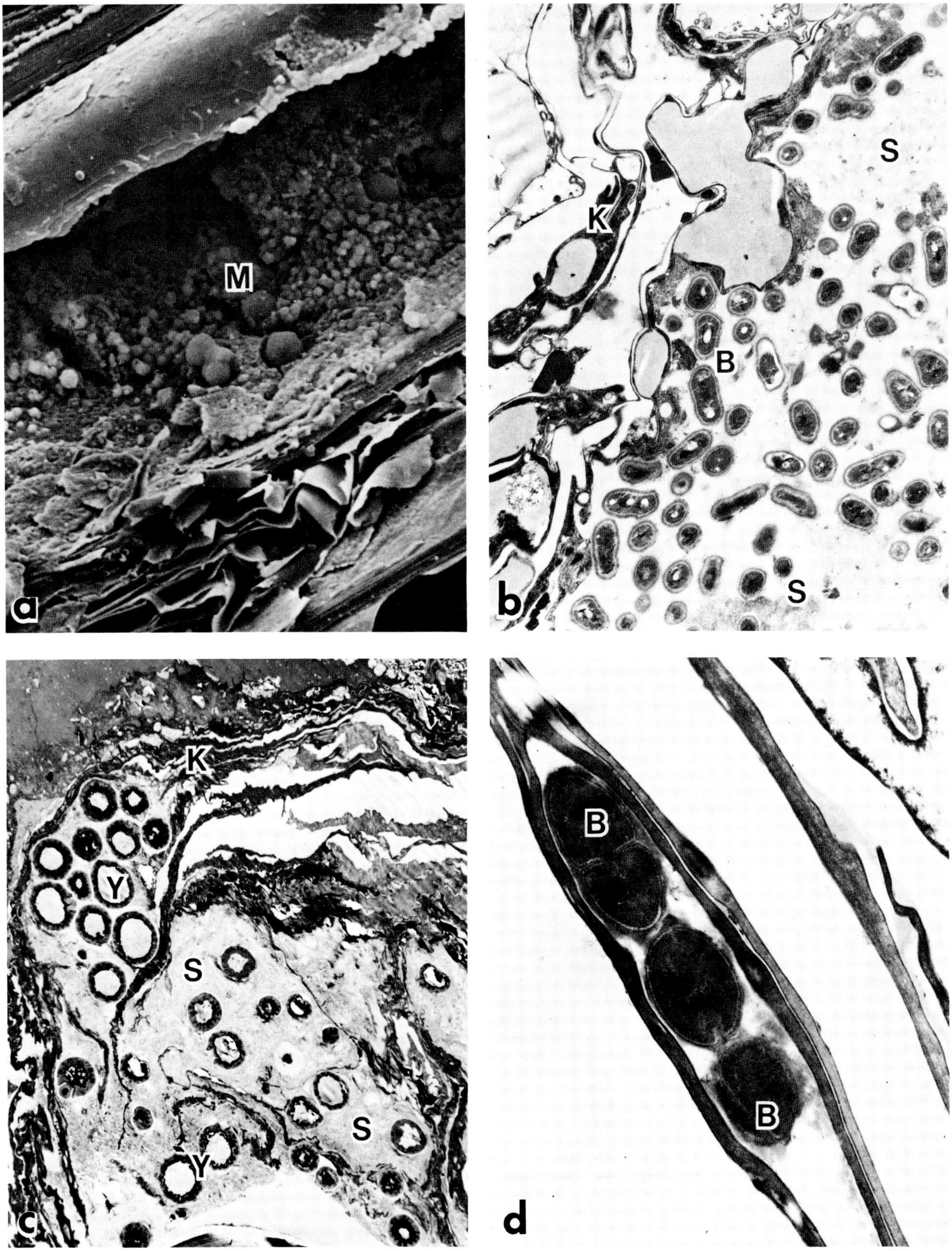

Figure 3–17. Cutaneous flora depicted by SEM and TEM.

a. *Profile of scales with microorganisms (M) in space between scales. SEM has shown that skin specimens from all parts of the body frequently contain microorganisms nestled among the spaces between lamellae of scales. ×420.*

b. *TEM, microcolony of bacteria (B) below the superficial layers of keratinized cells (K) of the scalp. The amorphous material is sebum (S). ×11,250.*

c. *TEM, microcolonies of yeasts (Y) in association with sebum (S) between the keratinized cells (K) of the scalp. ×1,850.*

d. *TEM, dividing bacteria (B) between scales of scalp. ×23,485.*

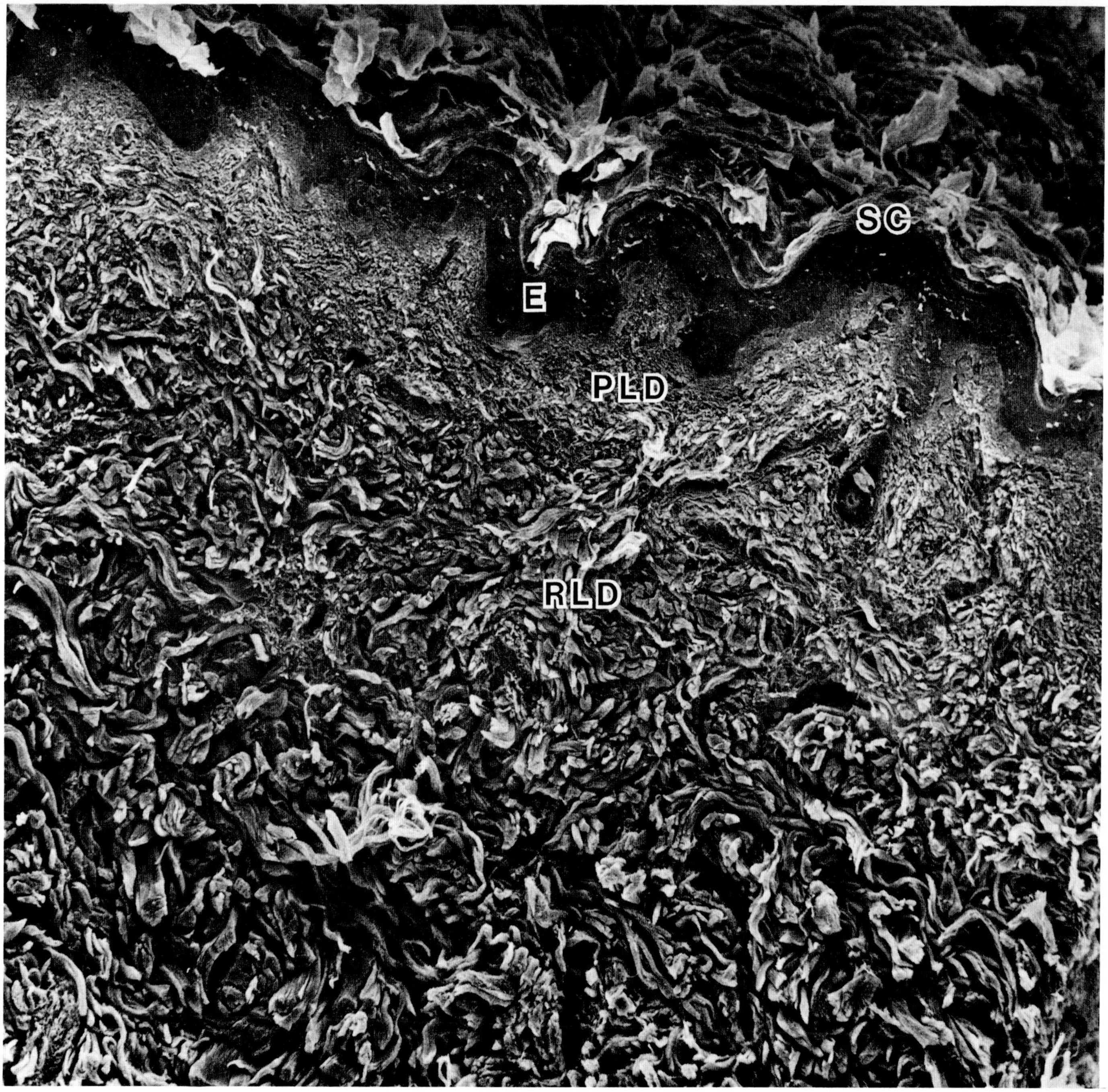

Figure 3–18. Thin skin in profile.

a. *Skin can be divided into two types, thin and thick, based on the thickness of the epidermis. In thin skin, the epidermis (E) which includes the stratum corneum (SC) varies in thickness from 0.07 mm to 0.12 mm. Thin skin is the general body skin; thick skin is found only on the palms and soles. In thick skin, the epidermis is several times thicker than in thin skin, measuring about 0.8 mm in the palms and 1.4 mm in the soles.*

The dermis can be divided into a papillary layer (PLD) and a reticular layer (RLD). Bundles of collagen of various sizes constitute the bulk of both layers. The papillary layer is the thinner of the two layers and its elevations form the dermal papillae that project between the ridges on the deep surface of the epidermis. The reticular layer is the deeper, thicker portion of the dermis. Here the bundles of collagen fibers are larger than in the papillary layer.

The dermis is usually 1–2 mm thick over most of the body. It is thinnest in the eyelids (0.6 mm or less) and thickest in the interscapular region (3 mm or more). ×265.

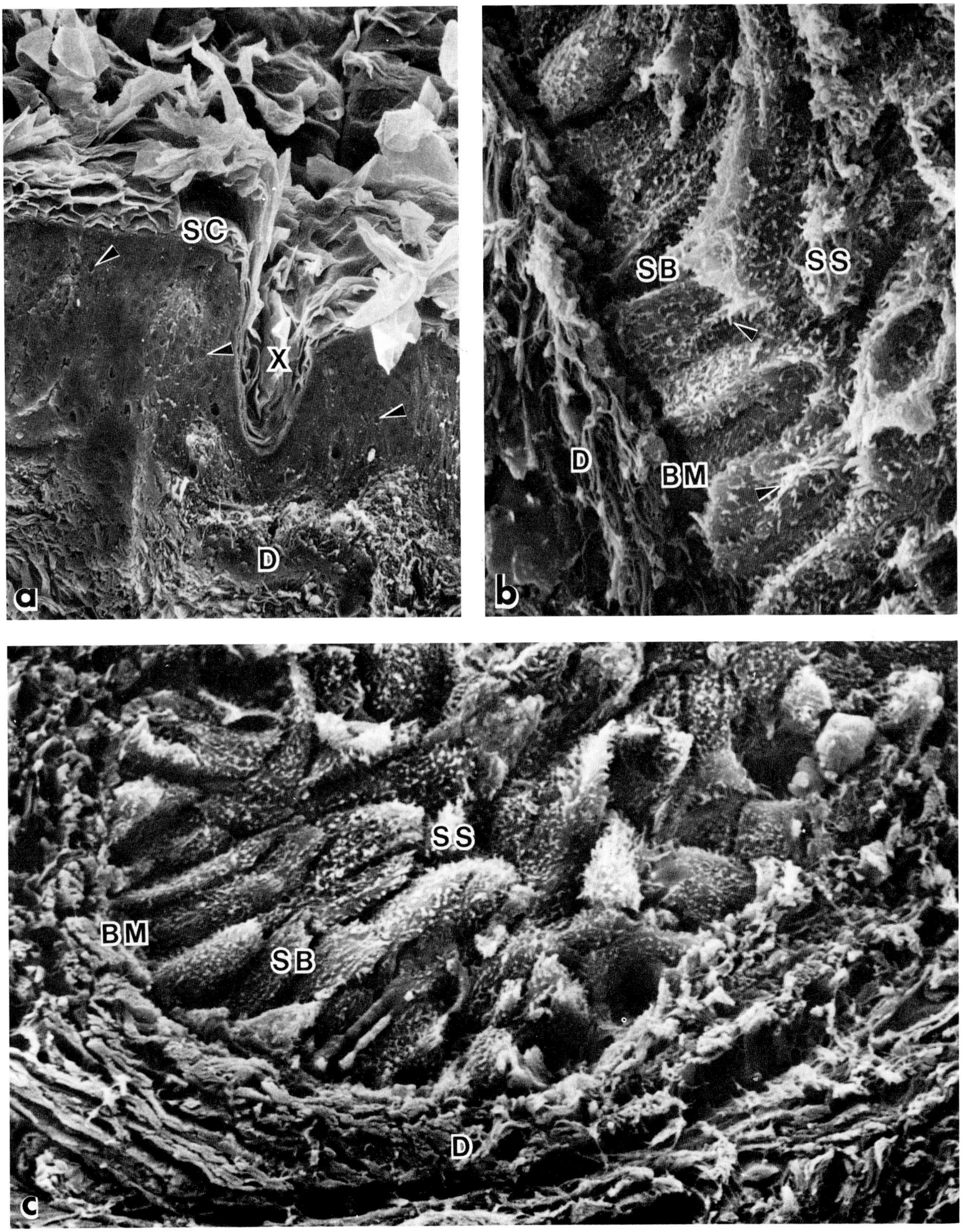

Figure 3–19. Sections of epidermis viewed by SEM.

a. Nuclear outlines (arrows) are visible in the strata of epidermis between the stratum corneum (SC) and dermis (D). The groove (X) is filled with scales. ×450.

b. Spinous processes (arrows) extend from keratinocytes of the stratum basale (SB) and stratum spinosum (SS). Note area of basement membrane (BM) and edge of dermis (D). ×1,760.

c. Rete ridge, basement membrane (BM), and dermis (D). Keratinocytes of the stratum spinosum (SS) have more processes than those of the stratum basale (SB). ×1,325.

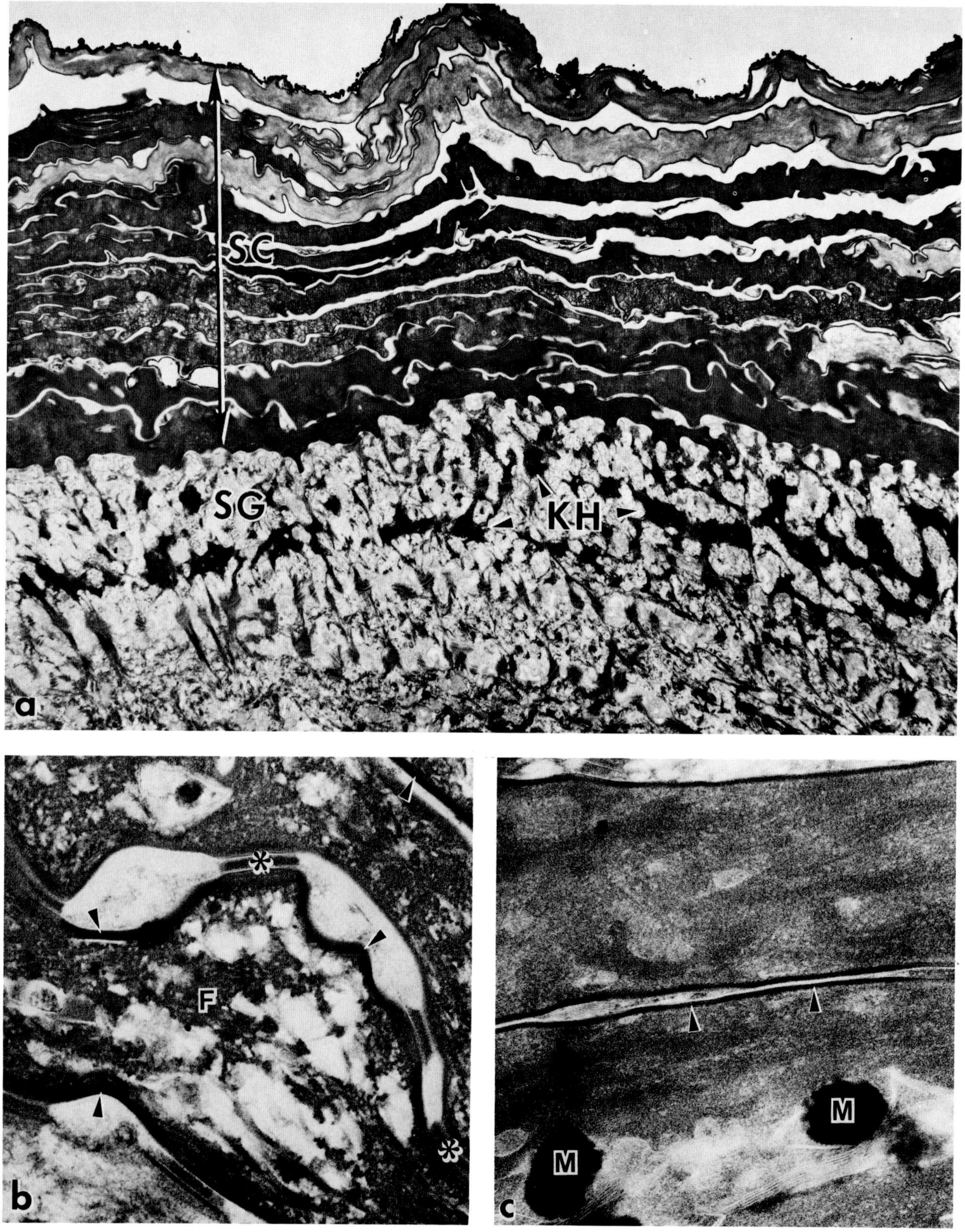

Figure 3–20. TEM, stratum corneum.

a. *The stratum corneum (SC) in this micrograph consists of 10 to 12 layers of dead cells. It overlies the stratum granulosum (SG) which contains irregularly-shaped keratohyalin granules (KH). Cells of the stratum corneum which are most superficial in position belong to the stratum disjunctum, a layer that undergoes continuous desquamation.* × *8,910.*

b. *Cornified cells show thickened cell membranes (arrows) and contain filamentous material (F) in various stages of keratinization. Organelles and inclusions characteristic of deeper strata are absent. Detached desmosomal remnants (*) are present in the intercellular spaces. Their detachment expedites exfoliation.* × *67,320.*

c. *Melanin pigment (M) is sometimes present in or between filament-filled keratinized cells whose cell membranes (arrows) are thickened.* × *76,950.*

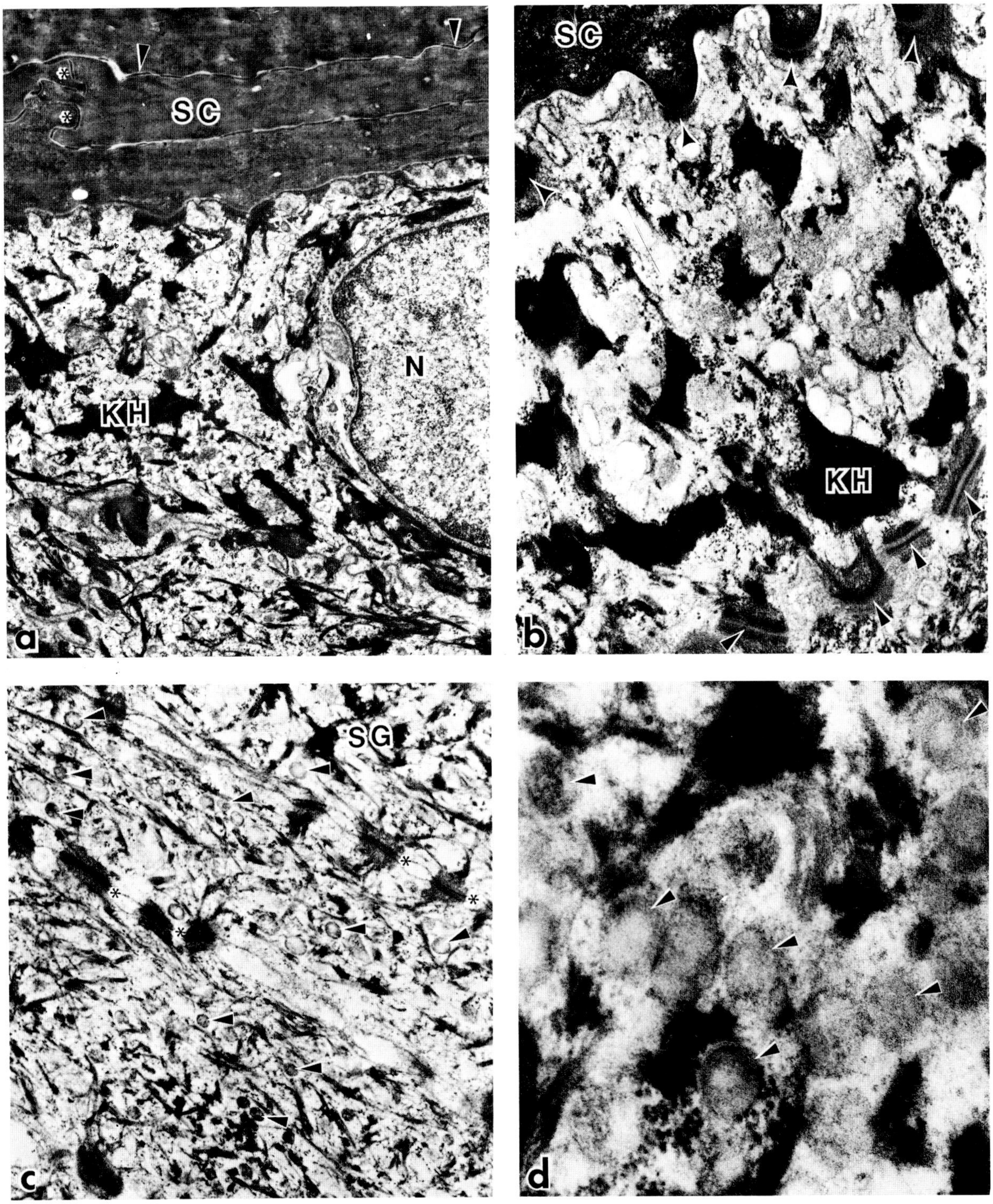

Figure 3–21. TEM, stratum granulosum and membrane-coating granules.

a. *Cells of the stratum corneum (SC) interdigitate (*), a feature that helps to bind them together. Thickened plaques (arrows) indicate former desmosomes. Note keratohyalin granules (KH) and edge of nucleus (N) in stratum granulosum. ×11,110.*

b. *Pleomorphic keratohyalin granules (KH) are shown in the uppermost cell layer of the stratum granulosum. Degenerating desmosomes (upper arrows) border the stratum corneum (SC); intact desmosomes (lower arrows) are present between the first and second cell layers of the stratum granulosum. ×27,450.*

c. *Membrane-coating granules (arrows) are most numerous in the upper part of the stratum spinosum and some are present in the stratum granulosum (SG). Intact desmosomes (*) are shown. ×20,570.*

Membrane-coating granules are also called lamellar bodies, keratinosomes, and Odland bodies. They are not limited to the epidermis, but they may be present in other stratified epithelia that have the potential to undergo keratinization. Arising as membrane-bound bodies from the Golgi complex, they migrate to the cell surface where they fuse with the cell membrane and empty their contents into the intercellular space. The released material is believed to seal the intercellular space and thereby prevent the passage of nutrients.

d. *Membrane-coating granules (arrows) at higher magnification. Ultrastructural and cytochemical studies have identified lipids, sugars, and hydrolytic enzymes in the granules. ×86,700.*

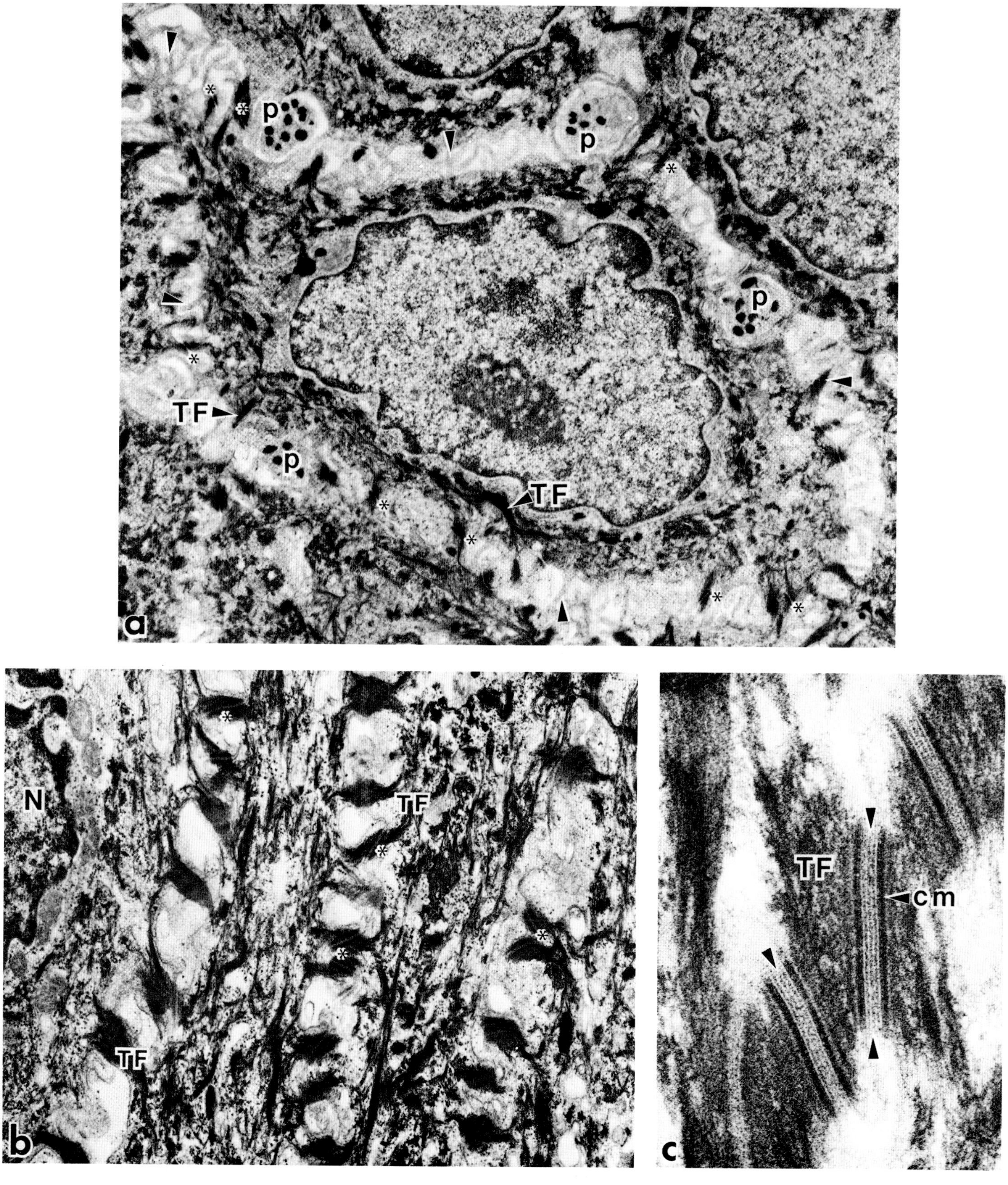
p
TF
a
N
b
cm
c

Figure 3–22. TEM, stratum spinosum.

a. *Skin from a black person. Melanocyte processes in the intercellular spaces of the skin of blacks are apt to contain pigment (p). Keratinocytes in the stratum spinosum of all races are known to have a spiny or prickly appearance when viewed with the light microscope. This electron micrograph shows that the spiny appearance is caused by the multitude of cytoplasmic processes (arrows) that project into the intercellular spaces. Tonofilaments (TF) are present in the processes. Bundles of tonofilaments are visible by light microscopy and are called tonofibrils. Desmosomes (*) occur where contact is made between spinous processes of adjacent cells. × 11,250.*

b. *Processes of keratinocytes in stratum spinosum, showing desmosomes (*) and tonofilaments (TF) associated with the processes. The processes were believed to be true intercellular bridges until TEM showed that desmosomes (*) joined the processes and prevented true intercellular continuity. Edge of nucleus, N. × 22.500.*

c. *Details of desmosome. Three desmosomes are shown. Components of a desmosome include part of the cell membrane (cm) of each adjacent cell, aggregates of tonofilaments (TF), and parallel dense lines (arrows) in the intercellular space. The cell membrane at sites of desmosomes is no thicker than elsewhere, but it may appear thicker because condensed cytoplasm occurs along the cell membrane. The intercellular space contains a sialic acid-rich mucoprotein that acts as an adhesive to anchor the two adjacent cell membranes. × 105,400.*

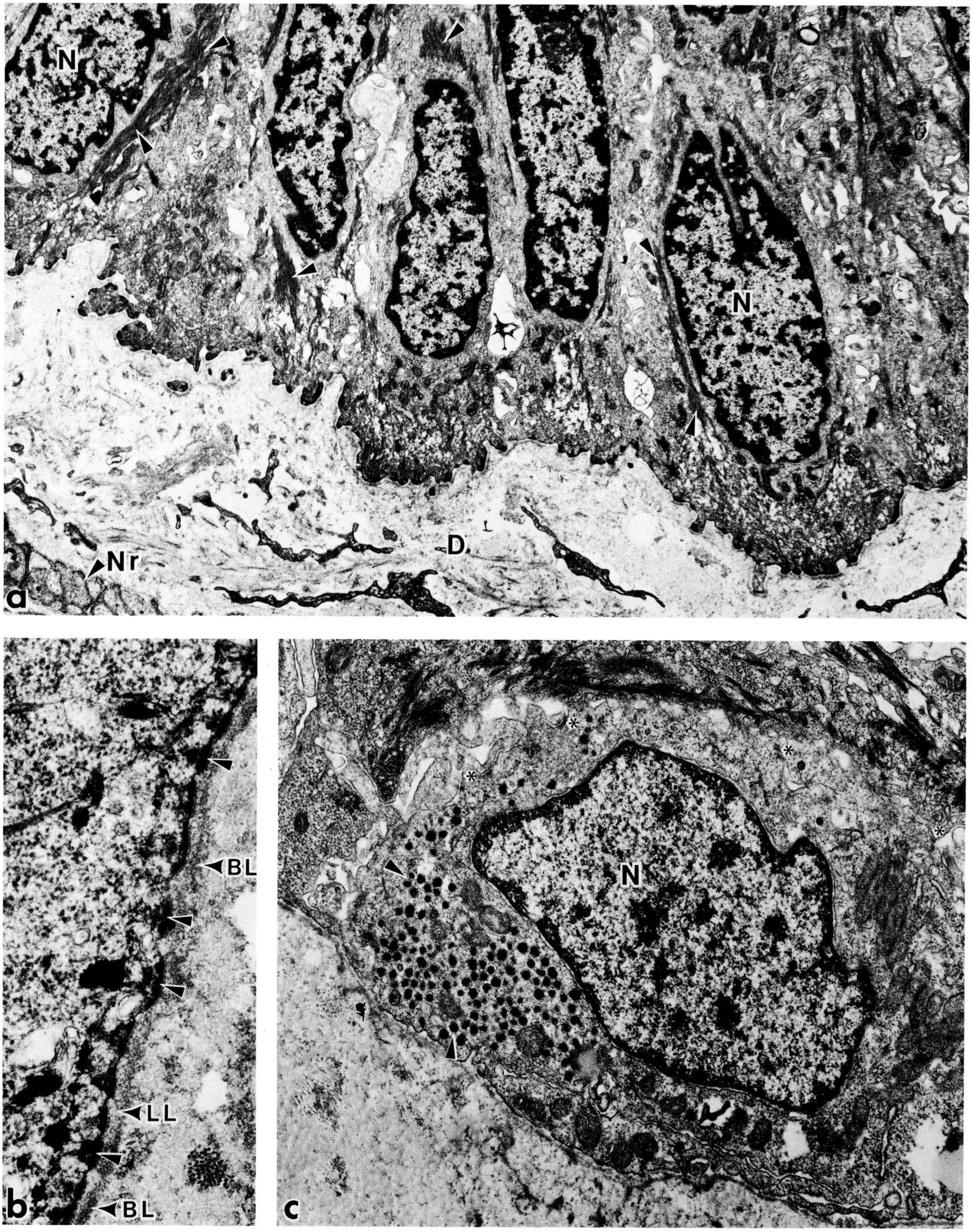
N
N
Nr
D
a
BL
LL
BL
b
N
c

Figure 3–23. TEM, stratum basale and basement membrane.

a. *Cells of the stratum basale (stratum cylindricum) are shown adjacent to the dermis (D). Basal cells range from cuboidal to columnar in height, rest on the basement membrane, and are mitotically active. The nucleus is large and the cytoplasm is rich in tonofilaments which may occur singly or in bundles (arrows). Tonofilaments are involved in the keratinization process. Part of a nerve (Nr) is shown in the dermis. ×9,690.*

b. *Basement membrane and hemidesmosomes. Hemidesmosomes (arrows) are formed by thickenings of the basal cell membrane and by the cytoplasmic filaments that are associated with the thickenings. Hemidesmosomes aid in binding the stratum basale to the dermis. The basement membrane consists of three parts: basal lamina, lamina lucida, and reticular lamina. The basal lamina (BL) is about 500 Å thick and is separated from the cell membrane by a 300 Å clear space called the lamina lucida (LL). The basal lamina is a product of the epidermal cells. It contains microfilaments with a diameter of about 20 Å embedded in a glycosaminoglycan matrix. The reticular lamina is the only part of the basement membrane that is visible by light microscopy. It contains reticular fibers. Reticular fibers are blackened by silver stains. These argyrophilic fibers also stain red with periodic acid-Schiff because polysaccharides coat their surfaces. ×22,500.*

c. *Merkel cell in stratum basale. Observe the electron dense granules (arrows) and nucleus (N). Desmosomes (*) attach Merkel cells to adjacent keratinocytes. The Merkel cell has no established function, but its association with unmyelinated axons of afferent sensory nerves suggests that the cell is concerned with sensory reception. ×10,650.*

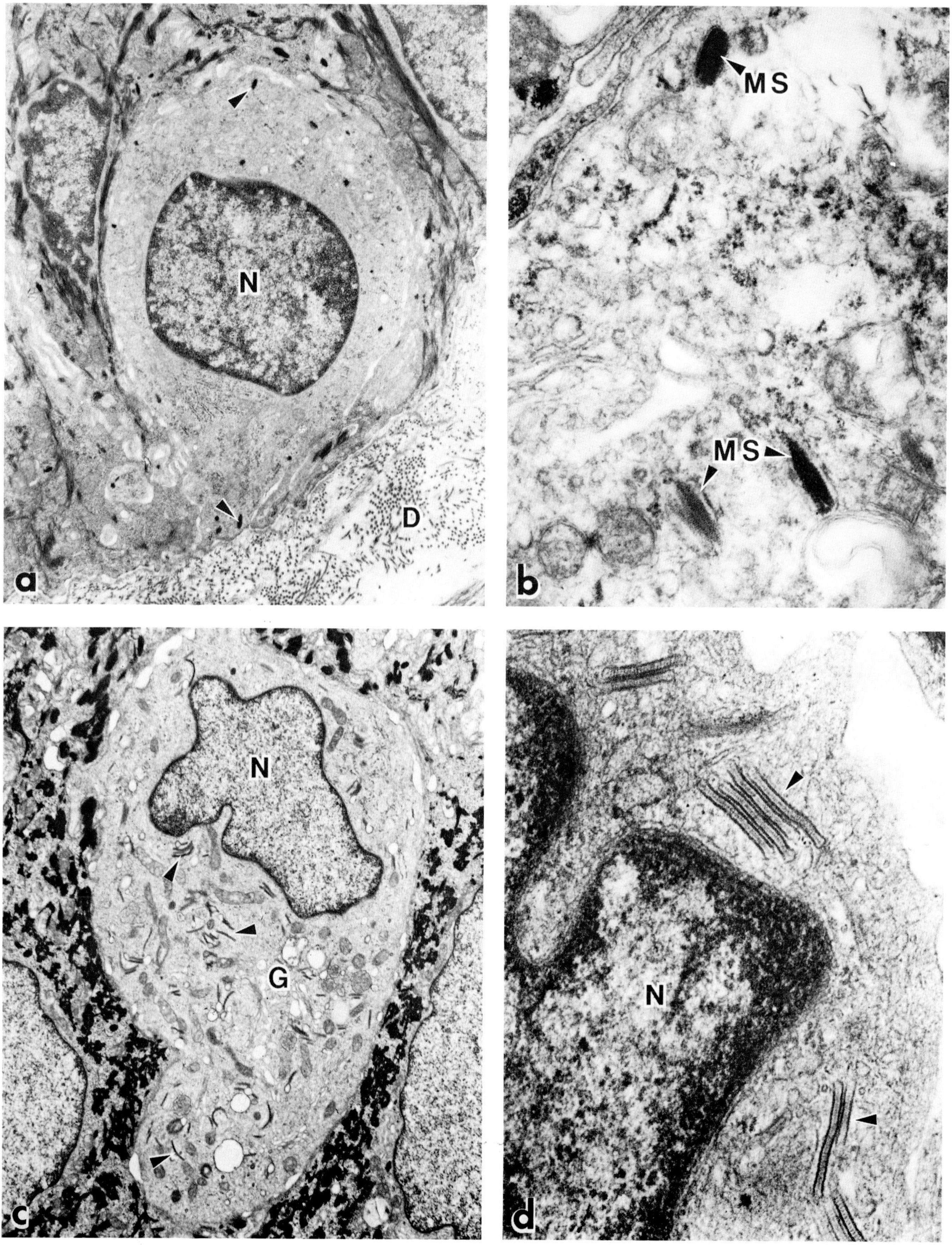
a
N
D
b
MS
MS
c
N
G
d
N

Figure 3–24. TEM, melanocytes and Langerhans cells in epidermis.

a. *Cell body of melanocyte in stratum basale. Desmosomal attachments are absent; few melanin pigment granules (arrows) are present; the nucleus (N) is large and round.* × 8,550.

b. *Dendritic process of melanocyte with three melanosomes (MS). Melanin synthesis takes place in melanosomes. In man, most of these bodies are elongated (about 0.2 μm by 0.6 μm) except in individuals with red hair where many are spherical. Melanosomes have a fibrillar or lamellar internal structure and exhibit periodicity in their early stages of development. These internal features become obscure as melanin accumulates. Dendritic processes of melanocytes course between keratinocytes and permit the transfer of pigment to the keratinocytes.* × 42,500.

c. *Body and typical irregular nucleus (N) of Langerhans cell. Granules (arrows) and Golgi membranes (G) are present; desmosomes are absent. Unlike melanocytes, Langerhans cells occur in about the same numbers in all regions of the body. They can synthesize DNA and divide, and they have some phagocytic ability. In histological sections viewed with the light microscope, Langerhans cells are DOPA-negative and gold chloride-positive. The use of gold chloride permits the visualization of the dendritic processes that extend from Langerhans cells.* × 13,000.

d. *Higher magnification of granules near the nucleus (N) of a Langerhans cell. The granules in this cell are rod-shaped, but granules of other shapes (e.g., racquet-shaped and boomerang-shaped) may occur in the same or different cells. The rod-shaped granules shown here have a periodicity of about 90 Å. Granules are approximately 400 Å wide and as much as 5,000 Å long.* × 57,000.

Langerhans cells are macrophages of a special type that migrate into the epidermis and phagocytose antigens that penetrate the skin. The cells play a key role in the development of contact sensitivity, an allergic response to certain substances that enter the skin.

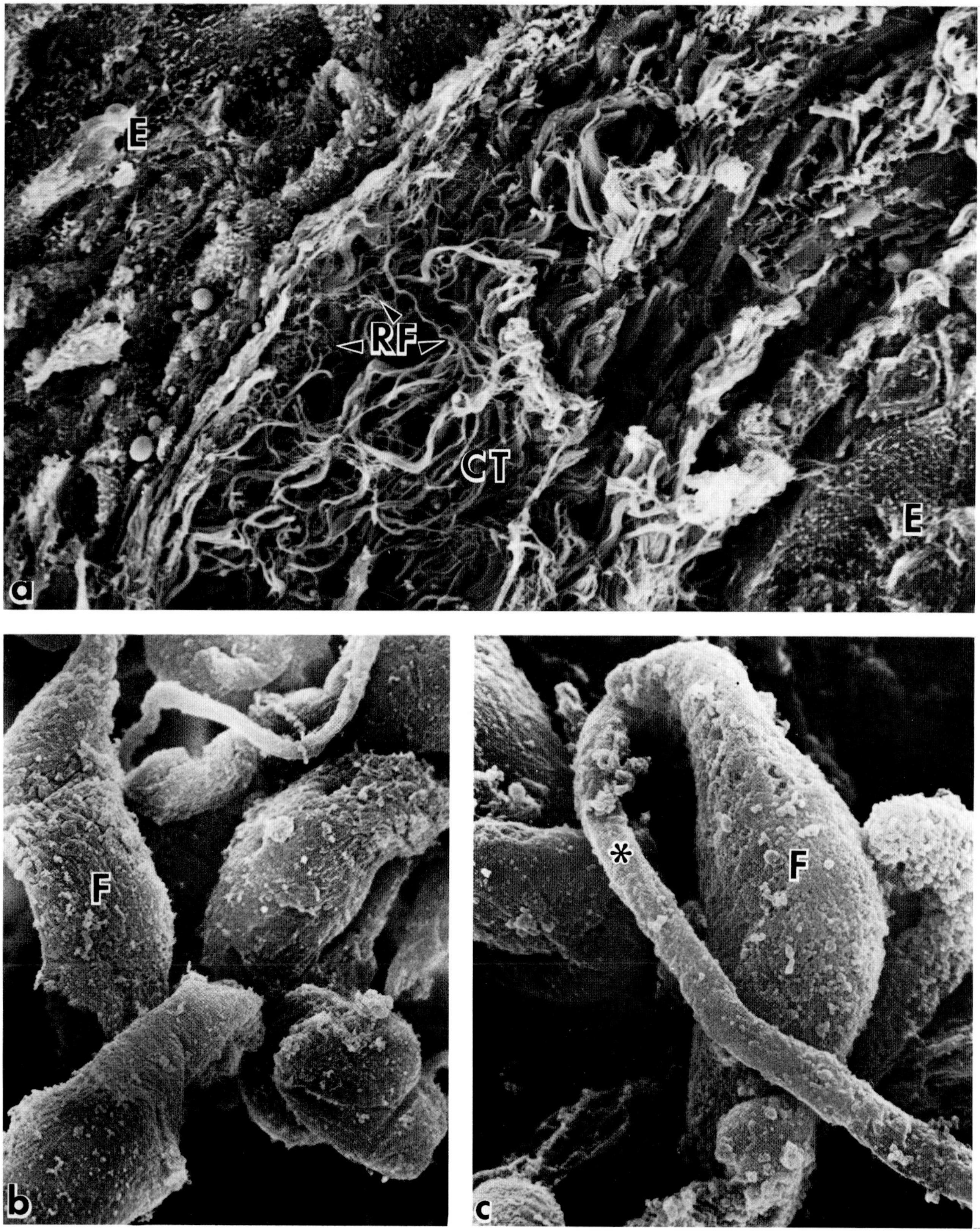

Figure 3–25. Papillary layer of dermis.

a. *Connective tissue (CT) of dermal papilla with epidermis (E) at sides of papilla. The papillary layer contains numerous, small reticular fibers (RF). ×1,175.*

b. *Elongated cell bodies of fibroblasts (F). Fibroblasts are the most abundant cells of the dermis. The connective tissue fibers they produce usually obscure them for study by SEM. ×2,760.*

c. *Cell body of fibroblast (F) with process (*) extending from cell body. Fibroblasts are generally spindle-shaped and contain the nucleus in the expanded portion of the cell. Globules of discharged cell products are shown on the cell body. ×5,520.*

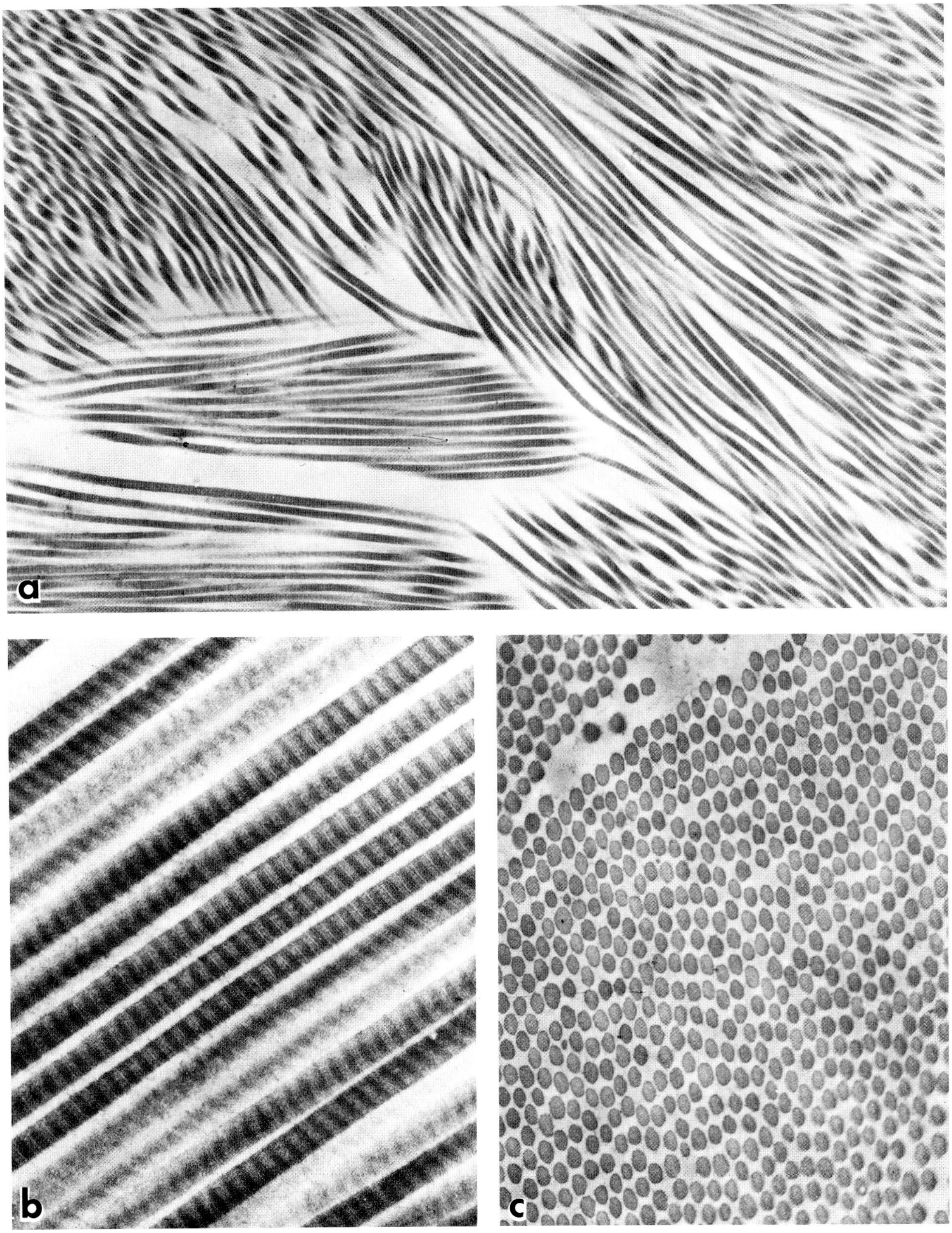

Figure 3–26. TEM, dermal collagen.

a. *Collagen fibrils course in different directions and their cross-striations are not pronounced at this magnification. The woven pattern of collagen contributes to the strength and pliability of the dermis.* ×3,175.

b. *Cross striations of fibrils result from the alignment of tropocollagen molecules of the fibril in a specific manner. A tropocollagen molecule is 2800 Å long and 15 Å wide. It consists of three polypeptide chains in the form of a coiled helix. During formation of a fibril, it is postulated that tropocollagen molecules line up end to end, but not touching; molecules of adjacent rows align themselves in a staggered fashion, overlapping by about 27% of their length. This results in the 640 Å to 700 Å periodicity that is characteristic of the collagen fibril.* ×6,900.

c. *Collagen fibrils in transverse section, showing their circular configuration and almost uniform diameter.* ×3,850.

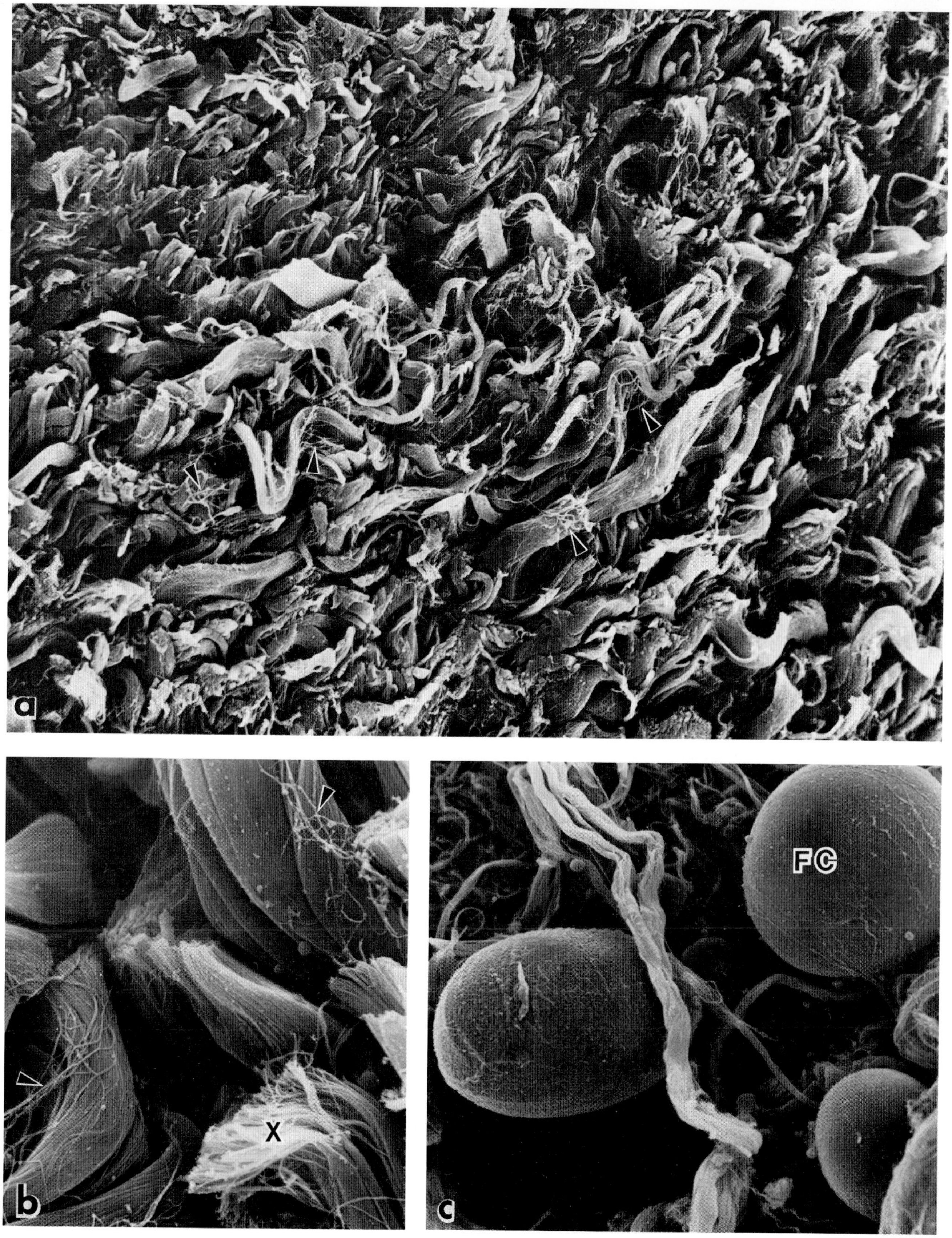

Figure 3–27. Collagen in papillary layer of dermis.

a. The fibers interlace extensively and run in different directions. They do not form the large bundles that are present in the reticular layer of the dermis. Elastic fibers (arrows) are the small branching fibers on and between the collagenous fibers. ×3,000.

b. Higher magnification shows the fibrils (X) in the collagenous fibers. Elastic fibers are indicated by arrows. ×4,560.

c. Large globular fat cells (FC) may occur as single or multiple cells anywhere in the dermis. Small reticular fibers often overlie the cell membranes of fat cells. ×525.

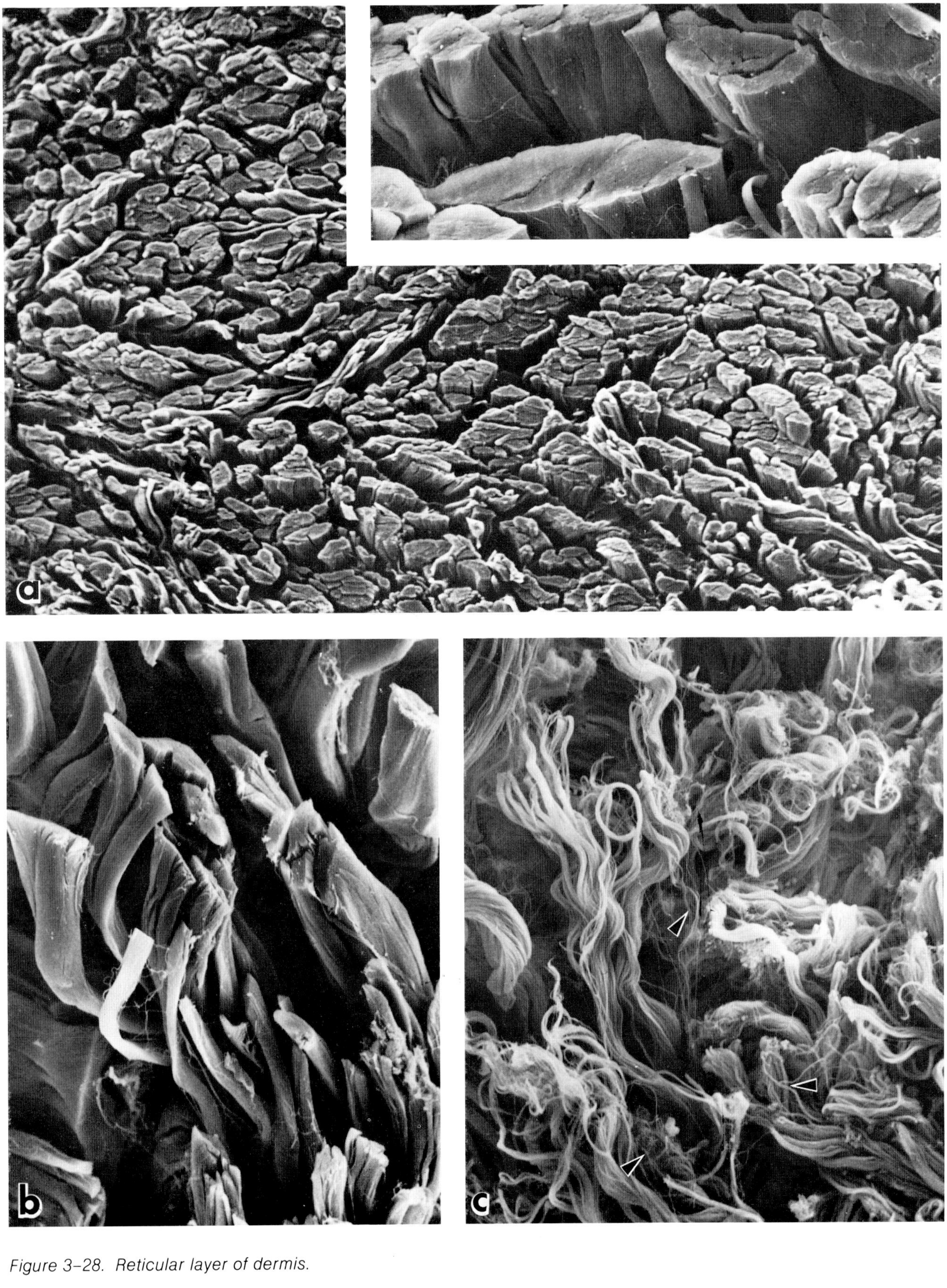

Figure 3–28. Reticular layer of dermis.

a. *Large, closely-packed bundles of collagenous fibers are present in the reticular layer of the dermis. They are sectioned transversely in this micrograph.* ×135.

Inset *shows the cut ends of collagenous fibers at high magnification. They resemble cables of various sizes.* ×780.

b. *Observe the "wavy" bundles of collagenous fibers. The fibers have great tensile strength but they are practically non-extensible.* ×780.

c. *The small collagenous fibers and networks of elastic fibers (arrows) shown here in the dermis serve as packing tissue that surrounds blood vessels, nerves, and sweat ducts.* ×390.

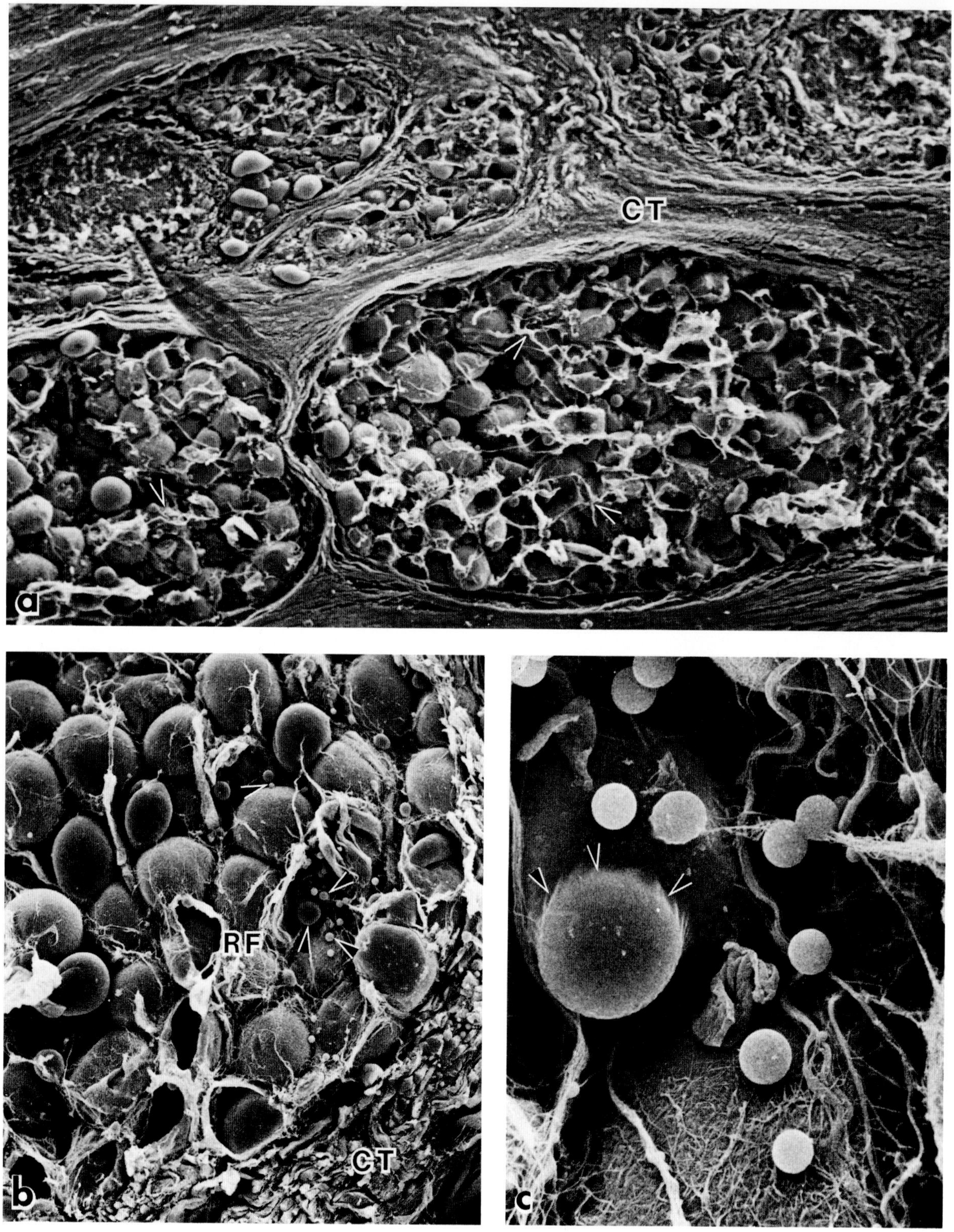

Figure 3–29. Fat in hypodermis.

a. *Fat cells occur in lobules which may form a thick layer in some parts of the body. Individual lobules are separated by septa of dense bands of connective tissue (CT). Reticular fibers (arrows) permeate the lobules and crisscross the fat cells.* × *125.*

b. *Edge of fat lobule and connective tissue septum (CT). Small droplets (arrows) are present on the surfaces of the fat cells. Some of the large spherical fat cells measure as much as 100 μm in diameter. Reticular fibers (RF) are associated with the surfaces of fat cells.* × *210.*

c. *Higher magnification of portions of two fat cells that were located at the edge of lobule in the previous micrograph. One of the fat cells shows a large protruding droplet (arrows) that is being released from the cell by the process of exocytosis. Exocytosis is clearly evident by the numerous droplets that are either associated with the cell surfaces or free between the cells. The droplets bud from the fat cells and become free in the subcutaneous tissue where sweat glands, hair follicles, and nerves are embedded.* × *1,530.*

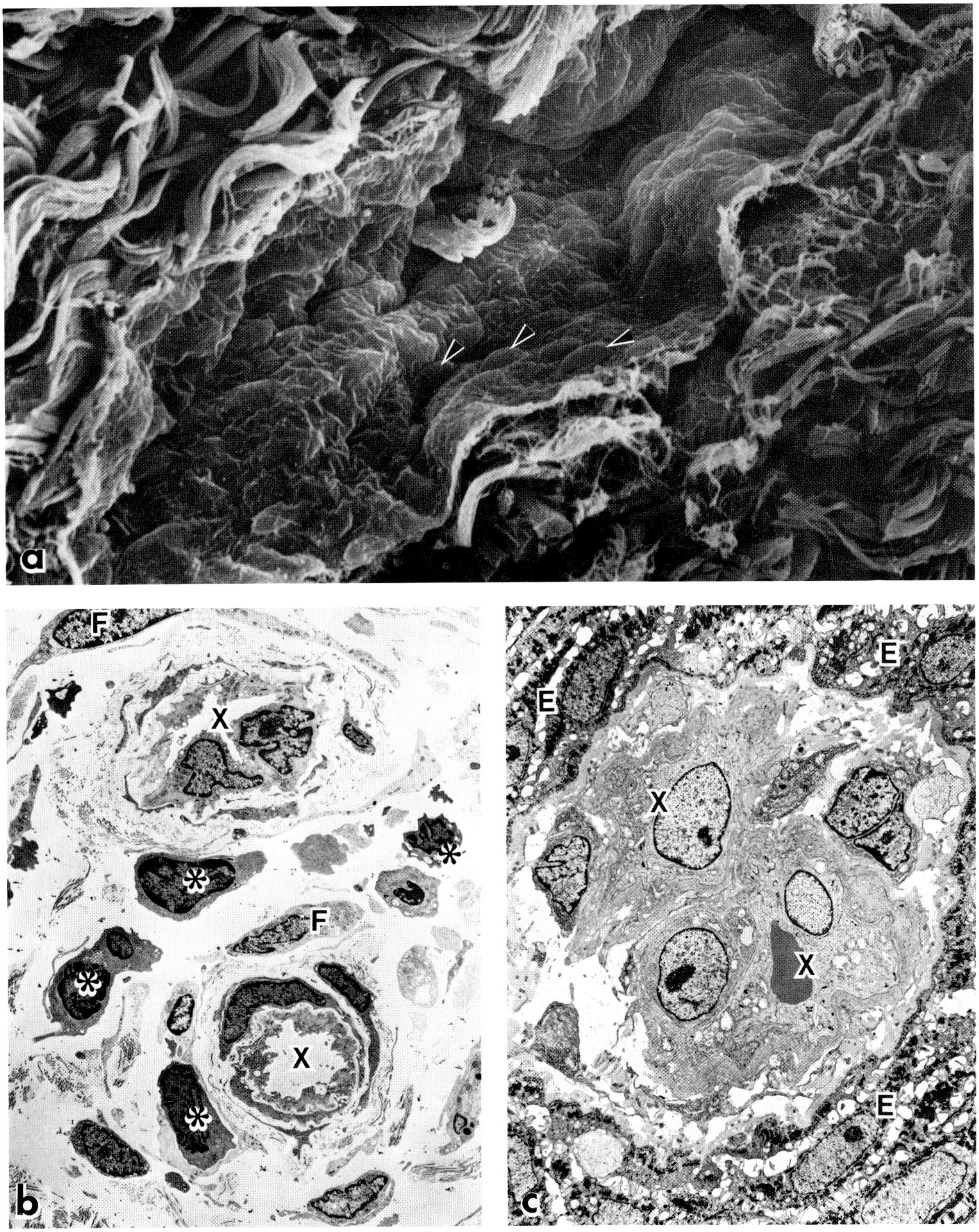

Figure 3–30. Dermal capillaries. Most dermal connective tissue is collagen, a relatively inert tissue that does not require extensive capillaries for nourishment. Accordingly, dermal capillaries are numerous at only three sites: immediately beneath the epidermis, surrounding hair follicles, and adjacent to sweat and sebaceous glands.

a. *Endothelium. The wall of this small blood vessel was removed during tissue preparation and the endothelium is exposed. The endothelial bulges (arrows) represent sites of nuclei. Dermal connective tissue fibers surround the vessel. × 1,600.*

b. *TEM, two capillaries (X) in papillary layer of dermis. Fibroblasts (F) and extravascular leukocytes (*) are near the capillaries. × 2,650.*

c. *TEM, portions of two capillaries (X) in dermal papilla. Since there are no capillaries in the epidermis, any nourishment to the epidermal cells (E) must be by diffusion from the dermal blood vessels. × 2,000.*

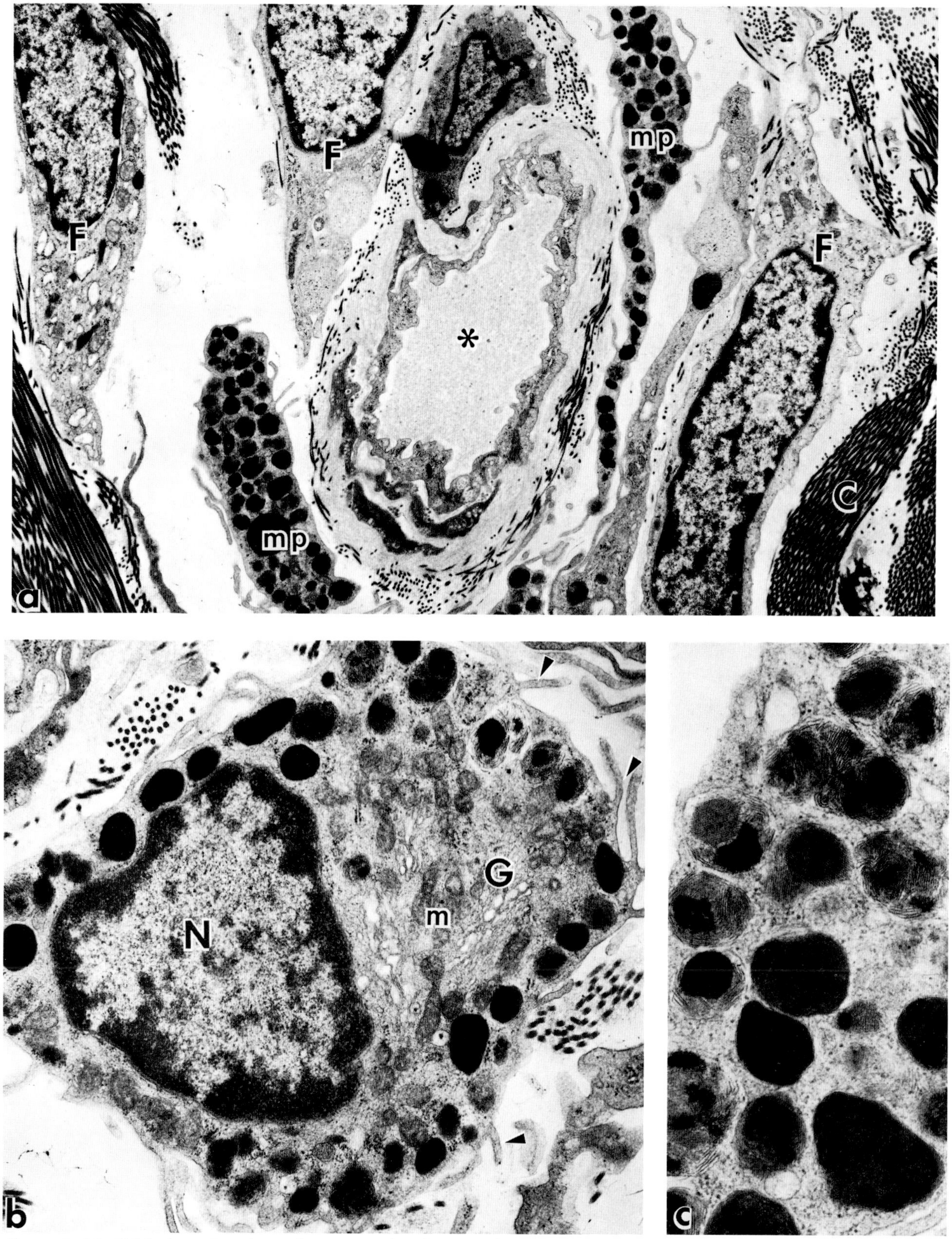

Figure 3–31. TEM, dermal perivascular connective tissue and mast cells.

a. *Capillary lumen (*) is surrounded by a thin endothelium. Note mast cell processes (mp), collagen (C), and fibroblasts (F) in the perivascular connective tissue. The number of mast cells in the dermis has been estimated to be 10,000/mm. The cells are most numerous adjacent to blood vessels. ×8,500.*

b. *Mast cell in perivascular connective tissue. Observe granules, Golgi membranes (G), mitochondria (m), nucleus (N), and cytoplasmic processes (arrows). ×20,800.*

c. *This micrograph shows the heterogeneity of the contents of mast cell granules. Lamellar bodies, whorls, and paracrystalline structures are often present in the granules. Granules contain heparin and histamine and stain metachromatically in appropriately prepared histological sections. Mast cells carry IgE on their surfaces. They are responsive to several conditions, including asthma, hay fever, urticaria, drug reactions, and anaphylactic shock. ×38,250.*

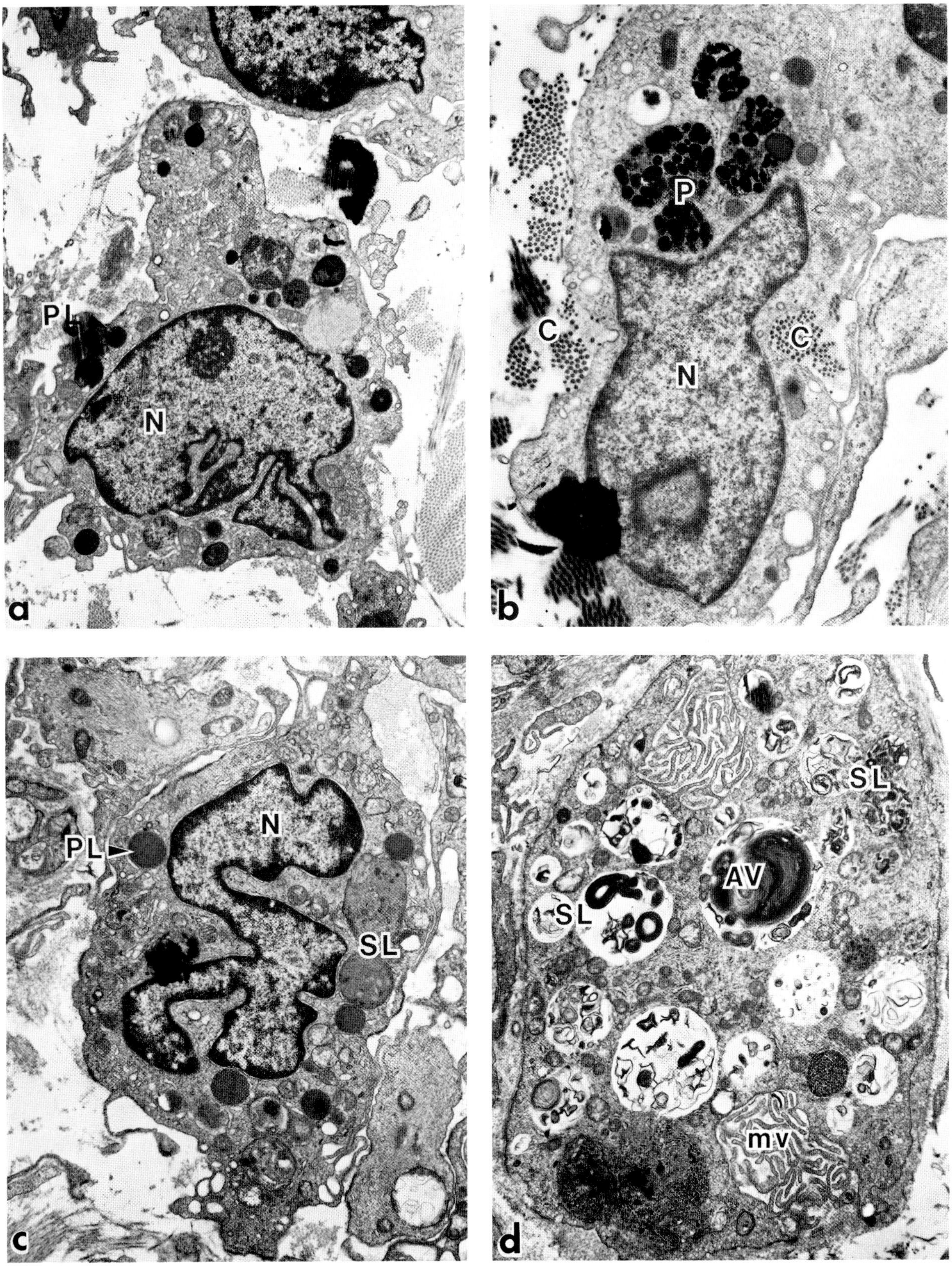

Figure 3–32. TEM, dermal macrophages. These cells are also called histiocytes, chromatophores, and melanophages. a. ×5,500; b. ×11,500; c. ×7,300; d. ×7,300.

An irregular nucleus (N) and cytoplasmic pigment (P) are features of most dermal macrophages. Some of the melanin produced by epidermal melanocytes normally passes through the basement membrane and enters the dermis where it is phagocytosed by the macrophages. Collagen (C) that comes into contact with the macrophage surface can be engulfed and degraded as part of the continuous remodelling process that occurs in dermal connective tissue. The primary lysosomes (PL), secondary lysosomes (SL), and autophagic vacuoles (AV) of macrophages contain lytic enzymes necessary to carry out the processes of intracellular digestion. Collagen fibrils in the macrophages indicate that collagen is being degraded. Collagen degradation by the macrophages is known to occur concomitantly with collagen synthesis by the fibroblasts. Processes that resemble microvilli (mv) line the invaginations in Figure 3–32d.

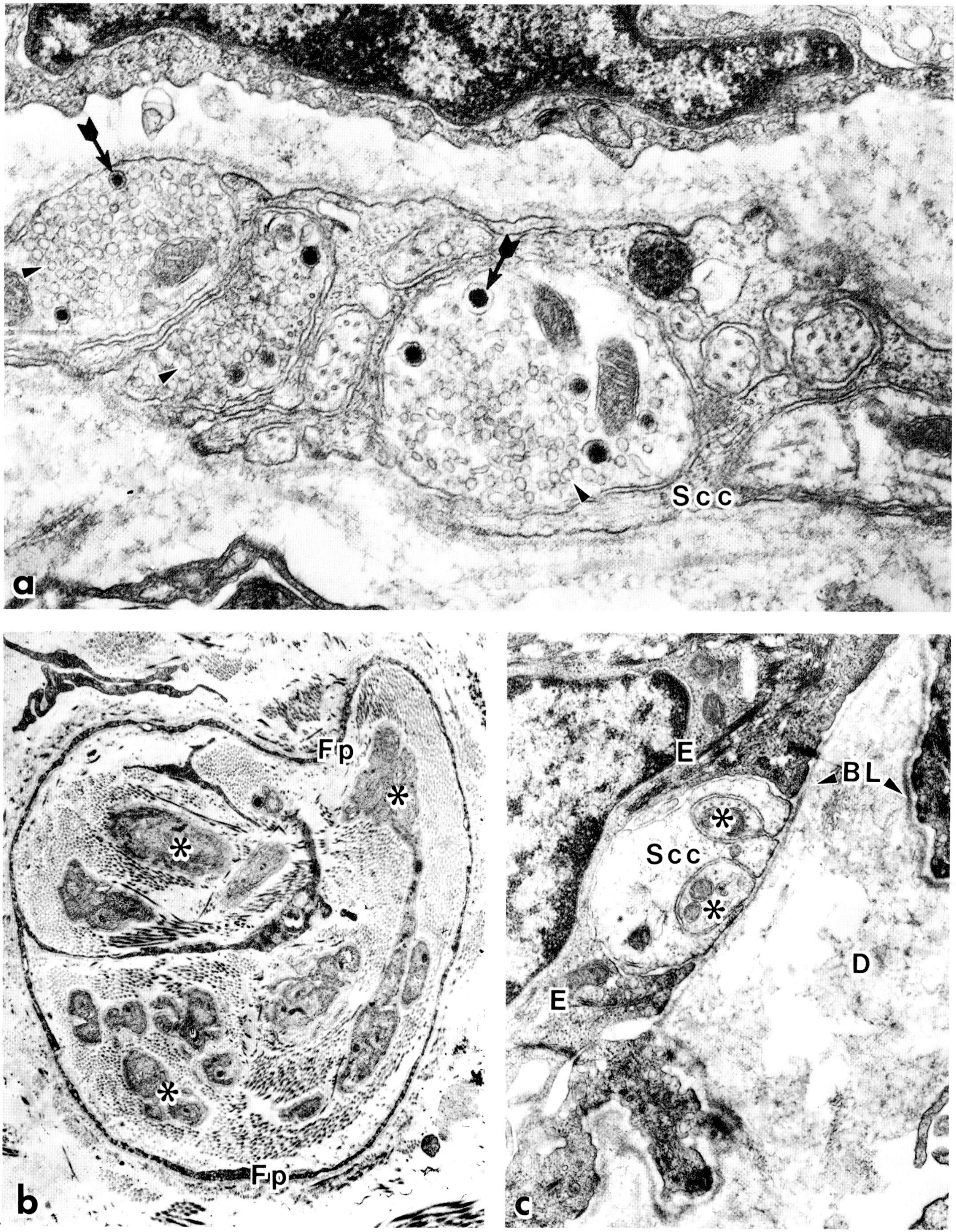
a
Scc
b
Fp
Fp
c
E
BL
Scc
D
E

Figure 3–33. TEM, nerves.

a. *Unmyelinated autonomic nerve (postganglionic sympathetic) in oblique section and located at the junction of dermis and hypodermis. Electron dense vesicles (large arrows) and electron lucent vesicles (small arrows) are present in the axonal swellings, which typify the terminal portions of autonomic axons. Some Schwann cell cytoplasm (Scc) surrounds the small axons. Two plexuses of nerves are formed by fibers that enter the skin from the hypodermis. The dermal plexus is found just below the epidermis. The nerve shown here belongs to the subcutaneous plexus that is located at the junction of dermis and hypodermis.* × 45,600.

b. *Small, unmyelinated nerve in dermis surrounded by processes of fibroblasts (Fp) and permeated by fine collagenous fibers. Individual fibers of the nerve (*) will eventually innervate specific cutaneous structures (e.g., vascular smooth muscle, glands, etc.).* × 6,750.

c. *Sensory nerve in epidermis. The nerve is a branch from the plexus in the superficial dermis (D). It occupies an invagination of the basal cell in the epidermis (E). The nerve consists of two axons (*) surrounded by Schwann cell cytoplasm (Scc).* × 24,200.

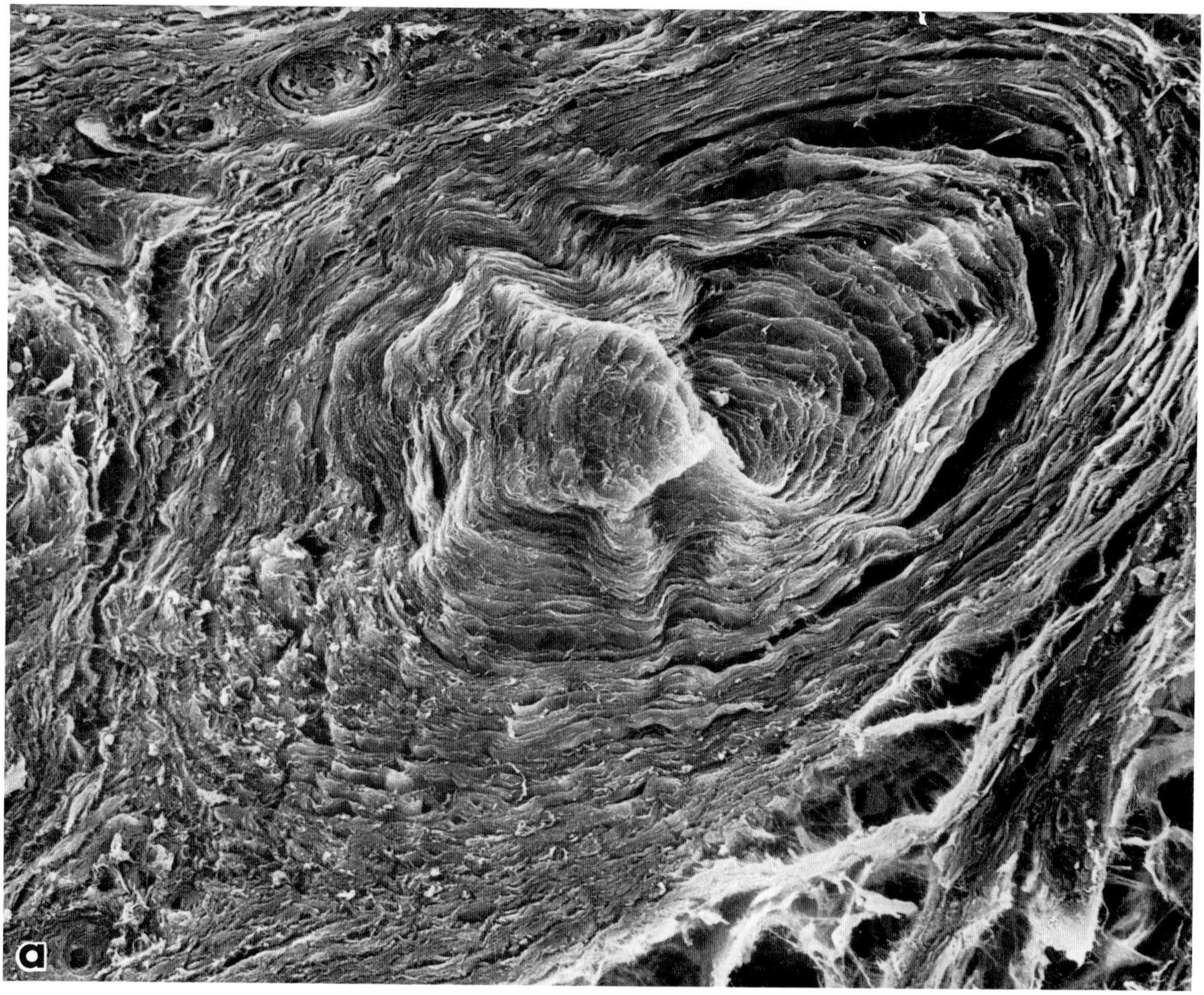

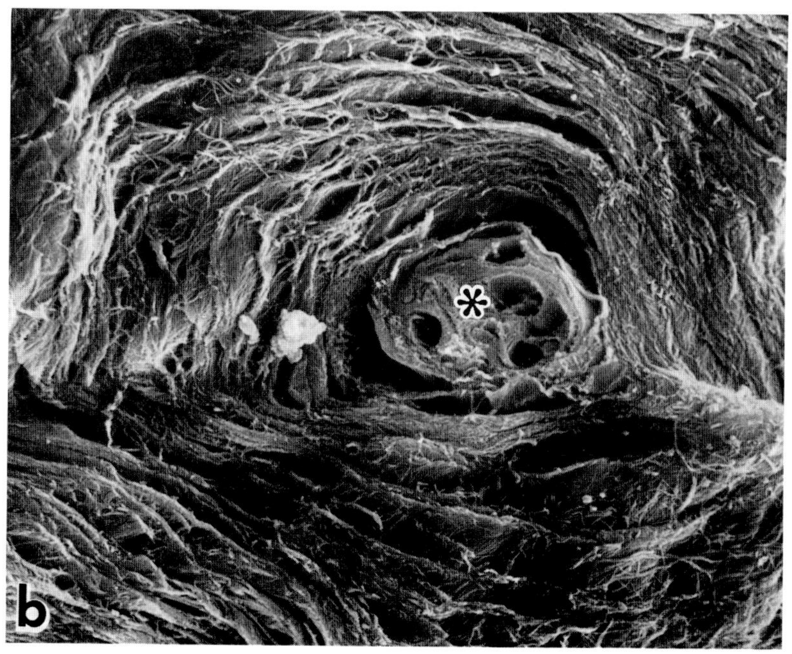

Figure 3–34. Pacinian corpuscle in hypodermis. See comments with Figure 3–7.

a. *The corpuscle is elliptical and composed of more than 30 concentric rings formed by the overlapping processes of several fibroblast-like cells. Each ring in life is separated from its neighbor by a fluid-filled space.* ×610.

b. *The central core of the Pacinian corpuscle contains a nerve fiber (*). Slight compression or distortion of a corpuscle initiates nerve impulses which are interpreted by the brain as pressure.* ×1,470.

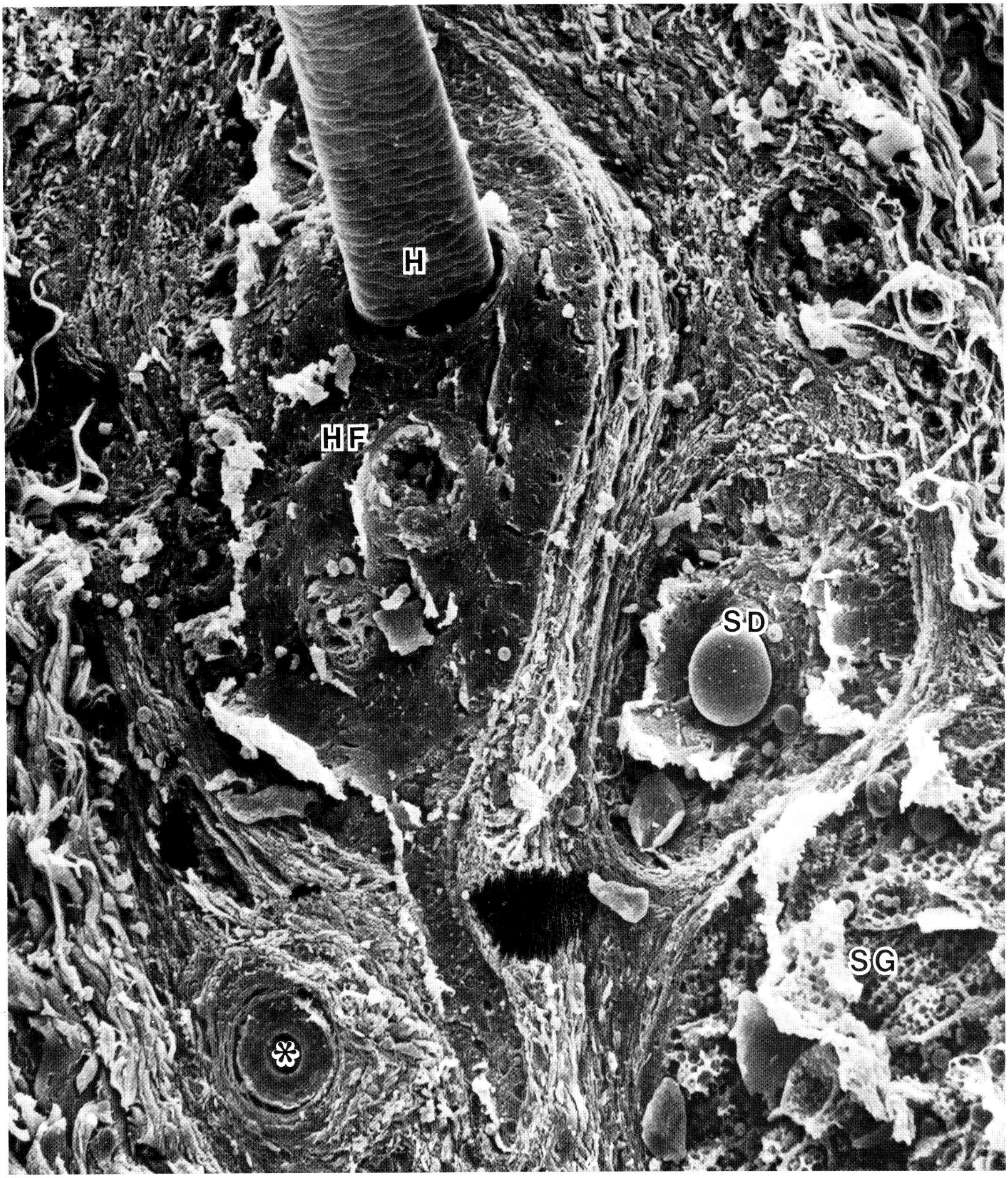

Figure 3–35. Dermis, axillary skin. Hair (H) in hair follicle (HF) is covered with a cuticle of overlapping scales; duct of sweat gland (*), sebaceous gland (SG), and duct of sebaceous gland (SD) with large sebum droplet in lumen. × 755.

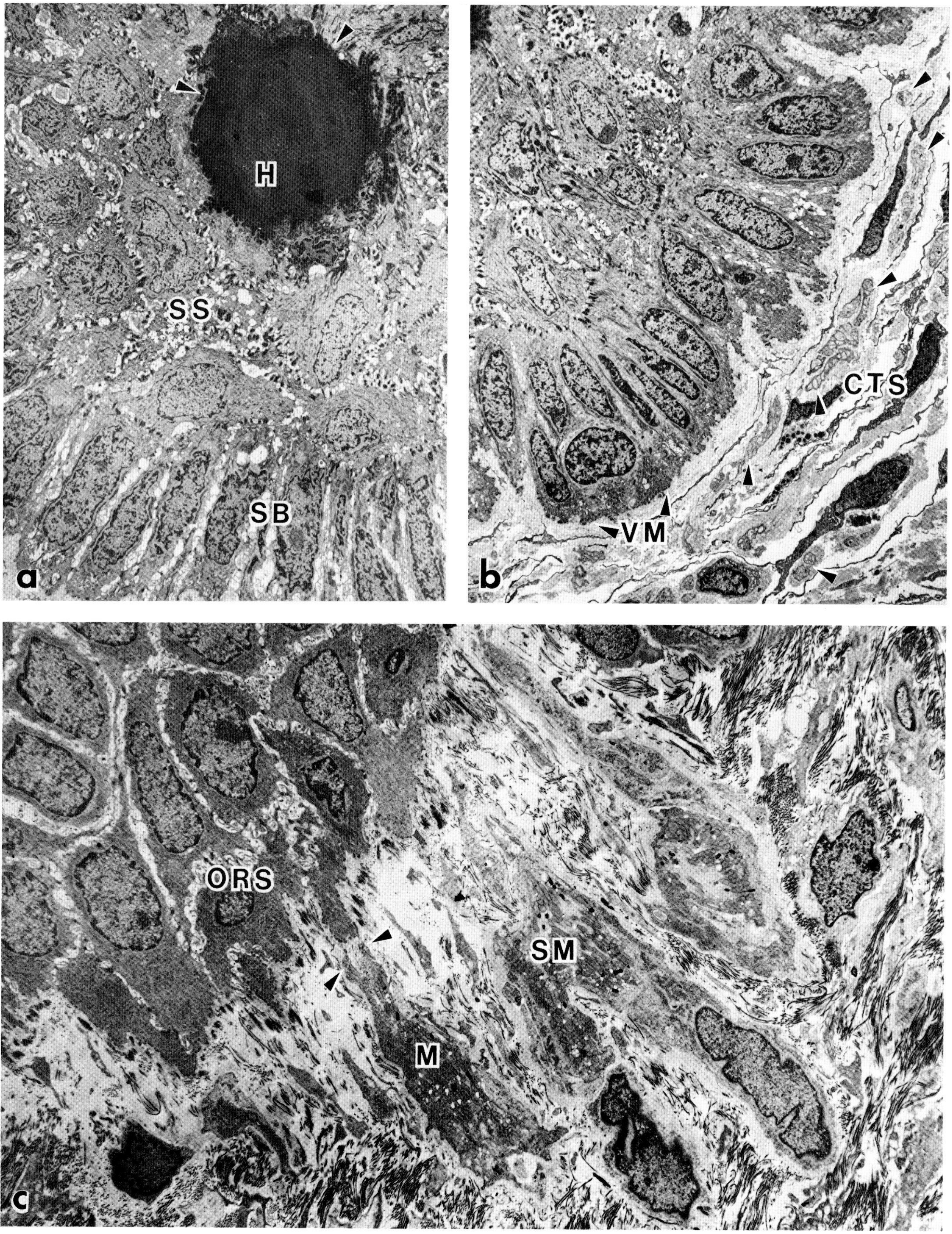
H
SS
SB
a
CTS
VM
b
ORS
SM
M
c

Figure 3–36. TEM, transverse sections of hair follicles. a *and* b *are above the entrance of the sebaceous duct and the inner epithelial root sheath is no longer present.*

a. *The cortex comprises most of the hair (H) at this level. The cuticle (arrows) of the hair is surrounded by the outer epithelial root sheath which contains a stratum spinosum (SS) and a stratum basale (SB). These two strata are continuous with corresponding layers of the epidermis. ×2,250.*

b. *Observe the vitreous membrane (VM) which is the narrow basement membrane that separates the stratum basale of the outer epithelial root sheath from the connective tissue sheath (CTS) of the follicle. Note the numerous axons (arrows) that surround the outer epithelial root sheath. ×2,250.*

c. *Outer epithelial root sheath (ORS) and connective tissue sheath of hair follicle at level where arrector pili muscle cells attach. The smooth muscle cells (SM) appear to traverse the connective tissue sheath and attach through long processes (arrows) to the outer epithelial root sheath. Mitochondria (M) are abundant in the muscle cells. Their internal structure•is difficult to recognize at this magnification. ×3,300.*

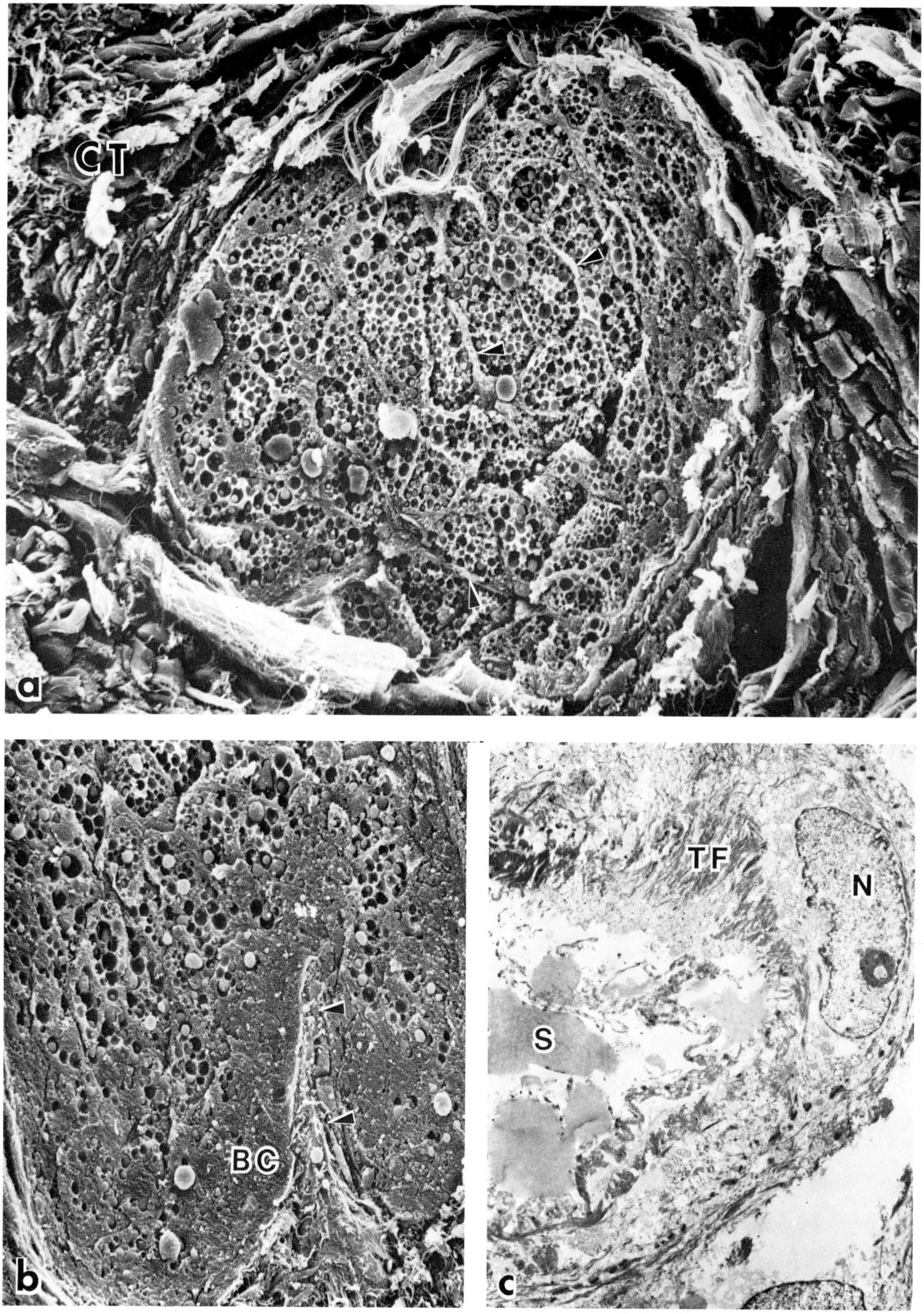
CT
a
BC
b
TF
N
S
c

Figure 3–37. Sebaceous glands.

a. *Connective tissue (CT) surrounds the alveolus which has a spongy appearance caused by the numerous, small lipid droplets in the alveolar cells. Some cell boundaries (arrows) are discernible. Sebaceous glands are classified anatomically as simple or branched alveolar glands, and their secretory units are called alveoli whose cells constitute the holocrine secretory product, sebum.* ×600.

b. *Part of an alveolus is shown with connective tissue (arrows) invaginating its periphery. The outermost layer of alveolar cells are the basal cells (BC). They rest on the basement membrane. Basal cells are smaller and contain less lipid than cells more central in the alveolus. They are able to divide and replace the central, lipid-laden cells that die, detach, and enter the duct of the gland. Sebaceous glands secrete by the holocrine mode characterized by the formation of a secretory product composed of dead, whole cells.* ×720.

c. *TEM, duct of sebaceous gland. Only the epithelium of the duct is shown. The cells are flattened, 2 to 3 cell layers thick, and rich in tonofilaments (TF). Sebum (S) is present in the lumen. Nucleus (N) of one cell is illustrated.* ×4,760.

Ducts of most sebaceous glands end in hair follicles. Sebaceous glands in a few areas of the body have ducts that empty directly onto the skin surface (e.g., those in the lips, nipple, glands and prepuce of penis, and labia minora). Sebaceous glands of the skin of the nose are very large. Their ducts open into very small hair follicles.

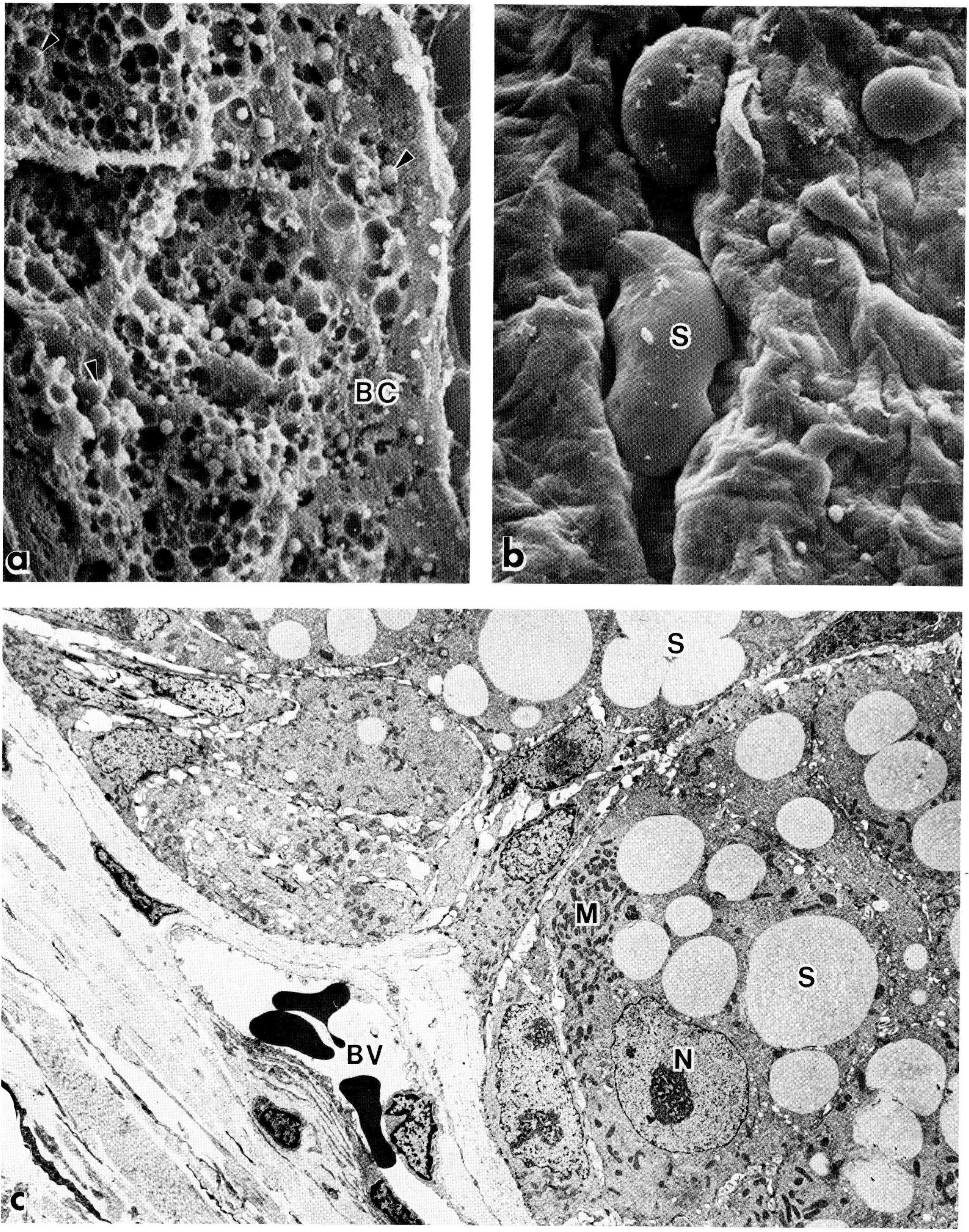
a
BC
b
S
c
S
M
S
N
BV

Figure 3–38. Sebaceous glands.

a. *Outpocketing of an alveolus, illustrating layer of basal cells (BC) and spherical lipid droplets (arrows).* ×960.

b. *Sebum (S) on skin surface and inside the crevice in center of micrograph. Sebum is known to spread over the skin surface after it leaves the orifices of hair follicles.* ×960.

c. *TEM, basal cells of an alveolus, depicting sebum droplets (S), nucleus (N), and mitochondria (M). The capillary (BV) is in the connective tissue just outside the basement membrane of the alveolus.* ×3,300.

Sebaceous glands become active in both sexes at puberty when blood levels of sex hormones become high. Continued activity depends on (1) proliferation of basal cells at periphery of alveoli, (2) movement of newly formed cells toward center of alveoli, (3) synthesis and accumulation of lipid droplets in cells as they move centrally, and (4) necrosis of central cells as they accumulate lipid and move away from their blood supply.

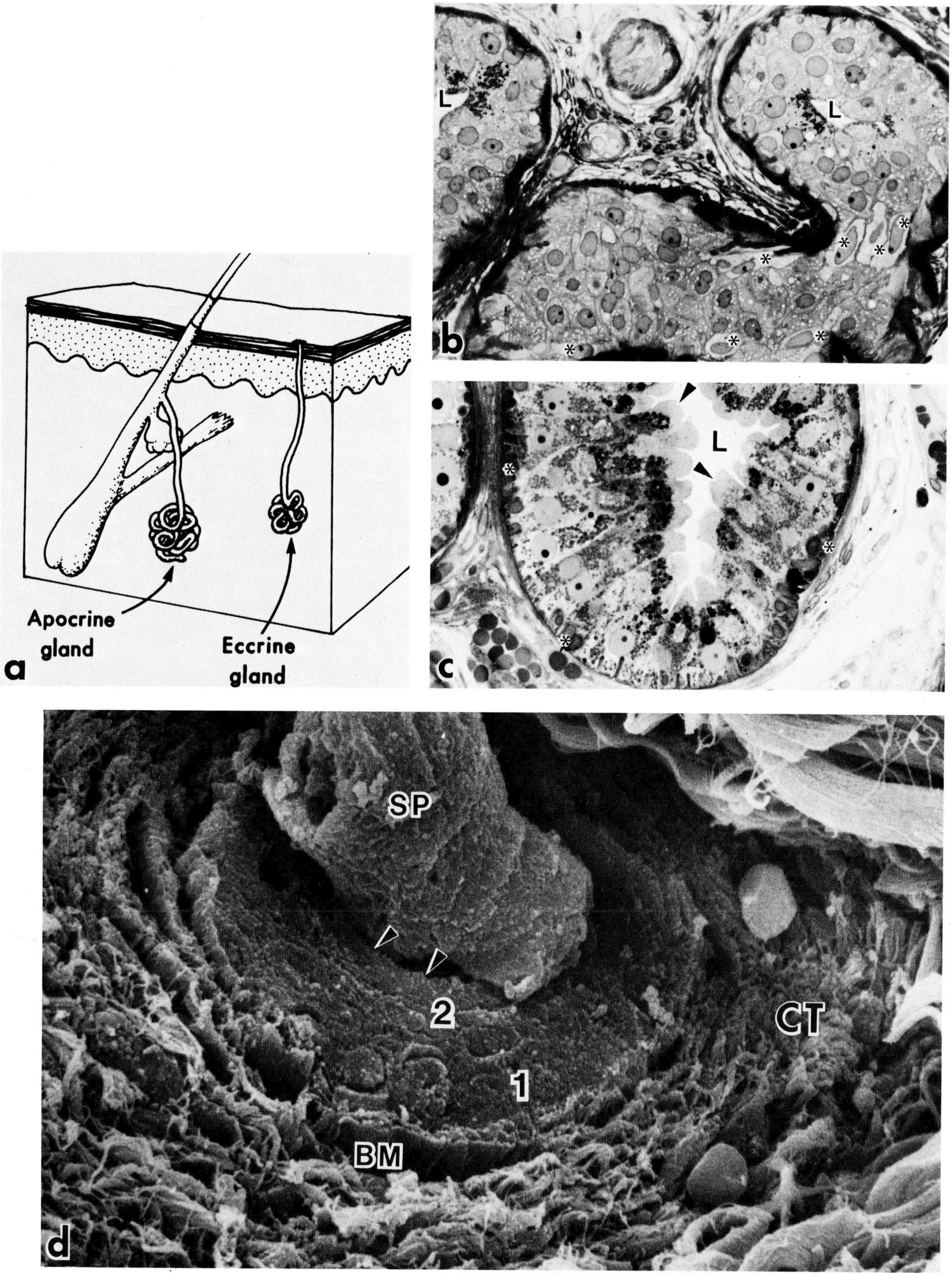
Apocrine gland
Eccrine gland
a
L
L
b
L
c
SP
2
1
CT
BM
d

Figure 3–39. Sweat glands.

a. *Diagrammatic representation of the two types of sweat glands. The duct of the apocrine sweat gland opens into a hair follicle superficial to the sebaceous gland and arrector pili muscle. The duct of the eccrine sweat gland opens onto the skin surface. The secretory portion of each type of gland is highly coiled and is located in the deep dermis or in the superficial portion of the hypodermis. Of the two gland types, apocrine glands tend to be somewhat more deeply located.*

b. *and* c. *Photomicrographs of secretory tubules of an eccrine gland (b) and an appocrine gland (c) for comparison of size. Myoepithelial cells (*) are present in both glands and are shown especially well where the eccrine tubule is cut obliquely. Note lumen (L), round apices (arrows) of secretory cells in the apocrine gland, and secretory granules in both glands. Granules in eccrine glands are found only in dark cells. ×1,200.*

d. *Duct of axillary apocrine sweat gland. Ducts of both types of sweat glands are lined by two layers of cuboidal epithelial cells. The outer cell layer (1) rests on a basement membrane (BM) which is continuous with the surrounding connective tissue (CT). The inner cell layer (2) has a cuticular border (arrows). The duct lumen contains secretory products (SP) contributed by secretory cells in the coiled portion of the gland. ×3,250.*

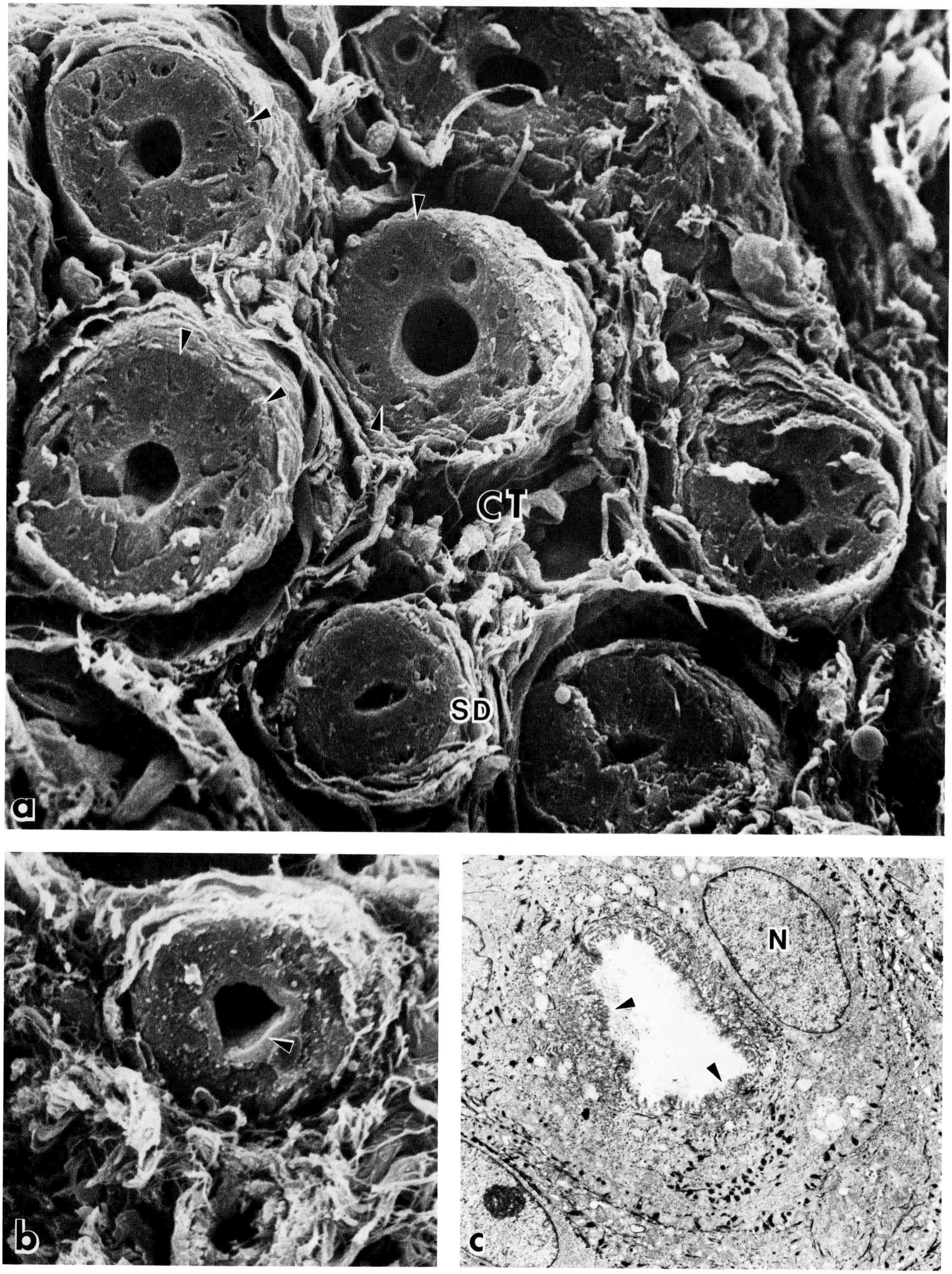
CT
SD
a
b
N
c

Figure 3–40. Eccrine sweat glands (sudoriferous glands).

a. *Cross sections of coiled secretory portion of an eccrine sweat gland and its duct (SD). The secretory portion is located at the junction of dermis and hypodermis. Although multiple glands appear to be present, all sections are through the same coiled gland. The coiled tubules of eccrine glands are about 10× smaller than tubules of apocrine glands, but ducts of both gland types have about the same diameter. Coils are separated by connective tissue (CT) and contain contractile myoepithelial cells (arrows) at their bases which aid in the expulsion of sweat.* ×9,020.

b. *Duct of eccrine sweat gland in dermis. The cuticular border (arrows) is shown.* ×1,540.

c. *TEM, duct of eccrine sweat gland. Microvilli (arrows) and tonofilaments are components of the cuticular border. Nucleus, N.* ×4,080.

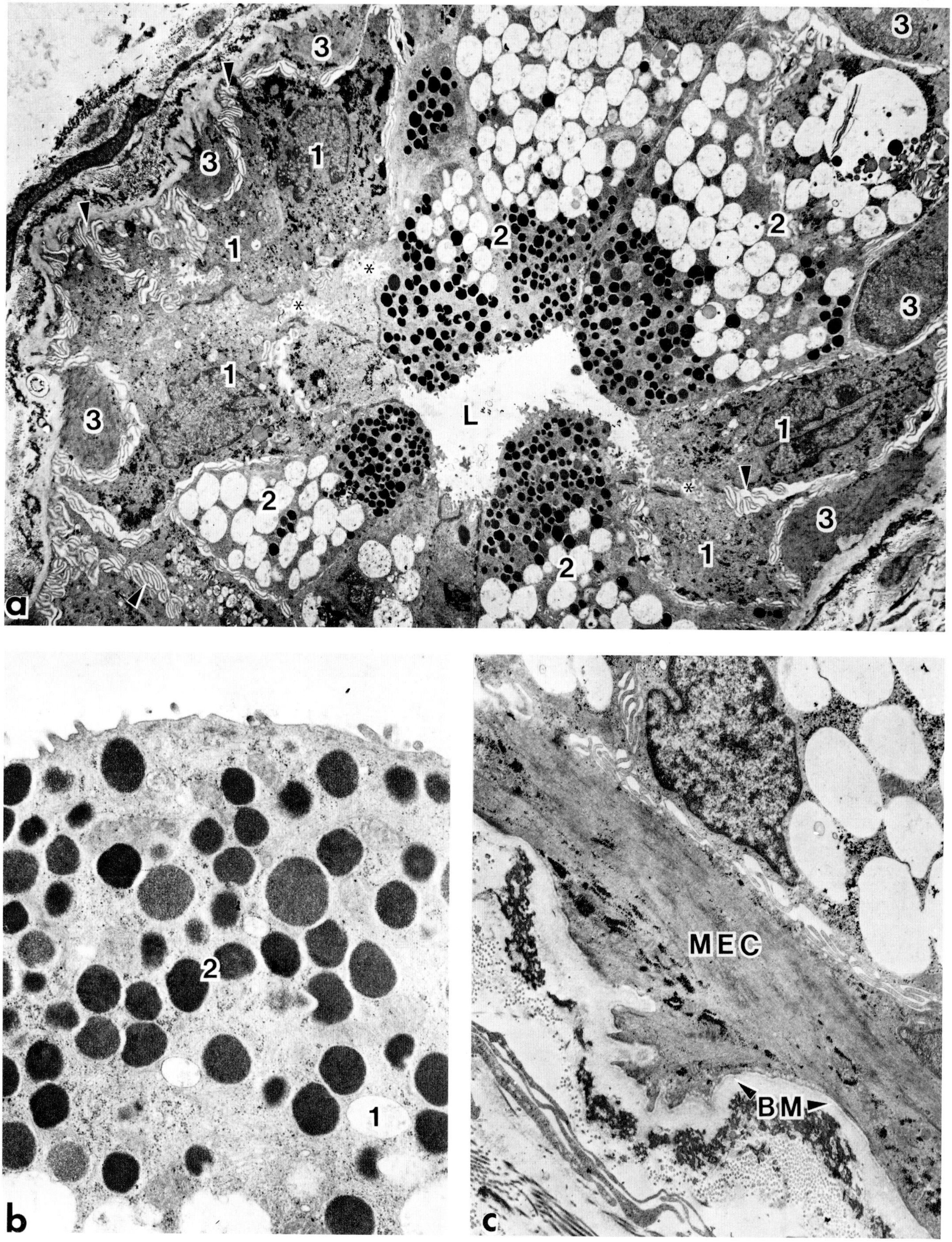
a
1
2
3
L
b
c
MEC
BM

Figure 3–41. TEM, cells in secretory portion of an eccrine sweat gland.

a. *Secretory tubule. About equal numbers of serous cells (1) and mucous cells (2) line the tubule. Both types of cells have myoepithelial cells (3) at their bases. Microvilli extend from apices of secretory cells into the lumen (L) of the tubule. ×4,320.*

Serous cells are also called clear cells. Their basal and lateral membranes (arrows) are folded and interdigitate elaborately. Intercellular canaliculi (*) course between serous cells and between adjacent serous and mucous cells. They are absent between adjacent mucous cells. Intercellular canaliculi are small channels that represent extensions of the gland lumen. Serous cells contain aggregates of glycogen and their endoplasmic reticulum is mainly of the smooth type. The Golgi apparatus is small. Serous cells produce the watery portion of eccrine sweat that contains sodium chloride. The primary secretion is hyperosmotic. It becomes hypoosmotic as it passes through the duct and sodium chloride is reabsorbed.

Mucous cells are also called dark cells. In comparison to serous cells, their cell membranes are far less folded. The cells are shaped like inverted pyramids, and their broad apices may overlie and obscure the much narrower apices of serous cells. The mucous cell varies in size and ultrastructural features with the phase of the secretory cycle through which the cell is passing. The cytoplasm contains abundant secretory granules of different densities. The largest granules are pale (electron lucent) and have flocculent material. The smallest granules are dark (electron dense); they are the older and more mature granules that are most numerous in the cell apices near the lumen (L). Granules contain the secretory product which is a PAS-positive, carbohydrate and protein complex that coats the surfaces of the duct cells once it is expelled. It has been proposed that this coating protects the duct cells from their own hydrolytic enzymes and aids in sodium reabsorption.

b. *Pale, immature secretory granules (1) and dark, mature secretory granules (2) in apex of mucous cell. Dark granules constitute the predominant type in the cell apices. ×22,500.*

c. *Process of myoepithelial cell (MEC) at base of mucous cell. Note basement membrane (BM) and nucleus (N) of mucous cell. Myofilaments fill the process of the myoepithelial cell. Myoepithelial cells are associated with secretory cells of glands derived from ectoderm. Their contractions help to expel the secretory products from the gland cells. ×8,550.*

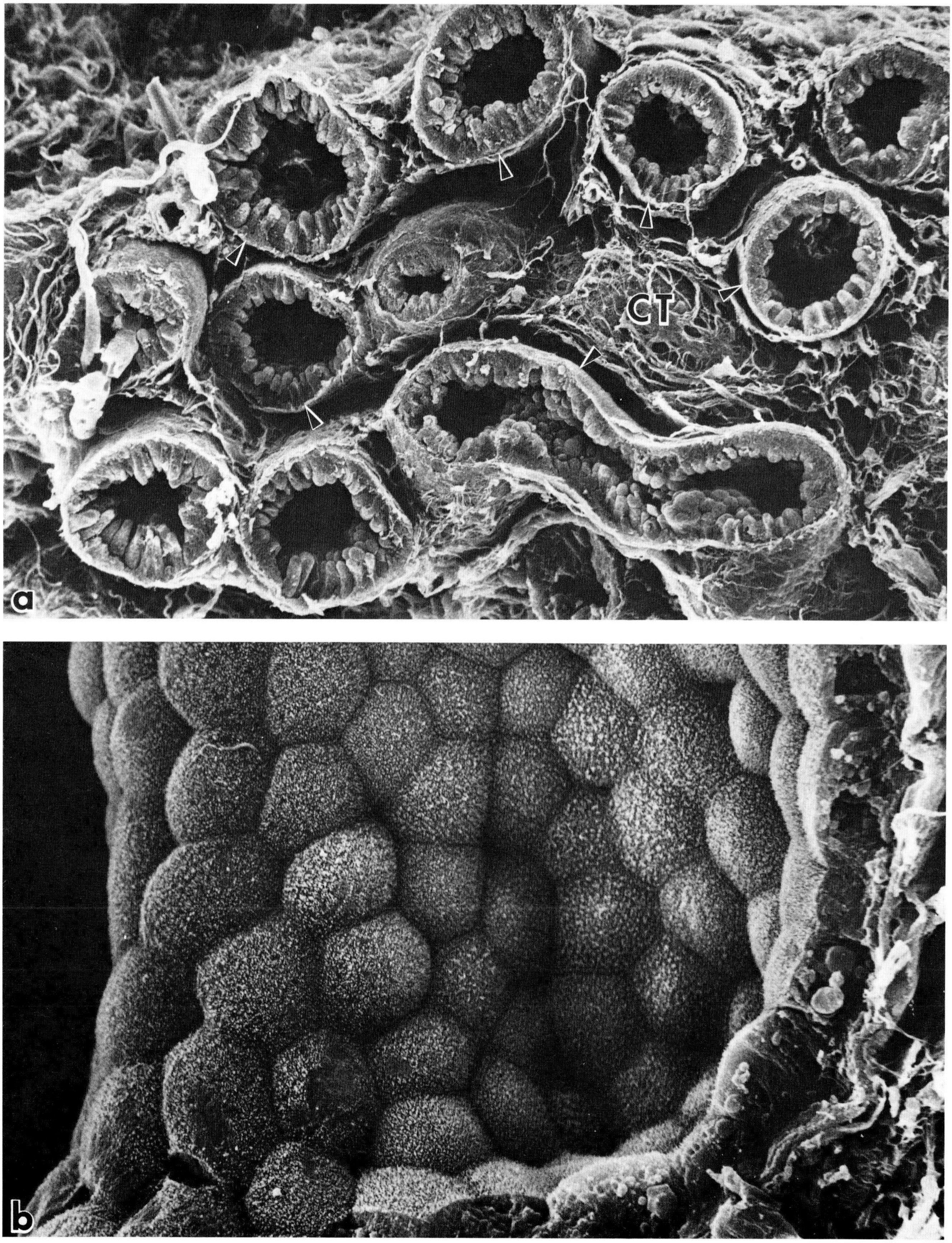

Figure 3–42. Axillary apocrine sweat glands.

a. *Low magnification of apocrine secretory tubules sectioned in various planes. Convex cell apices and large lumina of the tubules are shown. The basement membrane (arrows) on which the secretory cells rest is thin and relatively smooth. In this preparation it is often detached from the connective tissue (CT) that separates the tubules. Tubules range from 60 μm to 125 μm in diameter. ×350.*

b. *The convex cell apices belong to quiescent secretory cells of a tubule. Microvilli densely cover the slightly protruding cell apices. ×1,730.*

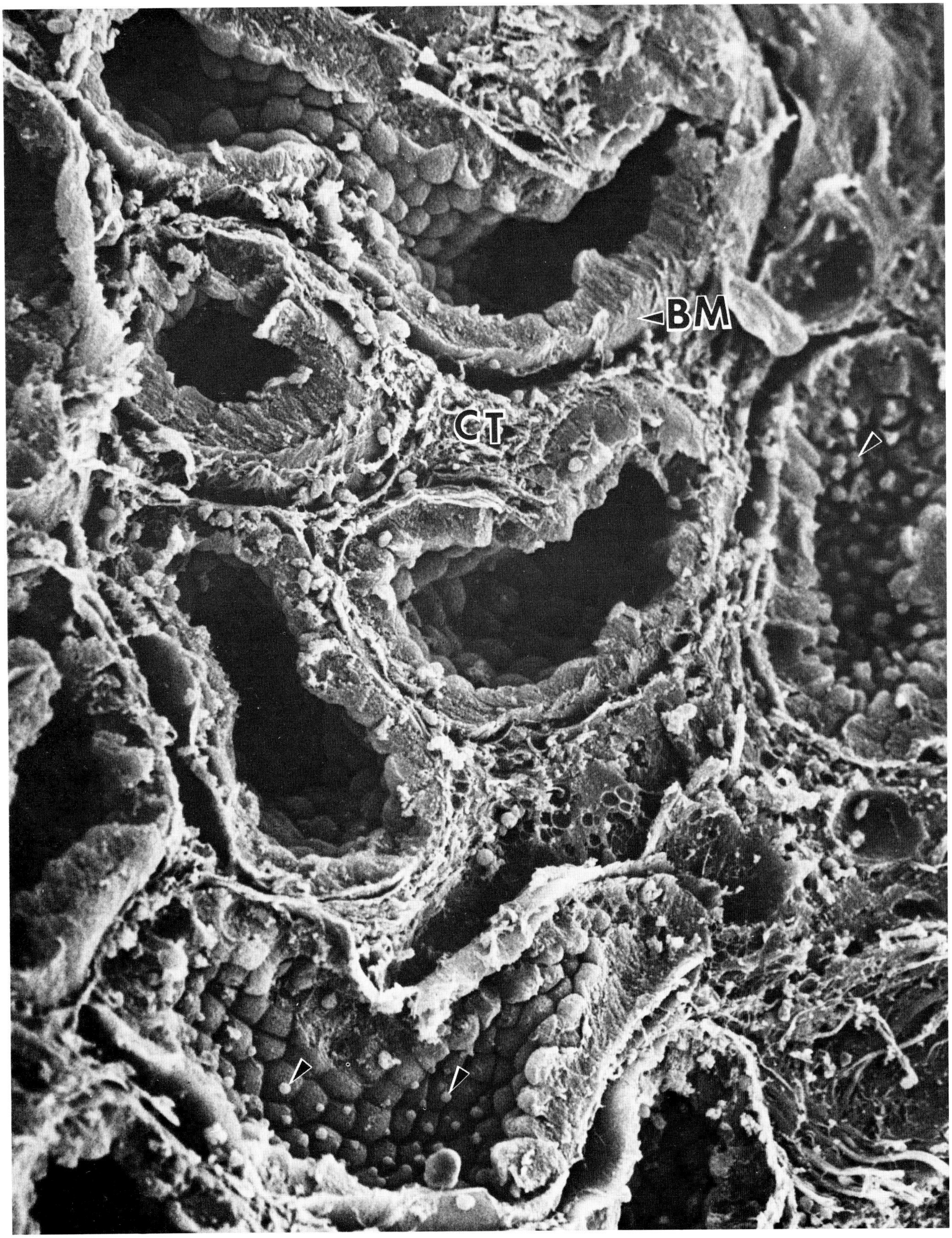

Figure 3–43. Axillary apocrine sweat gland, showing multiple sections of a single coiled secretory tubule. Droplets of secretory products (arrows) are attached to the convex apices of many of the secretory cells. Note basement membrane (BM) and connective tissue (CT) between the tubules. ×630.

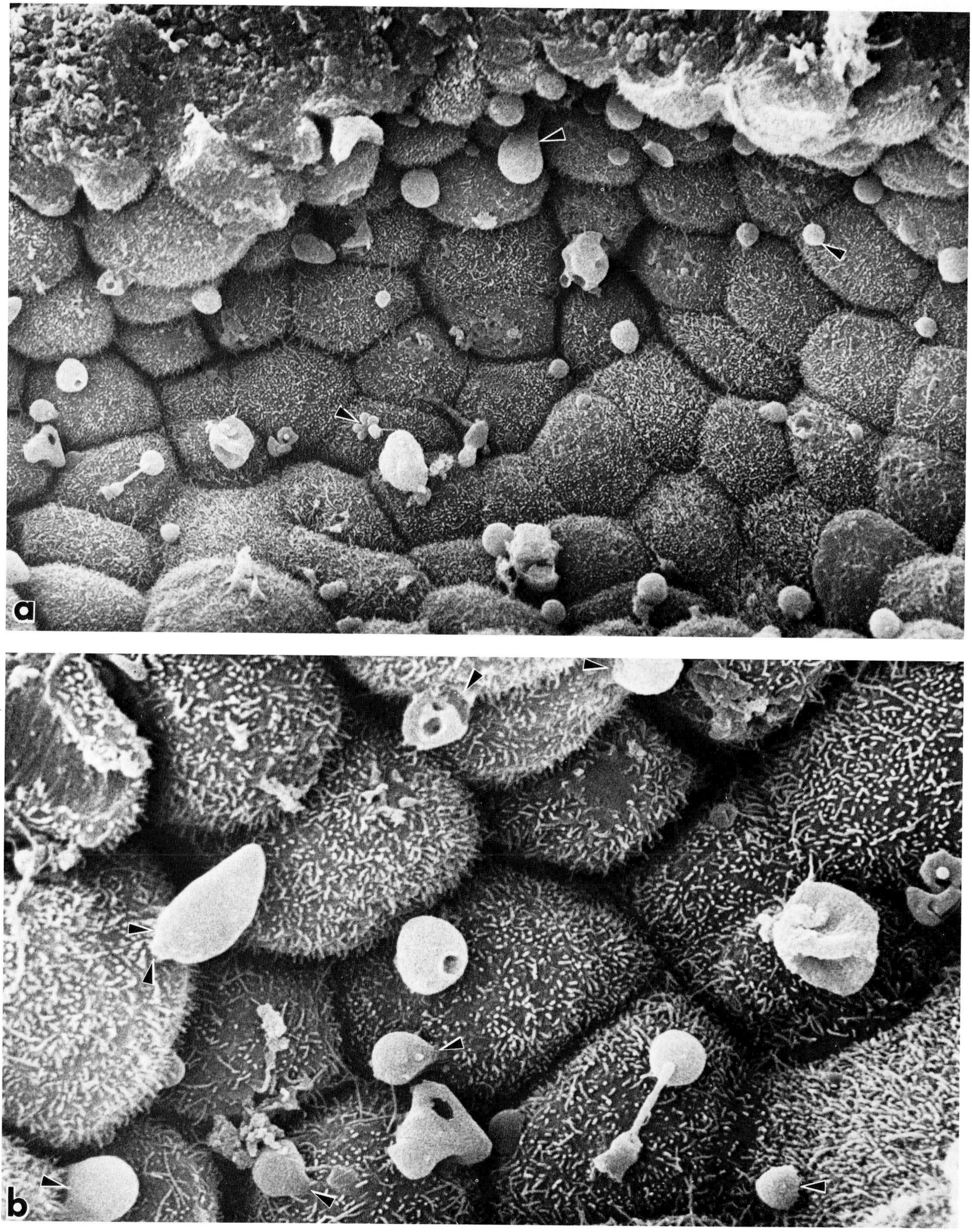
a
b

Figure 3–44. Secretory products at apices of secretory cells of axillary apocrine sweat glands.

a. *Secretory products (arrows) are attached to a small part of the apex of a secretory cell and the remainder is occupied by microvilli. A single cell apex may have multiple secretory protrusions that differ in size. The method of exocytosis that involves the formation and release of secretory products as small protrusions of the cell apex is called microapocrine secretion. × 2,290.*

b. *Higher magnification of microapocrine secretion. The protrusions range from 1 μm to 2.5 μm in diameter and they tend to become polyp-like Each is attached to the cell apex by a stalk (arrows). Microapocrine secretion, characterized by a pinching-off of secretory products along with a small portion of apical cytoplasm, is the predominant method of exocytosis in human axillary apocrine sweat glands. × 5,940.*

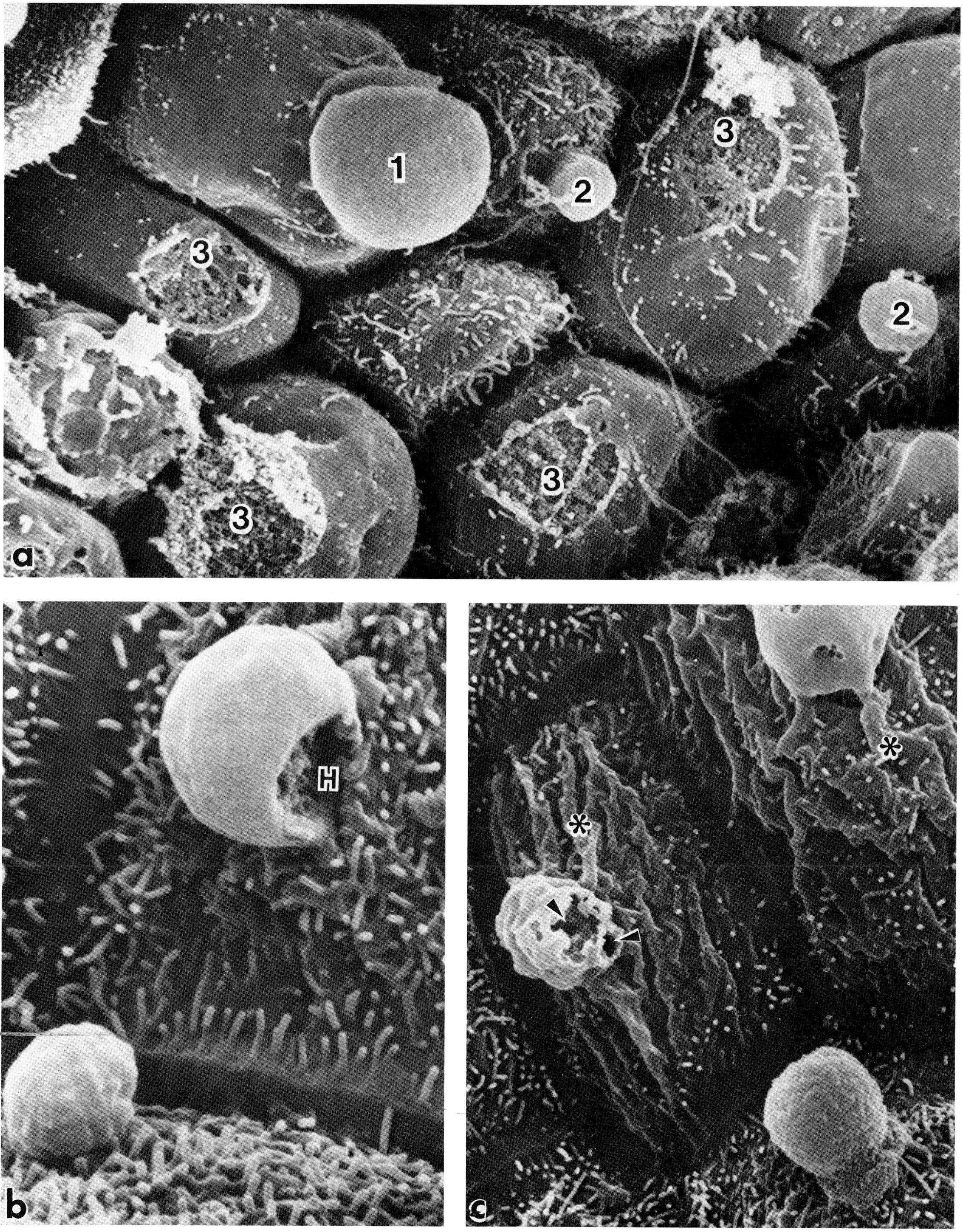
1
2
3
2
3
3
3
3
a
H
b
*
*
c

Figure 3–45. Apices of secretory cells of axillary apocrine sweat glands.

a. *One large (1) and two small (2) apical protrusions are illustrated. The large protrusion includes most of the cell apex and is representative of apocrine secretion. The major difference between apocrine secretion and the more frequently occurring microapocrine secretion is the size of the area that detaches. Apocrine secretion may involve the entire cell apex while microapocrine secretion involves a much smaller dimension of the cell apex (2.5 μm or less). The porous areas (3) are sites where protrusions have detached.* × *6,900.*

b. *Small protrusions of the cell apex have formed during microapocrine secretion. Cytoplasmic vesicles visible through the hole (H) illustrate that the protrusion is part of the cell, rather than an extraneous structure that overlies the cell. Note the smooth surface of the protrusion, and the microvilli on the remainder of the cell surface. Cleft near bottom of picture separates two cells.* × *7,140.*

c. *A small protrusion indicative of microapocrine secretion is on the apex of each of three cells. Ruffles (*) merge with the protrusions. Holes (arrows) are sites where secretory products have escaped.* × *7,140.*

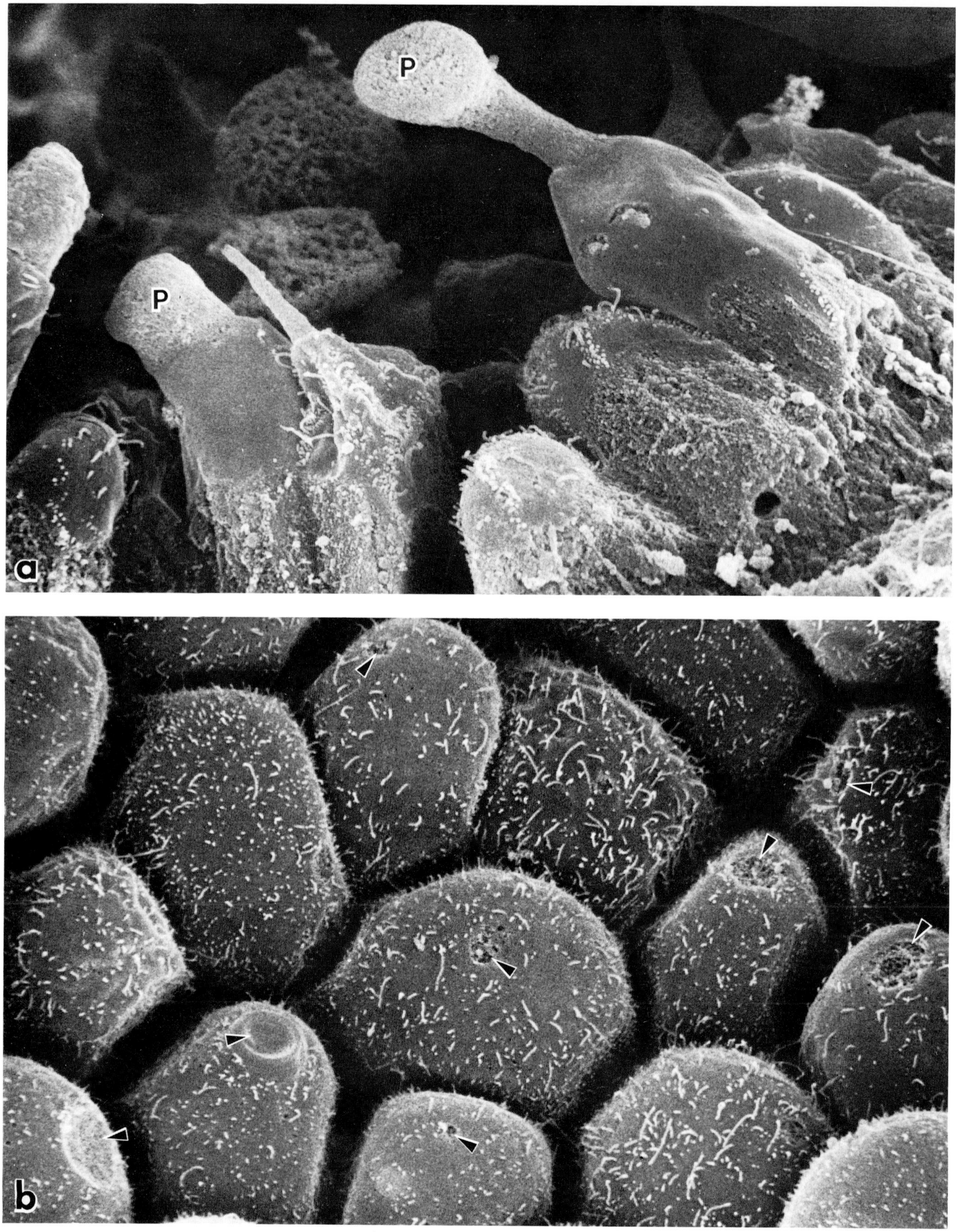

Figure 3–46. Secretory cell apices of axillary apocrine sweat glands.

a. *Protrusions (P) of different sizes are shown in profile for comparison with previous "head on" views.* ×4,370.

b. *Porous areas (arrows) on cell apices differ in size. Each porous area indicates where a protrusion of secretory product has detached.* ×6,500.

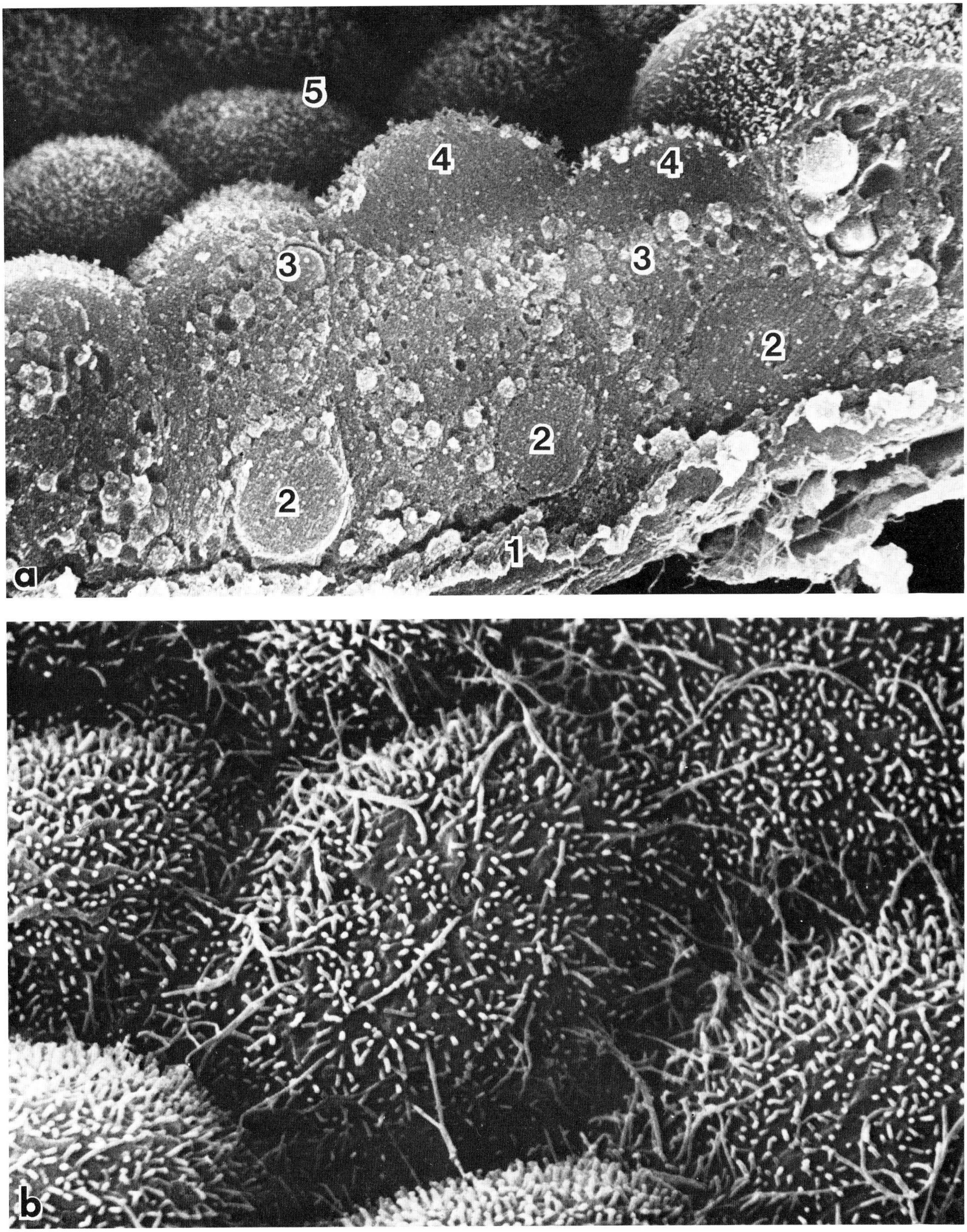

Figure 3–47. Secretory cells of axillary apocrine sweat glands.

a. *The secretory tubules were fractured after freezing with liquid nitrogen, and the cytoplasm of the secretory cells is shown. Observe basement membrane area (1), nucleus (2), secretory granules (3) of various sizes, apical cytoplasm (4), and lumen of tubule (5) with microvilli covering the cell apices.* $\times 3{,}840$.

b. *Convex apices of secretory cells and lumen of secretory tubule. Microvilli are of unequal length and some extend between adjacent cell apices. Unusually long microvilli, such as the ones shown here, can be found on the secretory cells of women during the luteal phase of the menstrual cycle.* $\times 17{,}600$.

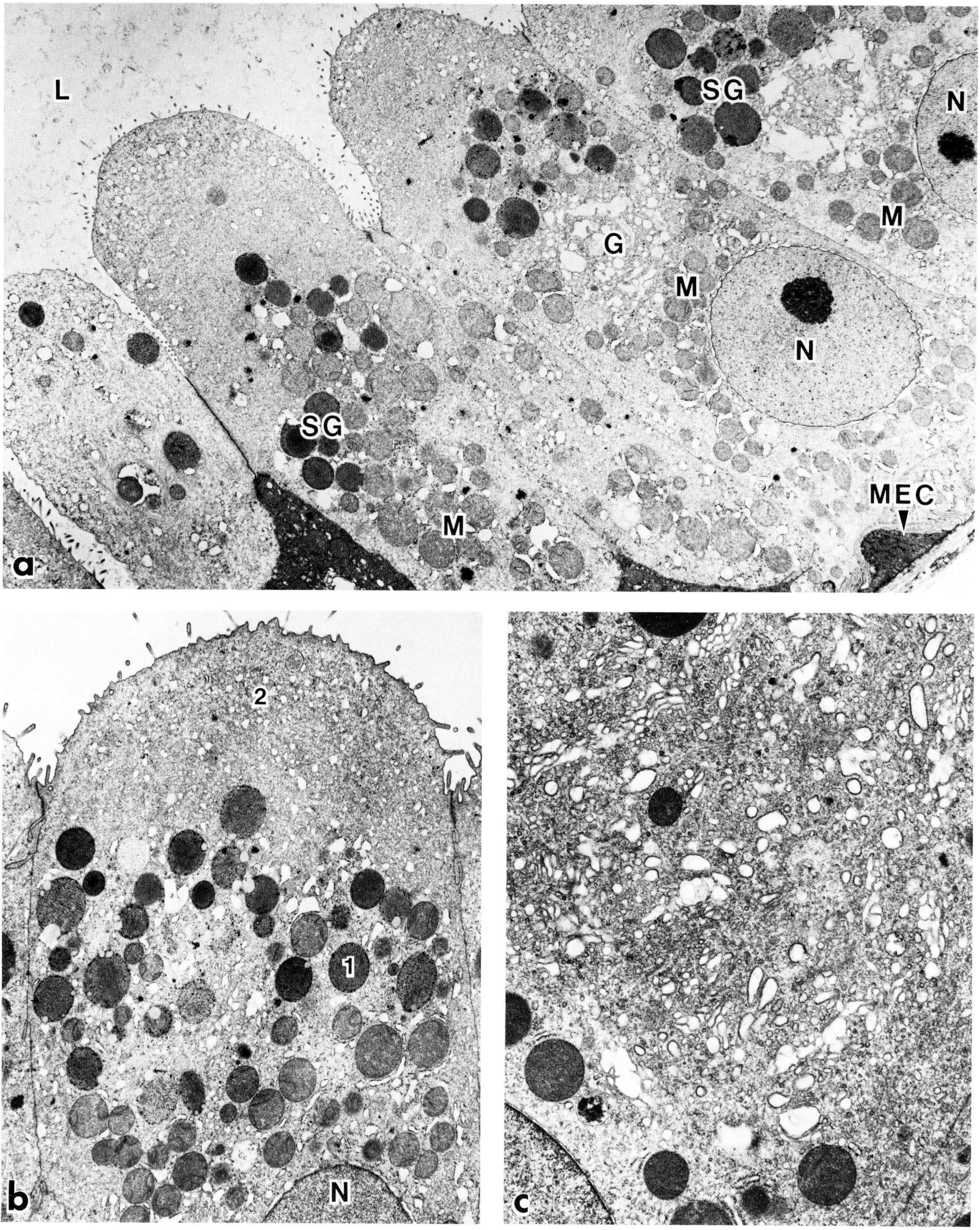
L
SG
N
M
G
M
N
SG
MEC
M
a
2
1
N
b
c

Figure 3–48. TEM, secretory cells of axillary apocrine sweat glands.

a. *Note lumen (L) of tubule, the round cell apices lined by microvilli, secretory granules (SG) of various sizes and densities, the nucleus (N) with prominent nucleolus, and membranes of the Golgi apparatus (G). Small, electron lucent granules or vesicles are concentrated in the apical cytoplasm. Mitochondria (M) are abundant and exhibit the characteristically sparse cristae. The dark, contractile processes of myoepithelial cells (MEC) occur at the bases of secretory cells. × 4,180.*

b. *Two chief types of granules are present above the nucleus (N) of the secretory cell: electron dense (1) and electron lucent (2). × 6,750.*

c. *In this illustration of a secretory cell, the Golgi apparatus occupies most of the area above the nucleus. Electron lucent and electron dense granules emanate from the Golgi apparatus. × 11,400.*

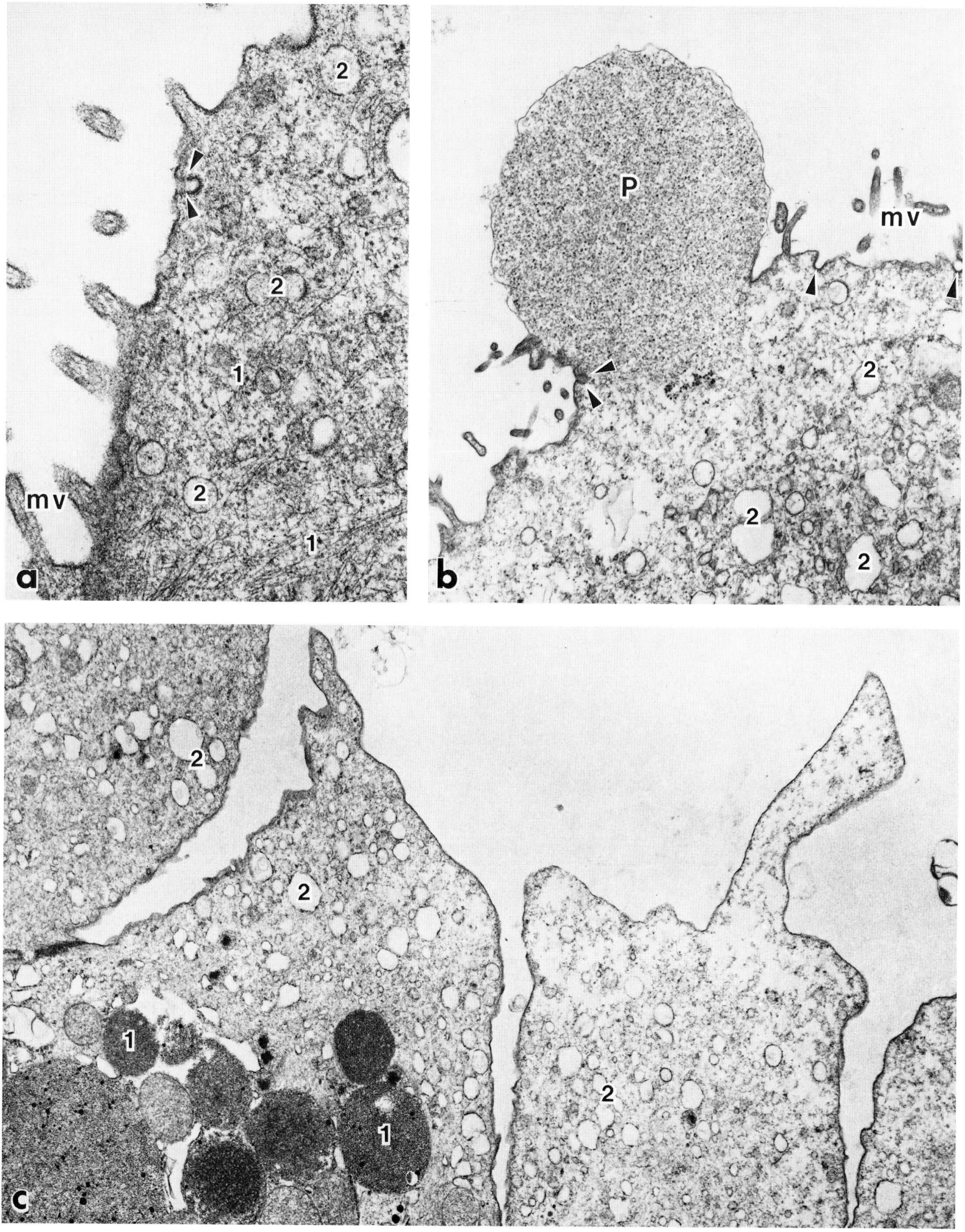
a
2
2
1
2
1
mv
b
P
mv
2
2
2
c
2
2
1
1
2

Figure 3–49. TEM, secretory cells of axillary apocrine sweat glands.

a. *The secretory cell apex is rich in microfilaments (1) and electron lucent secretory granules (2). Microfilaments contribute to the cytoskeleton of the cell and extend into the microvilli (mv). Electron lucent granules (arrows) may fuse with the apical cell membrane and release their contents by the merocrine method. ×45,000.*

b. *Projection (P) extends from part of the secretory cell apex where microvilli (mv), electron lucent granules or vesicles (2), and sites of merocrine secretion (arrows) are also present. Projections correspond to apical protrusions observed by SEM. ×22,000.*

c. *Secretory cell apices with projections and electron dense (1) and electron lucent (2) secretory granules. ×24,000.*

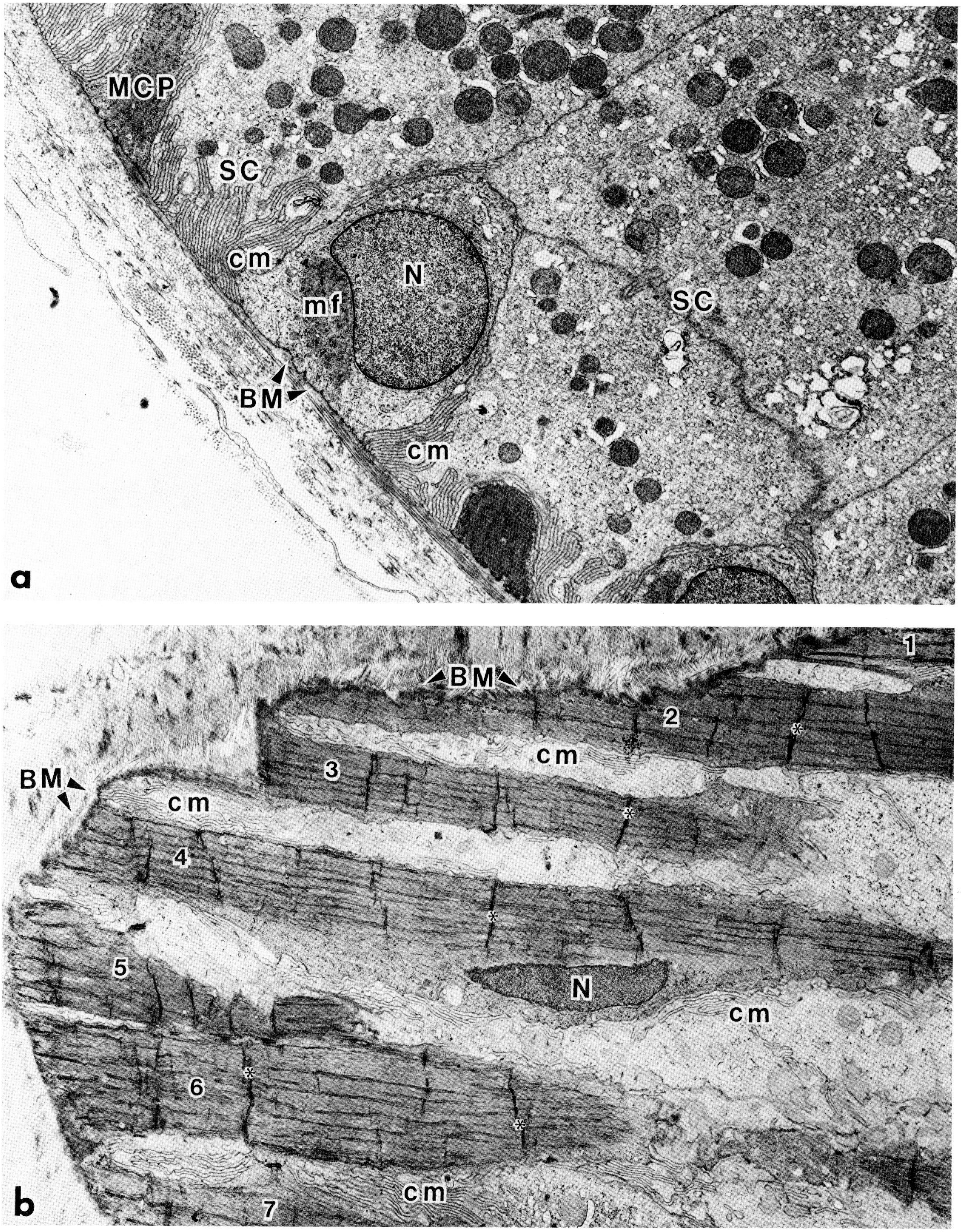
a
MCP
SC
cm
N
mf
BM
SC
cm
b
1
BM
2
cm
BM
3
cm
4
5
N
cm
6
cm
7

Figure 3–50. Myoepithelial cells and their processes at base of secretory cells in axillary apocrine sweat glands.

a. *Myoepithelial cells in apocrine glands and eccrine glands are similar ultrastructurally. They form an incomplete layer between the basement membrane (BM) and the bases of the secretory cells (SC). The thickest region of the myoepithelial cell contains the nucleus (N). Most cell organelles and inclusions are located in the perinuclear cytoplasm. Some myofilaments (mf) are present in the perinuclear cytoplasm, but each myoepithelial cell process (MCP) is filled with myofilaments. Cell membranes (cm) of secretory cells are highly folded between the myoepithelial cells. × 7,480.*

b. *Portions of seven myoepithelial cells (labelled 1 through 7) are shown in a section made through the base and diagonally to the axis of a secretory tubule. The cells extend from the basement membrane (BM) and are separated by the folded cell membranes (cm) of secretory cells. The nucleus (N) and perinuclear cytoplasm are shown in one myoepithelial cell (4). Note the longitudinal bundles of myofilaments and the dense lines (*) where myofilaments end. Contraction of the basket-like network of myoepithelial processes can squeeze the secretory cells and result in the expulsion of secretory products. × 5,500.*

ACNE 4

The primary lesion of acne vulgaris is the comedo. Comedones commonly develop on the face, chest, and back mainly during adolescence, the age at which the disease flourishes and affects 100% of the population to various degrees.

The comedo arises when a hair follicle and the excretory duct of its sebaceous gland become plugged with sebum, keratinized cells, and microorganisms. The comedo may have a wide opening (open comedo) or a very narrow opening (closed comedo). The closed comedo is covered with a black dot (blackhead) due to oxidation of the sebum at the follicular orifice. Closed comedones may rupture and release sebum and keratinized material into the dermis.

The material for this study consisted of approximately 150 comedones removed by comedo extractor or punch biopsy from 20 acne patients, 10 males and 10 females, who ranged from 18–30 years in age. Approximately one-half of the comedones came from the face, and the remainder from the back. Whole, bisected, and squashed comedones were processed for SEM. Representative SEM specimens were carefully removed from the stubs after they had been photographed. These were processed for TEM. Observations made on these samples were correlated with data obtained by SEM.

SEM clearly revealed five main components of the comedonic plug: scales, hairs, sebum, bacteria, and yeasts. Scales constituted the bulk of the lesion. Cultures of comedones from the same patients that provided the lesions for microscopy showed that *Propionibacterium (Corynebacterium) acnes* and *Pityrosporum ovale* were the two main microorganisms in the comedo. Although these microorganisms alone do not cause acne, they are important components of the acne lesion. The vast majority of microorganisms are extracellular, but the fact that some are within the scales helps to explain the effectiveness of keratolytic agents used for the treatment of acne.

References

Marples, R. R., K. J. McGinley, and O. H. Mills. Microbiology of comedones in acne vulgaris. J. Invest. Dermatol. 60: 80–83, 1973.

Montes, L. F., and W. H. Wilborn. Fine structure of Corynebacterium acnes. J. Invest. Dermatol. 54: 338–345, 1970.

Montes, L. F., and W. H. Wilborn. Scanning electron microscopy of comedones. Scanning Electron Microscopy, Vol. II, 1978, SEM Inc., Chicago, IL, pp. 253–258.

Montes, L. F., W. H. Wilborn, and A. D. Flanagan. Electron microscopic assay of a topical ance treatment: Benzoyle peroxide acetone gel. Scanning Electron Microscopy, Vol. III, 1979, SEM Inc., Chicago, IL, pp. 185–188 and 195–196.

Plewig, G., and A. M. Kligman. Acne. Morphogenesis and Treatment. Springer-Heidelberg-New York, 1975.

Weary, P. Comedogenic potential of the lipid extract of Pityrosporum ovale. Arch. Dermatol. 102: 84–91. 1970.

Wilborn, W. H., L. F. Montes, and B. M. Hyde. Scanning electron microscopy of hairs in comedones. *In:* Hair Research. Orfanos, Montagna, and Stutten, eds. pp. 446–455, Springer, Berlin-Heidelberg-New York, 1981.

Wilborn, W. H., L. F. Montes, R. E. Lyons, and G. W. Battista. Ultrastructural basis for the assay of topical acne treatments. Transmission and scanning electron microscopy of untreated comedones. J. Cut. Path. 5: 165–183, 1978.

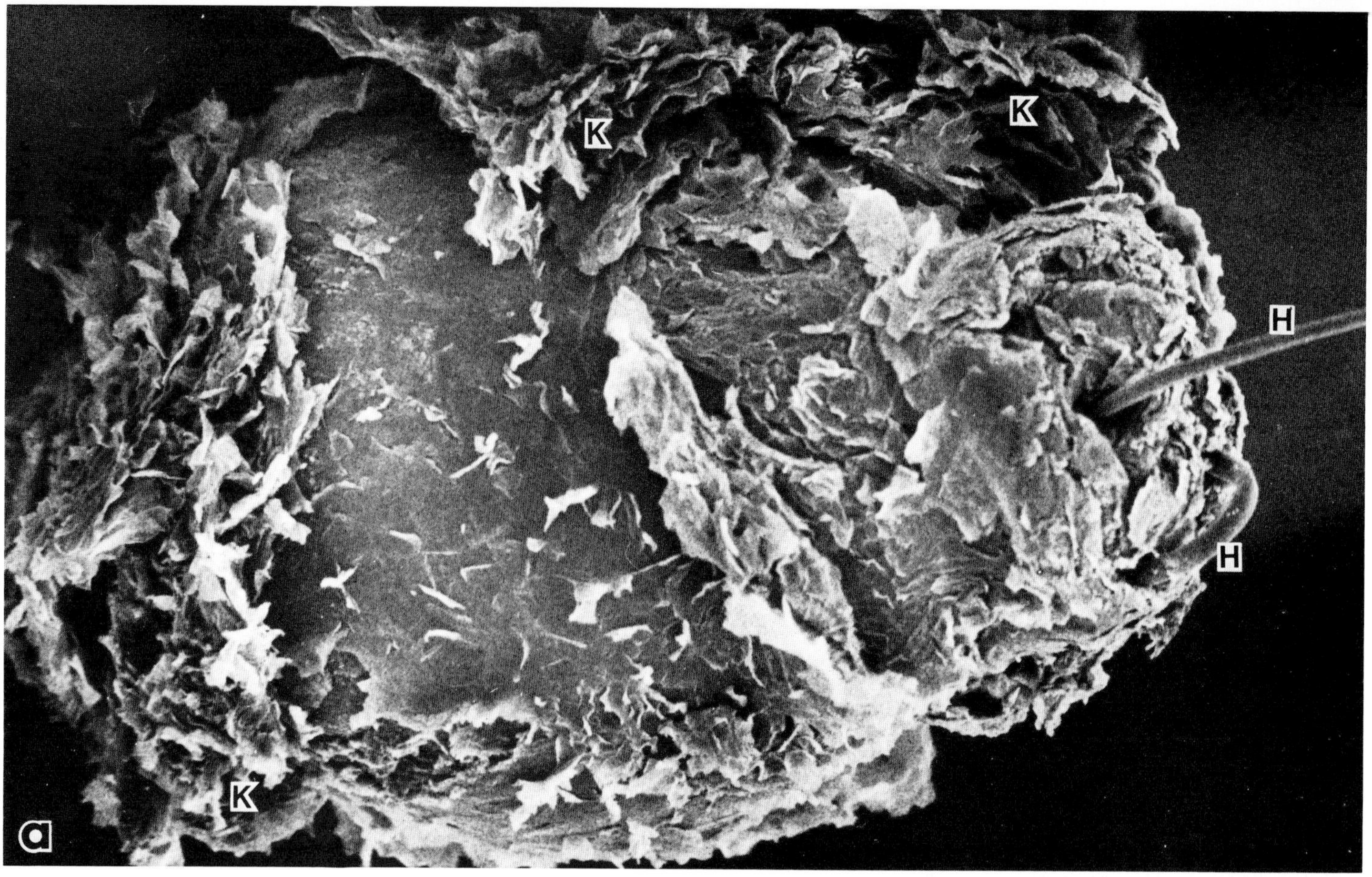
K
K
H
H
K
a

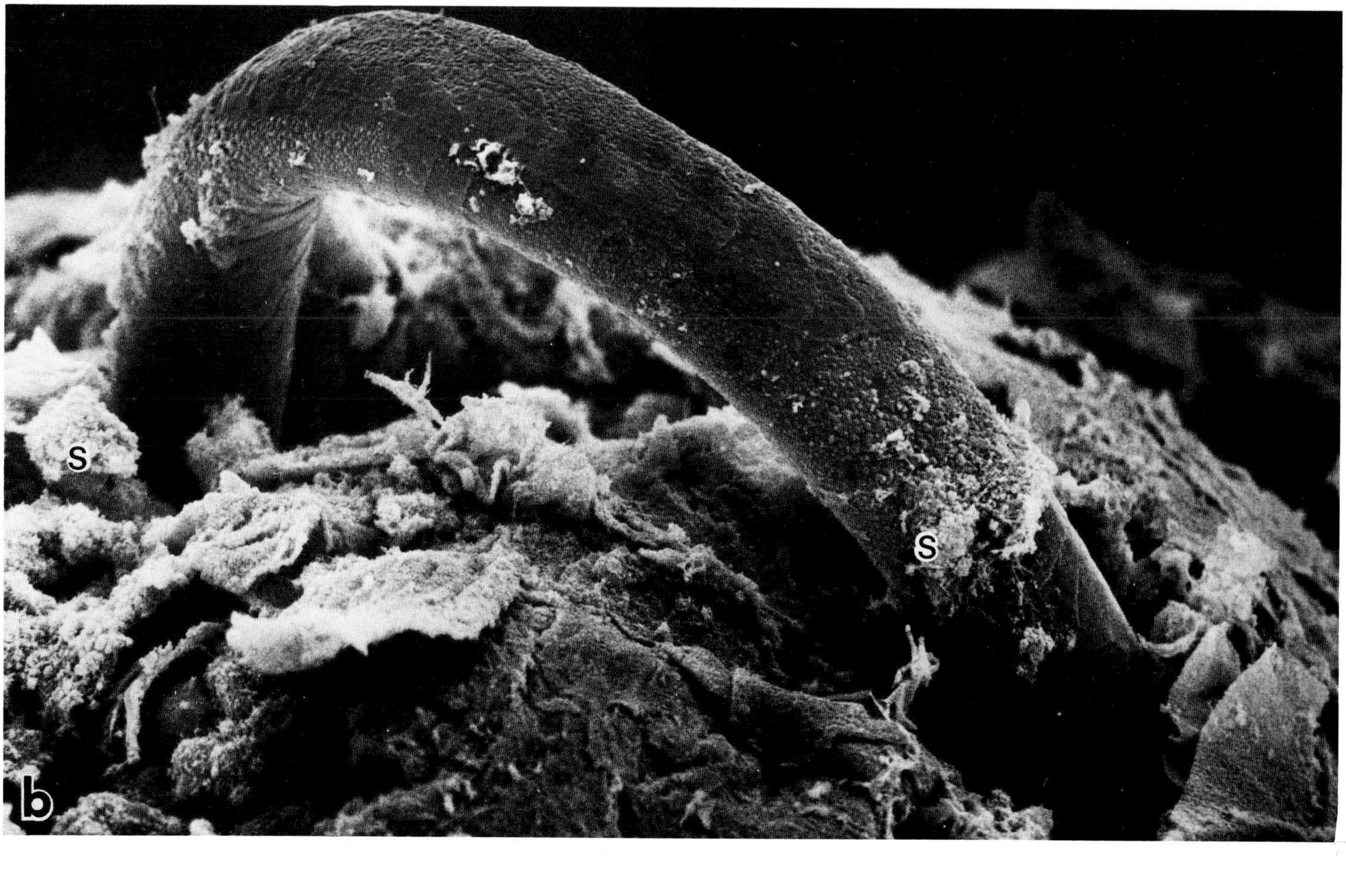
S
S
b

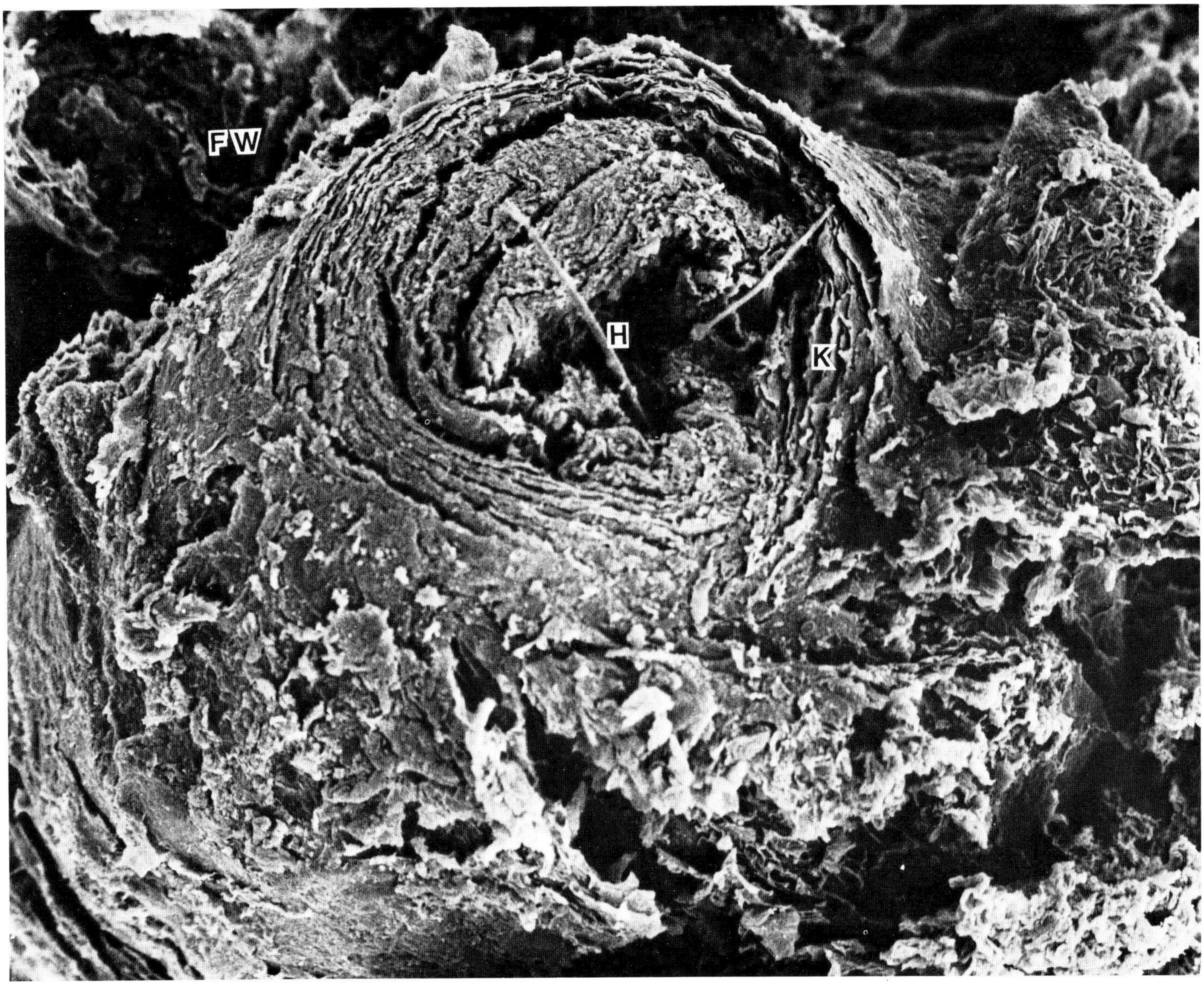

Figure 4–2. The apex of the intact comedo is surrounded by the dilated follicular wall (FW). Concentric lamellae of scales (K) circumscribe the two vellus hairs (H) that emerge from the central pit. Detaching scales and sebum occupy the periphery of the cabbage-like comedo. ×180.

Figure 4–1. a. *Comedones are often elongated with layers of loosely arranged scales (K) on their outer walls and hairs (H) that project from their distal ends. There are numerous shallow grooves and deep crevices or pits between the scales. These give the keratinous plug an uneven appearance. ×120.*

b. *One hair in Figure 4–1a is shown at higher magnification to illustrate the tendency of a hair to bend and re-enter the comedonal mass instead of terminating at the distal free surface. Droplets of sebum (S) cover portions of the hair and some of the comedonal scales. Sebum is a ubiquitous component of comedones and varies in amount from scanty to abundant. Sebum droplets may coalesce to form berry-like aggregates. ×925.*

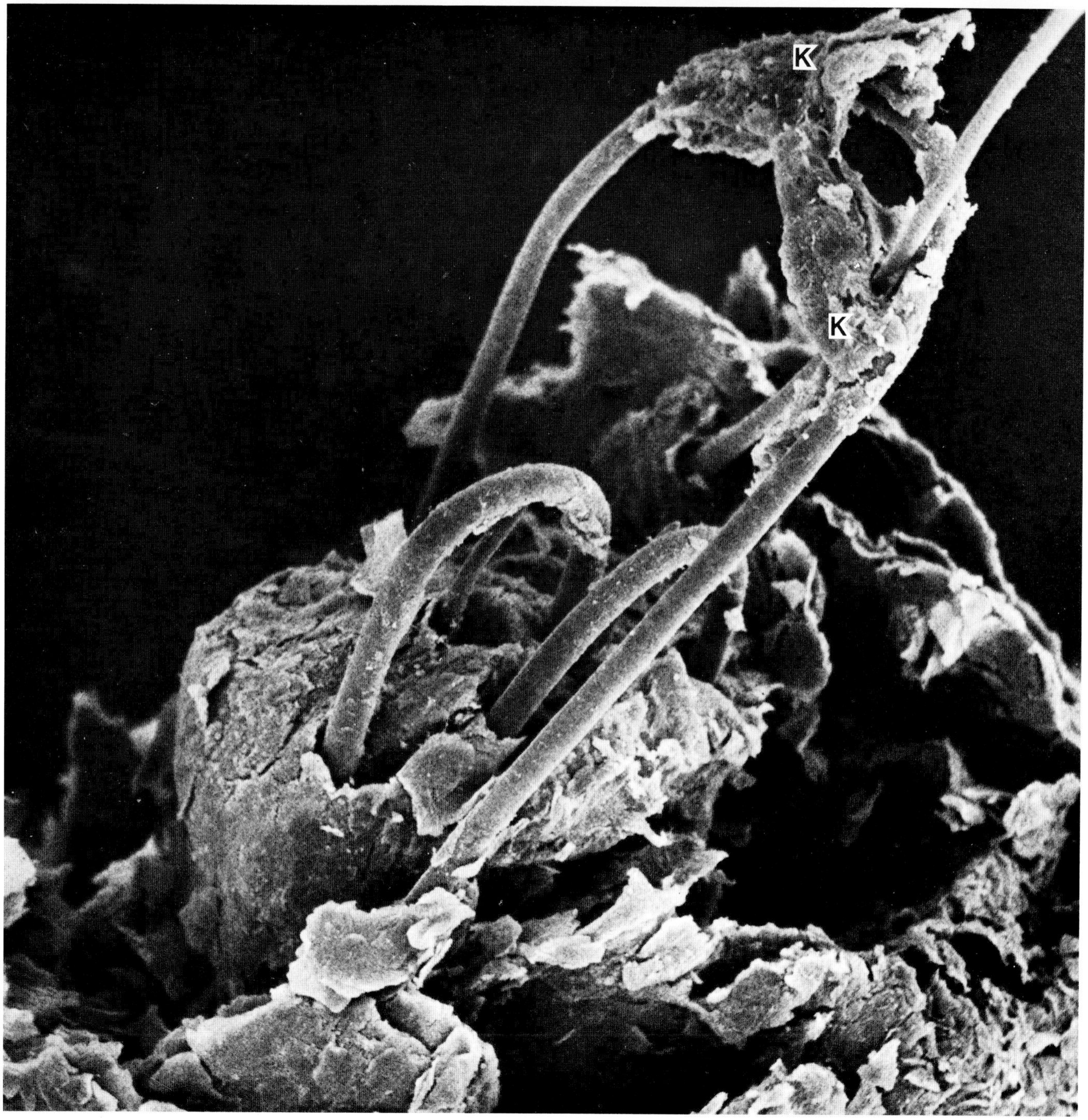

Figure 4–3. Some scales have been removed to expose the multiple hairs that ramify and intertwine extensively in the comedo. Portions of hairs remain encrusted with scales (K). A comedo may contain as many as 5–6 hairs that project from the surface and then bend to re-enter the comedo. Hairs are more abundant in comedones of the face than those of the back, but their prevalence is not dependent on patient age, sex, or senility of the comedo. Measurements were made of 50 hairs in comedones. These data showed that hairs averaged 22.4 μm in diameter and ranged from 5.5–41.7 μm in diameter. Thus, some hairs found in comedones were too large to be of the vellus type which averaged about 10 μm in diameter. × 240.

Figure 4–4. a. *Two or more small hairs (H) of the vellus type often course adjacent to each other in the comedonal mass. The overlapping, shingle-like cuticular scales constitute the most prominent feature of the hairs.* × 840.

b. *Yeasts (Y), identified by culture and TEM as* P. ovale, *are able to invade the hair cuticle which, as shown here, is partially enveloped in comedonal scales (K).* P. ovale *is lodged in a hole, a result of keratolytic activity.* × 5,000.

c. *The cuticle is riddled with holes (arrows) of various sizes. Holes indicate sites of previous keratolytic activity by microorganisms.* × 1975.

d. *The hair is matted with sebum (S) and microorganisms (M). Both bacteria and yeasts tend to congregate in sebum-rich areas where they may invade the cuticle. Yeasts are two or three times larger than bacteria.* × 5,040.

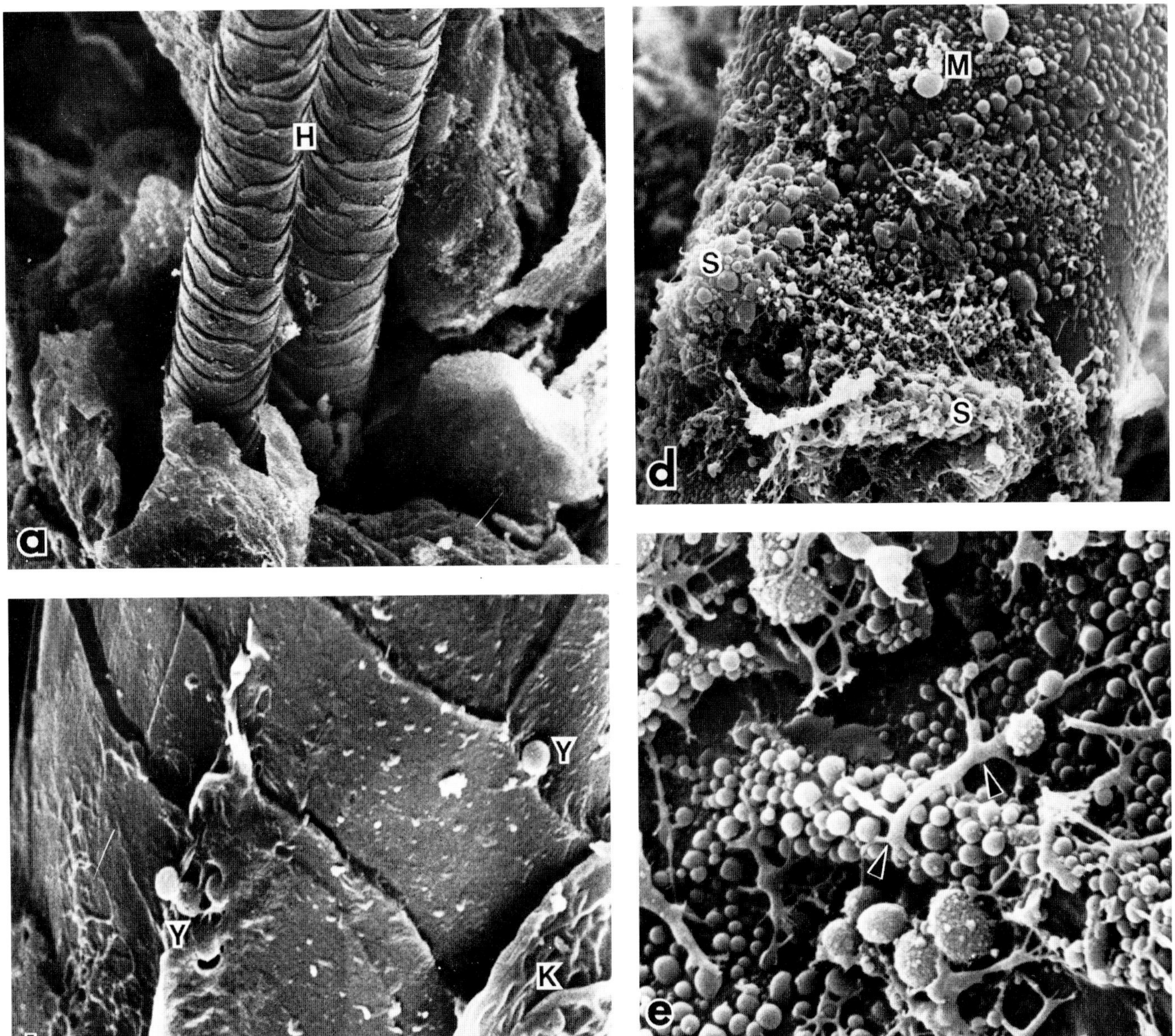

e. *Morphologically, two types of yeasts can be identified in comedones,* P. ovale *and* P. orbiculare. P. ovale *is by far the most common of the two types.* P. orbiculare, *in contrast to* P. ovale, *may form hyphae (arrows) as shown here associated with the hair cuticle. ×9,240.*

f. *The "weathered" hair has many holes and deranged scales. ×990.*

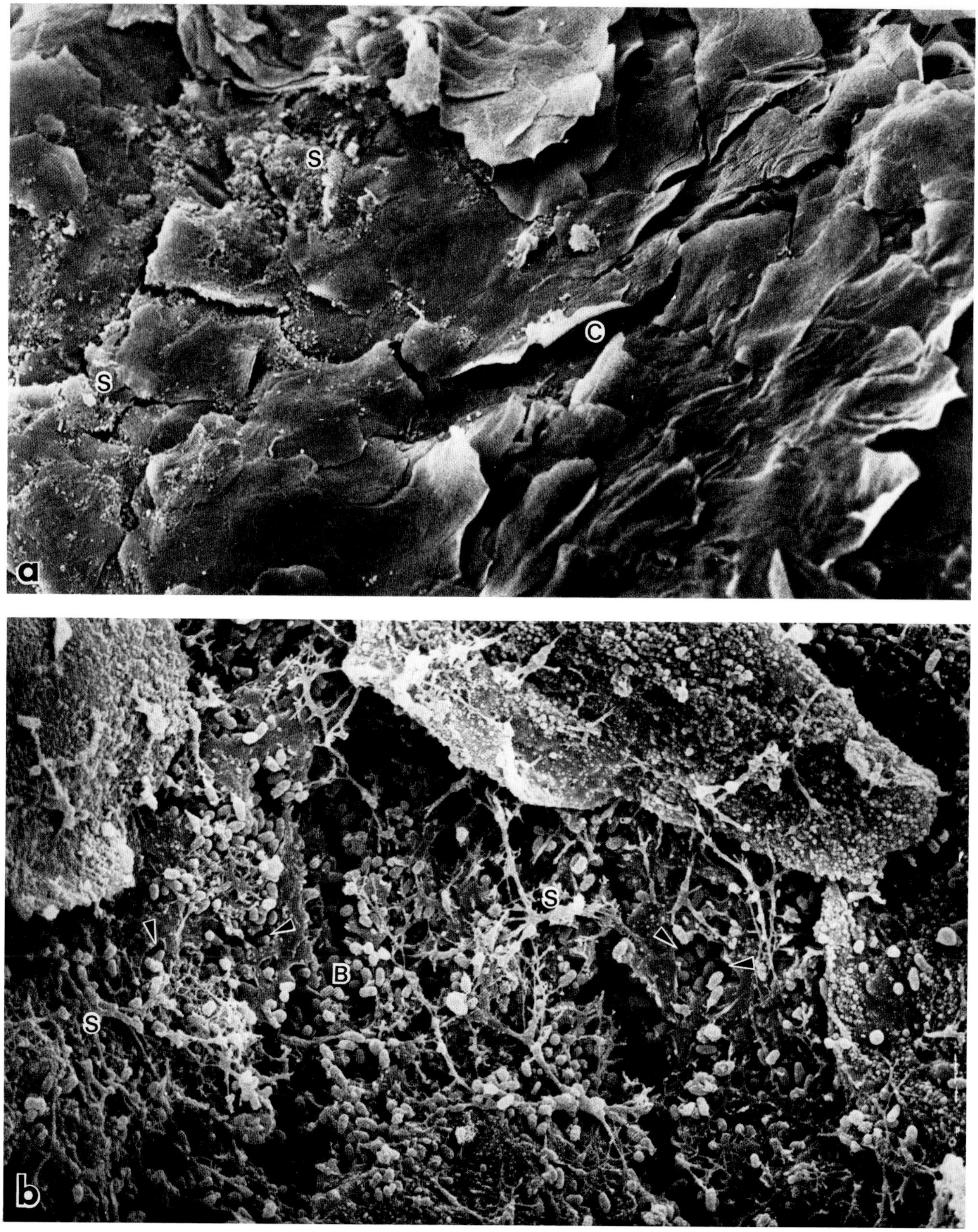

Figure 4–5. a. *Sebum (S) is unevenly and rather sparsely distributed over the superficial scales at the distal end of the comedo. Pocket-like cavities (C) are present below the elevated free borders of the scales. Microorganisms have a propensity for such pockets where they are hidden until the scales detach.* × *485.*

b. *A mixture of bacteria (B) and sebum (S) coat the deep portion of the comedo whose distal, more superficial portion was shown at lower magnification in Figure 4.5a. Droplets and strands of sebum cover the scales (K). Most bacteria that inhabit comedones, as confirmed by culture techniques and TEM, are* P. acnes. *They produce keratinase, an enzyme which permits microorganisms to perforate and penetrate the keratinized cells. Holes (arrows), with and without bacteria, in the keratinized cells mark present and former sites of bacterial invasion. Intracellular bacteria can be clearly visualized only by TEM.* × *3,170.*

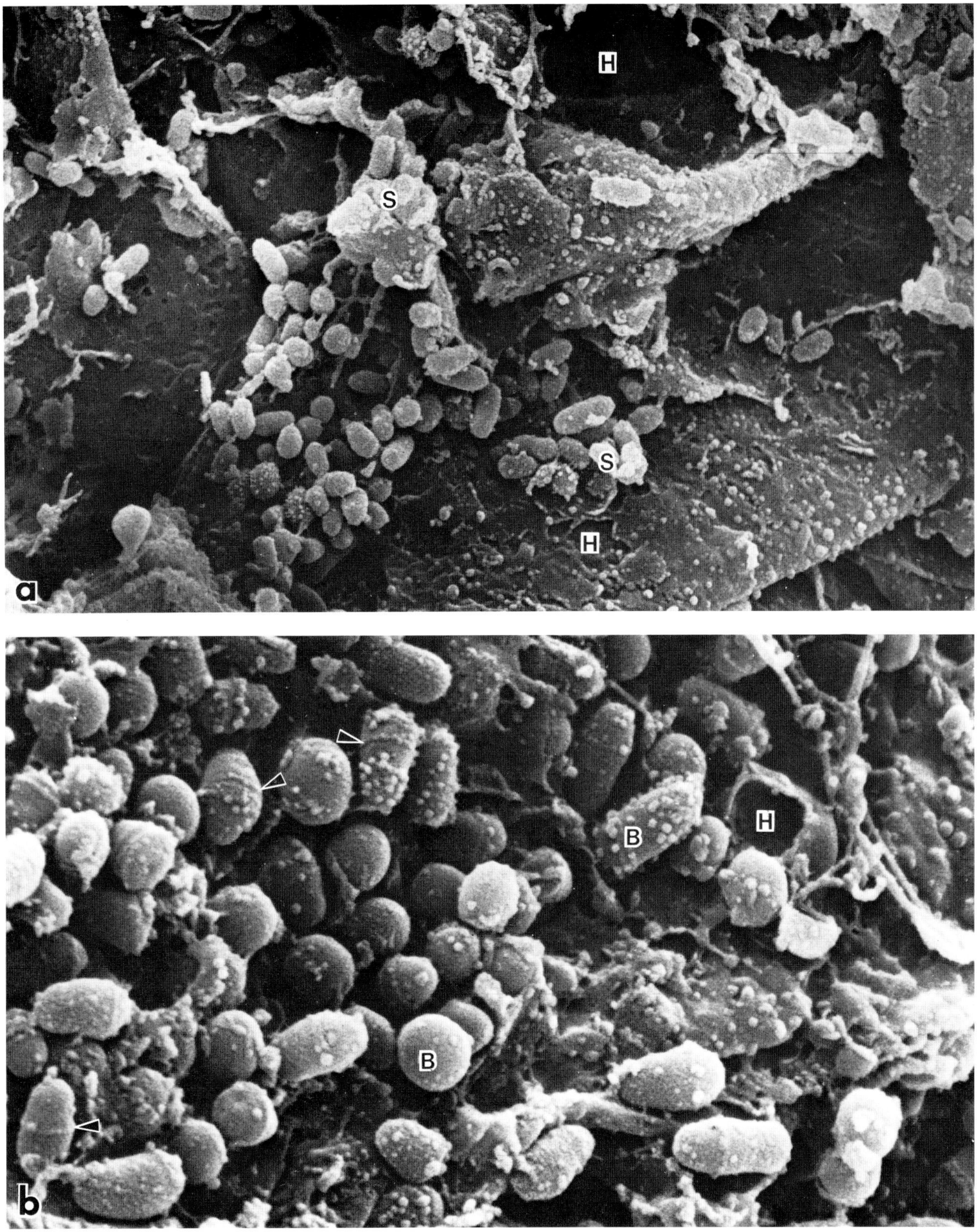

Figure 4–6. a. P. acnes *on the deep scales of the comedo are somewhat enlongated but lack the chain arrangement and round shape of cocci. Some bacteria are covered with sebum (S) and others have sebum droplets on their surfaces. Holes (H) indicate the potent keratolytic ability of the bacteria.* $\times$ *7,920.*

b. *Higher magnification of the deep portion of comedo shown above reveals the large number of sebum droplets that adhere to* P. acnes *(B). Dividing bacteria with surface bands (arrows) are common and indicate the prolific nature of* P. acnes *in the acne lesion. The hole (H) in the keratinized cell approximates the size of a single bacterium. Close association of sebum and bacteria signifies that* P. acnes *utilizes for fuel the fatty acids that are derived from sebum.* $\times$ *15,840.*

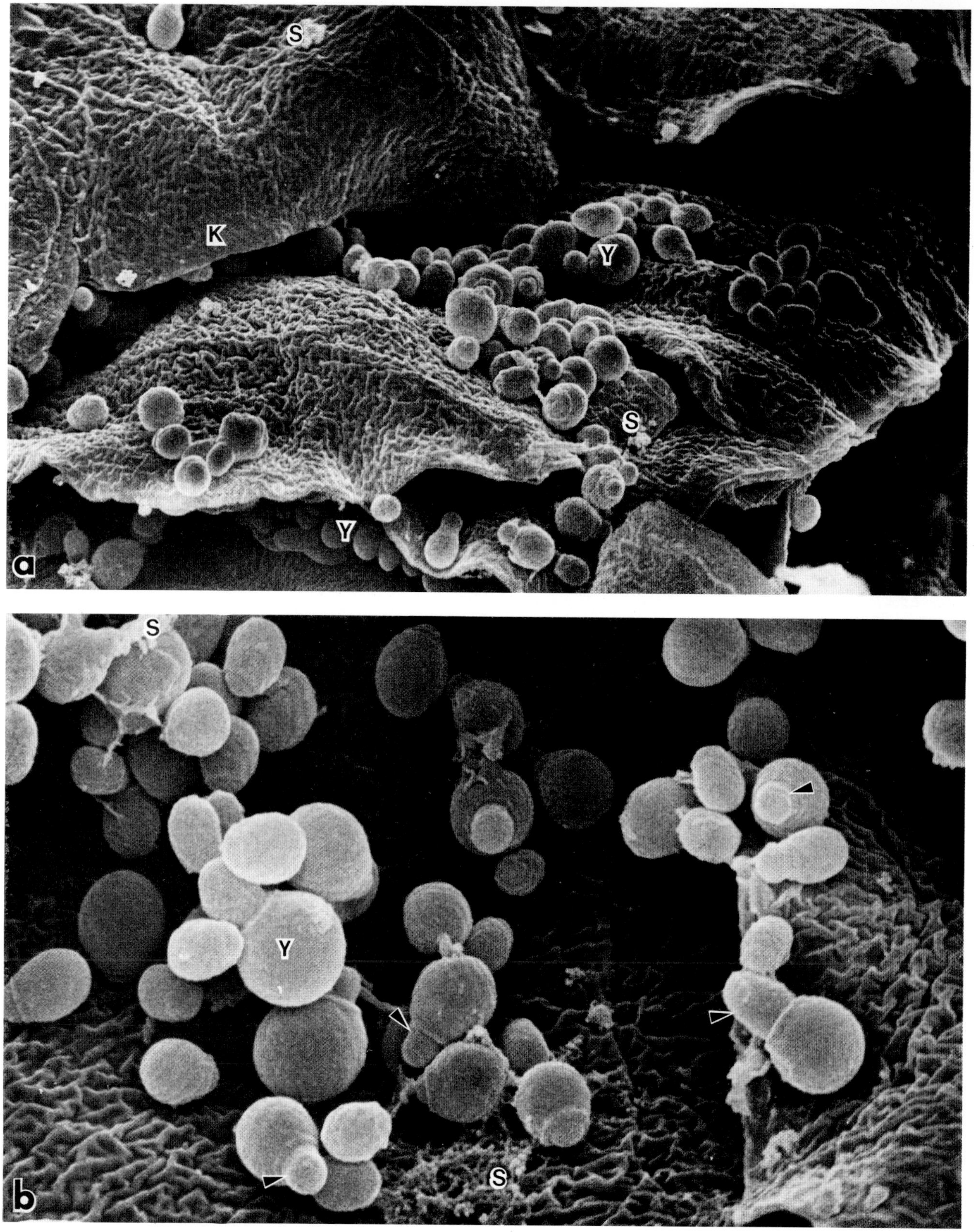

Figure 4–7. a. *Numerous yeasts (Y), readily identifiable by their shape, size and surface features as* P. ovale, *are located on the scales and among the sebum droplets. Yeasts have smooth surfaces unless covered by sebum. The fact that yeasts tend to be more superficially located than bacteria in the comedonal mass agrees with the respective aerobic and anaerobic nature of these yeasts and bacteria. Yeasts have a propensity for sites where scales (K) overlap and within pits and depressions. The ruffled surface of scales is due to the multitude of alternating microridges and microgrooves which enhance the entrapment of sebum (S). ×4,140.*

b. *Reproduction of yeasts (Y) is manifested by the formation of bud-like extensions (arrows). Surfaces of yeasts may be free of sebum (S) or wholly or partially covered with the fatty material. Some yeasts, as confirmed by TEM, may penetrate the scales and become intracellular.* P. ovale *also have the ability to form lipids which induce comedo formation and to elaborate free fatty acids from triglycerides. In general, open comedones have more yeasts and bacteria than closed comedones. ×8,280.*

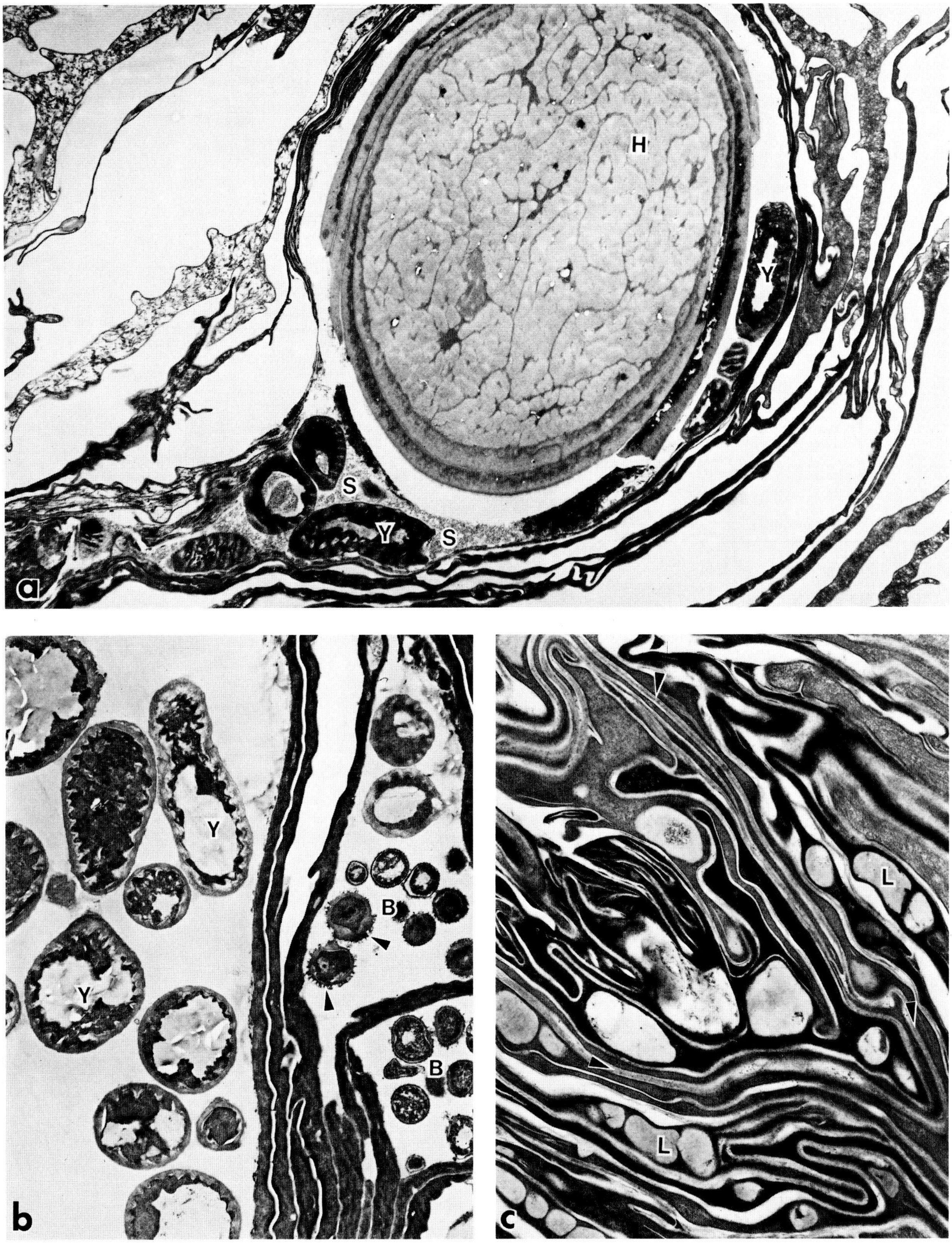

Figure 4–8. a. *TEM, distal end and central portion of comedo. Yeasts (Y) lie outside the hair (H) and among the thin scales. Large spaces separate many scales. One osmiophilic and granular, sebum-rich area (S) is present, but most of the sebum and other lipids were dissolved during tissue processing.* ×*6,510.*

b. *TEM, midregion and central portion of comedo. Yeasts (Y) and bacteria (B) tend to coexist in the midportion of the comedo. Bacteria are several times smaller than yeasts and have rough surfaces where sebum has adhered (arrows). Groups of microorganisms often lie in pocket-like spaces between the scales (K).* ×*6,445.*

c. *TEM, tightly-packed scales at periphery of comedo. Keratinized cells from the hard skeleton of the comedo. The peripheral comedonal scales are younger and more closely packed than scales in the center of the lesion shown in* a *and* b *(Fig. 4.8). Lipid droplets (L) of various sizes are characteristic of comedonal scales. The narrow intercellular spaces contain a cement-like substance (arrows) which contributes to the cohesiveness of the scales.* ×*12,440.*

PSORIASIS 5

Psoriasis affects about 2% of the population. It is genetically transmitted and usually does not become fully apparent until after puberty. Psoriasis has been called the scaling disease. Patients develop plaques of various sizes that are reddish in color but characteristically covered by silvery scales that are shed continuously. When psoriasis becomes highly active, the plaques undergo enlargement and confluence to cover wide areas of the skin. Patients then feel uncomfortable because of the dryness, itching, and fissuring of the skin and the accompanying serious cosmetic problems. Mental stress and emotional problems may develop and pose serious problems for psoriatics.

The removal of scales from plaques by scraping or superficial curettage results in small bleeding points (Auspitz's sign). Friction or rubbing of the skin leads to the development of psoriatic lesions (Koebner or isomorphic phenomenon). This explains why the elbows and knees most frequently show lesions in patients with psoriasis.

A main feature of psoriasis is acceleration of the renewal of the epidermis. This abnormality helps to explain many clinical features of the disease and the microscopic alterations of the skin. When studied with the light microscope, the affected skin reveals definite thickening of the stratum spinosum (acanthosis), increased mitotic activity, retention of nuclei in the stratum corneum (parakeratosis), elongation of the rete ridges, and increased amounts of glycogen in the epidermis. The dermis is also altered in psoriasis as shown by edema, discontinuity of the basement membrane, dilated capillaries with increased permeability, extravasation of blood cells which invade the epidermis (exocytosis), and infiltrates of lymphocytes and histiocytes. An interesting phenomenon is the migration of blood cells through the epidermis and their concentration in foci or microabscesses at the level of the stratum corneum (Munro abscesses, or Munro-Sabouraud abscesses).

It is noteworthy that patients with psoriasis frequently suffer from arthritis, diabetes, cardiovascular disorders, and elevated levels of uric acid and triglycerides in the blood. Thus, psoriasis can be considered a systemic disease with its primary manifestation in the skin. A generalized form of psoriasis with involvement of the entire skin sometimes develops. This is known as exfoliative dermatitis or psoriatic erythorderma and may carry a serious prognosis.

References

Brody, I. The ultrastructure of the horny layer in normal and psoriatic epidermis as revealed by electron microscopy. J. Invest. Dermatol. 39: 519–527, 1962.

Brody, I. The ultrastructure of epidermis in psoriasis vulgaris as revealed by electron microscopy. V. The noncornified layers in hyperkeratosis. J. Ultrastruct. Res. 8: 566–605, 1963.

Cox, A. J. The dermal-epidermal junction in psoriasis. J. Invest. Dermatol. 53: 428–435, 1969.

Gordon, M., and W. C. Johnson. Histopathology and histochemistry of psoriasis. I. The active lesion and clinically normal skin. Arch. Dermatol. 95: 402–407, 1967.

Montes, L. F., W. H. Wilborn, and I. Brody. Low strength anthralin in psoriasis. J. Cut. Path. 6: 445–456, 1979.

Van Scott, E. J. Tissue compartments of the skin lesion of psoriasis. J. Invest. Dermatol. 59: 4–6, 1972.

Weinstein, G. D., and McCullough, J. L. Cytokinetics in diseases of epidermal hyperplasia. Ann. Rev. Med. 24: 345–352, 1973.

Wilborn, W. H., and L. F. Montes. Ultrastructural changes in psoriatic epidermis following anthralin therapy. J. Cut. Path. 1: 132–150, 1974.

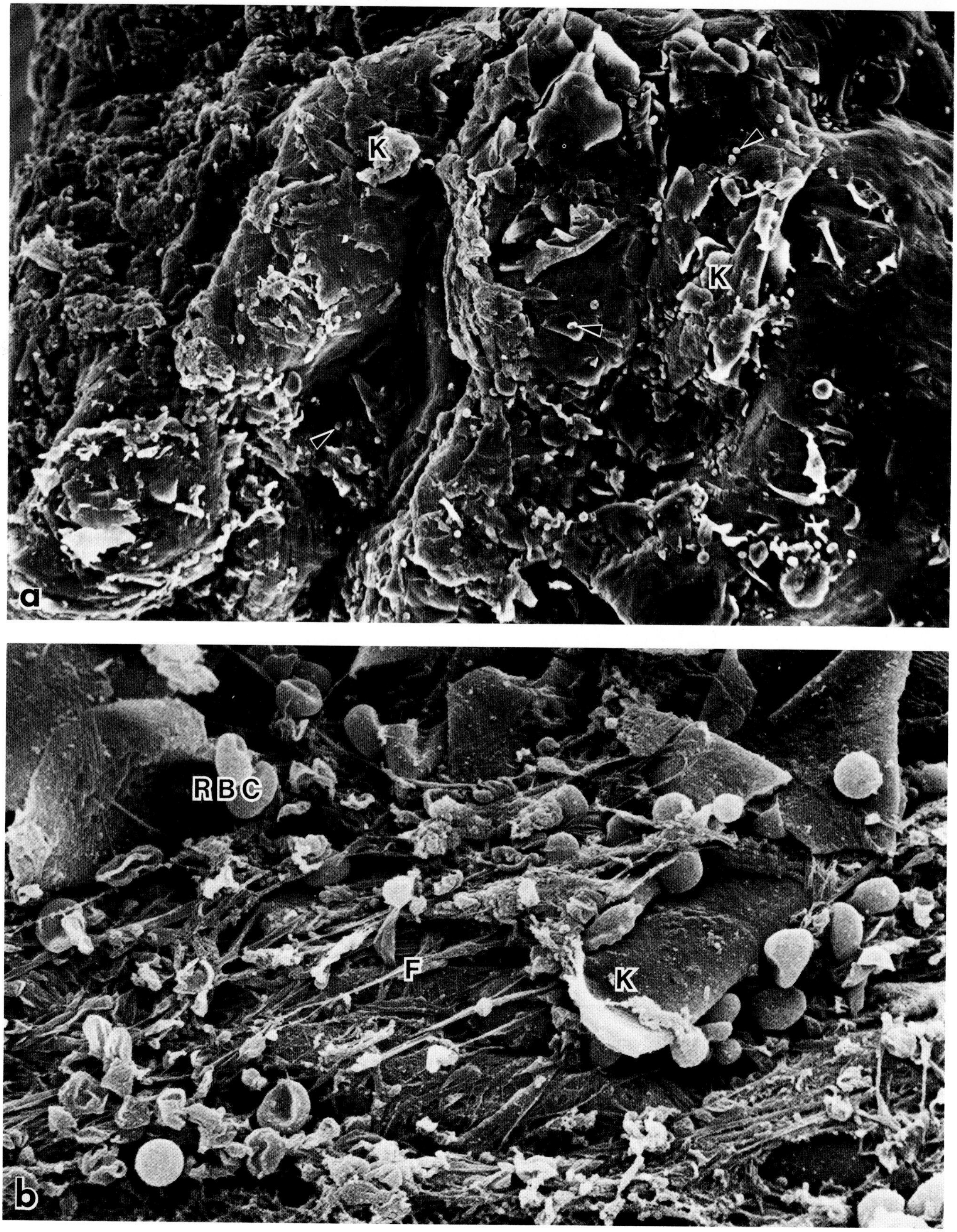

Figure 5–1. a. *Low magnification of the free surface of a psoriatic plaque reveals pits, depressions, and exfoliating scales (K). Erythrocytes and other formed elements of the blood (arrows) are randomly distributed over the surface of the scales. ×340.*

b. *At higher magnification, the psoriatic plaque shows red blood cells (RBC) mixed with strands of fibrin (F) lying above and beneath the loosely arranged keratinized cells (K). ×1,510.*

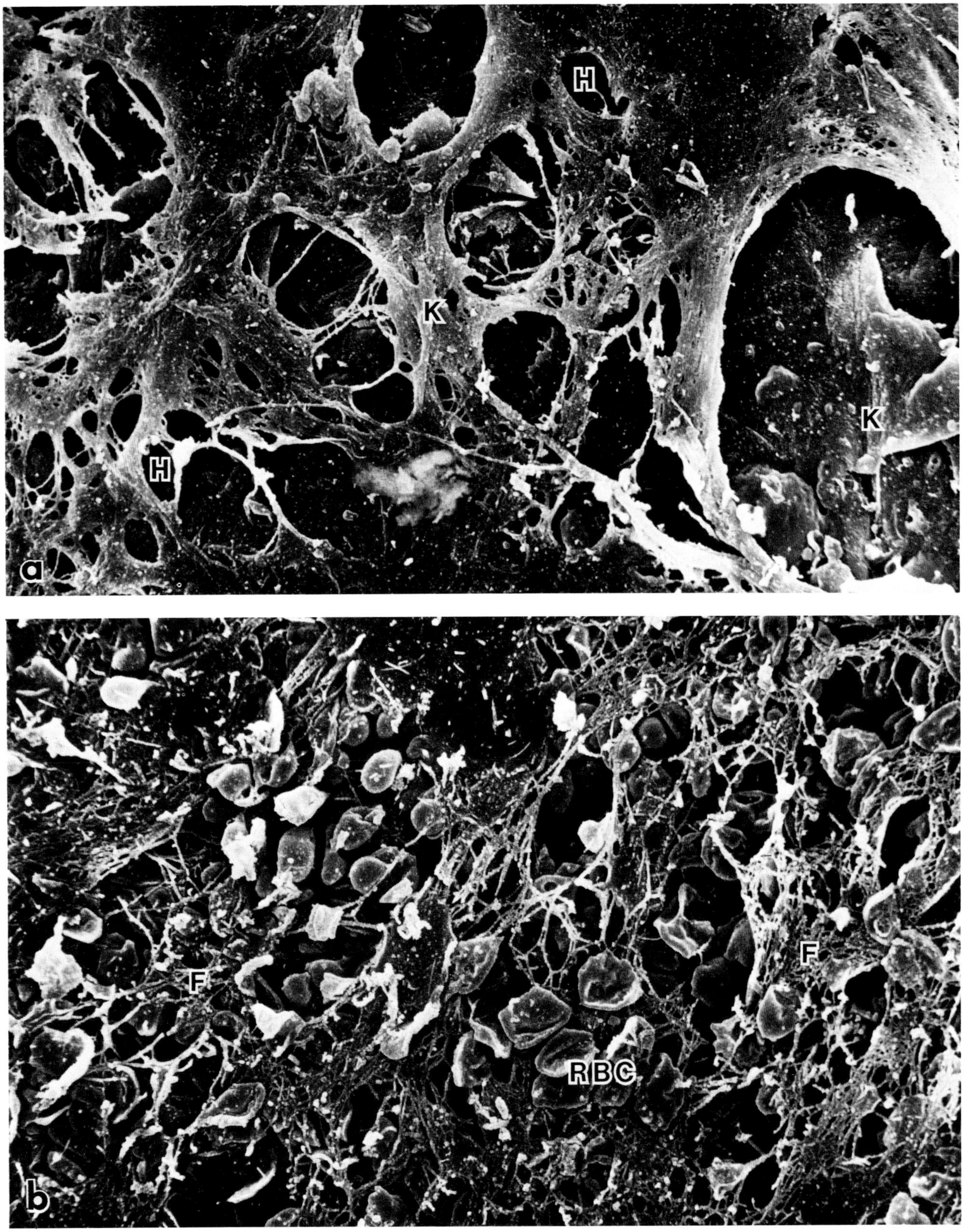

Figure 5–2. a. *Some keratinized cells (K) of the psoriatic plaque are extremely thin. Such squames appear to anastomose because they lack the distinct cell boundaries characteristic of scales that are formed during the normal keratinization process. Holes (H) of various sizes perforate the abnormal scales. ×1,530.*

b. *A psoriatic excoriation containing red blood cells (RBC) and fibrin (F) covers the surface of the scales. The source of the blood is from leaky blood vessels located in the connective tissue papillae that deeply indent the epidermis. ×2,485.*

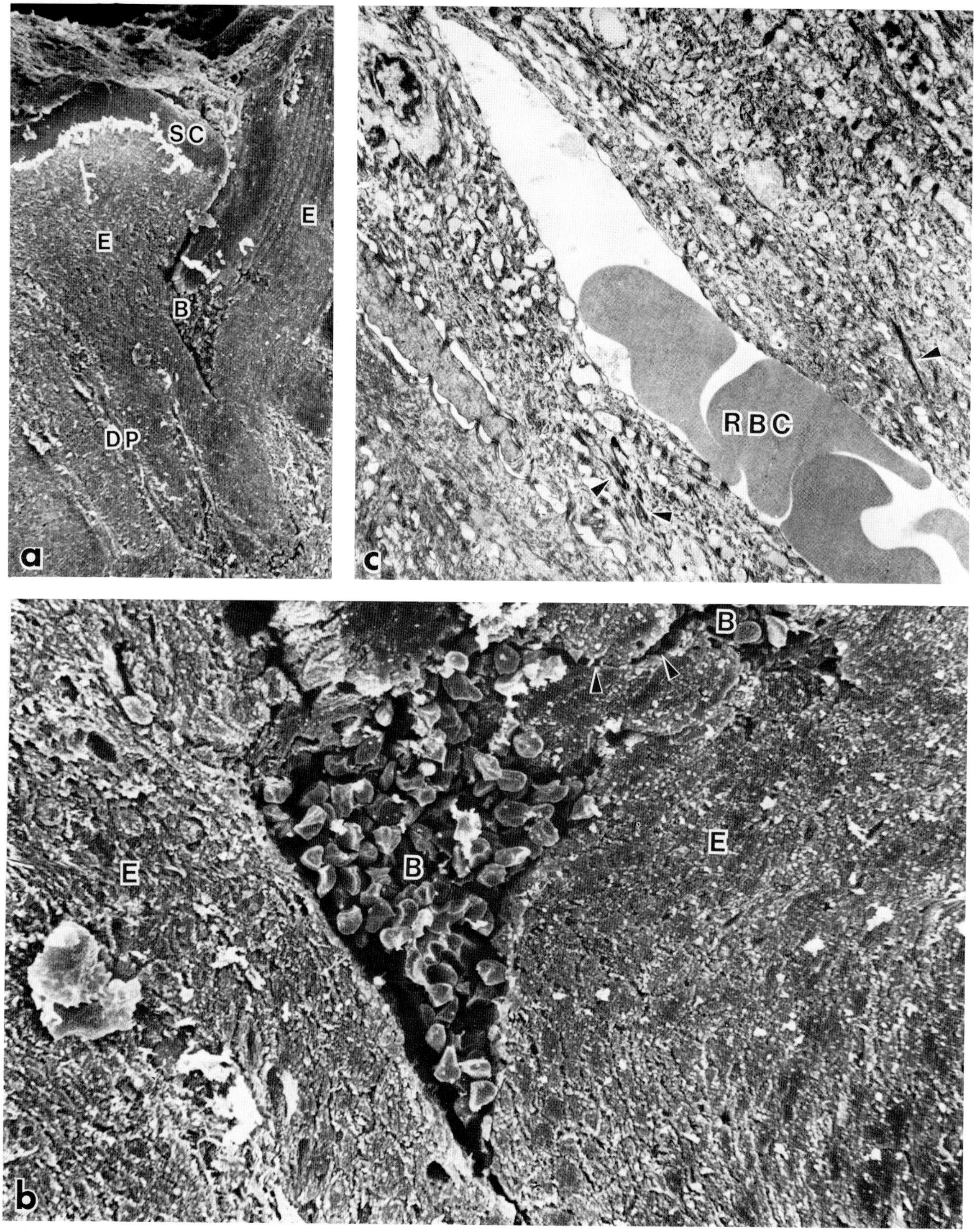

Figure 5–3. a. *Lakes of blood (B) from leaky blood vessels have formed in epidermal recesses beneath the stratum corneum (SC) of the psoriatic lesion. The acanthotic epidermis (E) is indented by tall connective tissue papillae (DP).* ×235.

b. *Higher magnification of a blood lake (B) in the thickened epidermis (E). Small channels (arrows) between the epidermal cells interconnect multiple lakes of blood.* ×1,185.

c. *A channel that courses between keratinocytes is illustrated by TEM. The channel contains red blood cells (RBC) but is not lined by endothelium. Keratinocytes in which the tonofilaments and tonofibrils (arrows) are reduced in number are characteristic of psoriatic skin.* ×5,755.

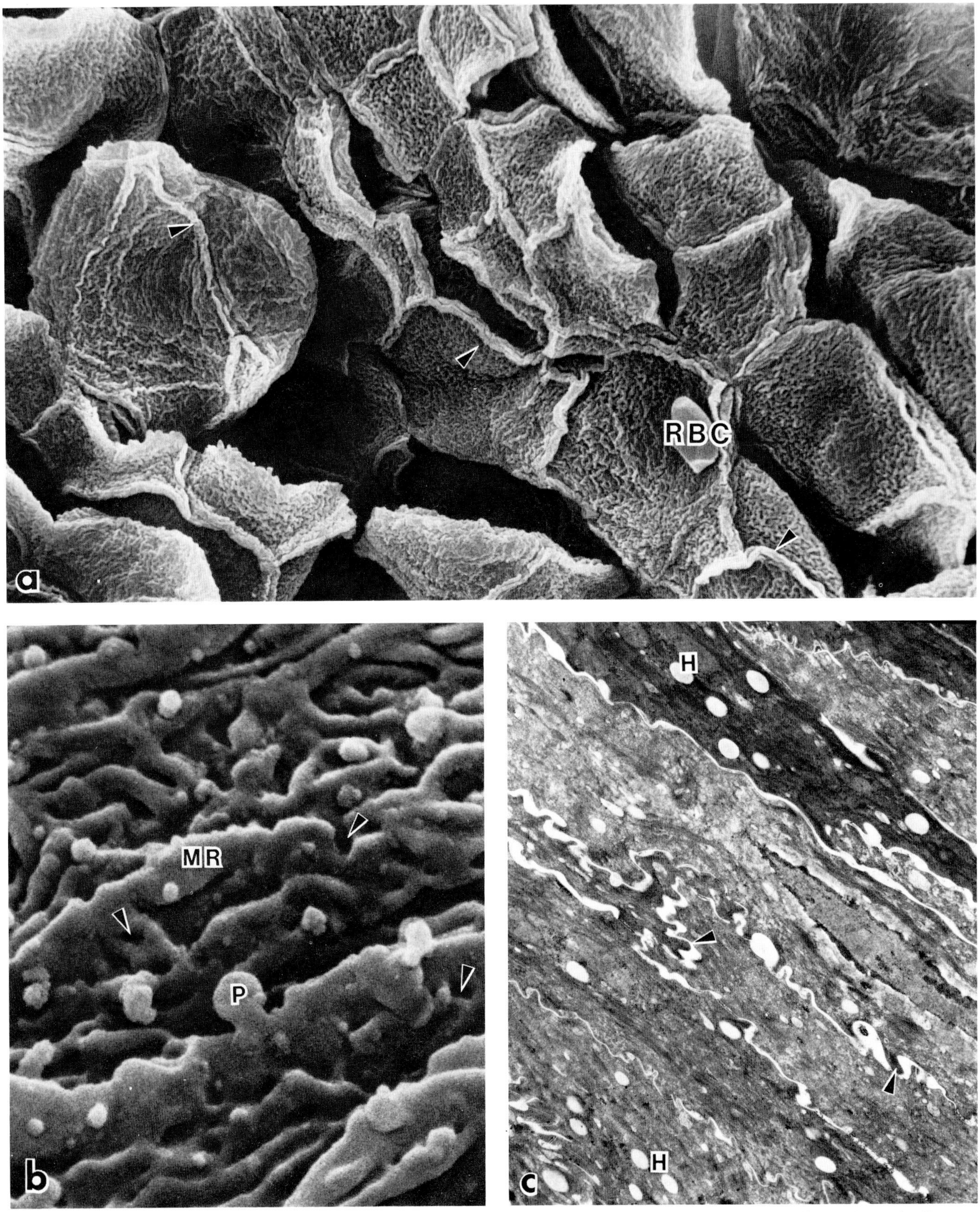

Figure 5–4. a. Newly formed keratinized cells (K) of psoriatic lesions have a "spongy" appearance. The free edges of adjacent squames form prominent ridges (arrows) where they overlap. Small microridges and microgrooves occupy the free surface of the scales between the overlapping cell borders. The remains of a red blood cell (RBC) is present near the cell border of one squame. ×3,460.

b. When viewed at high magnification, the microridges of psoriatic scales show knob-like protuberances (P). Similar protuberances were observed on fetal scales and scales of certain tumors. Some microridges (MR) contain pits (arrows) which are smaller than the microgrooves. ×15,200.

c. Psoriatic scales appear to contain holes (H) in ultrathin sections viewed by TEM. Correlative observations by SEM show that the holes correspond to pits in the microridges. The larger processes (arrows) of the scales represent the projections that were observed by SEM. ×13,490.

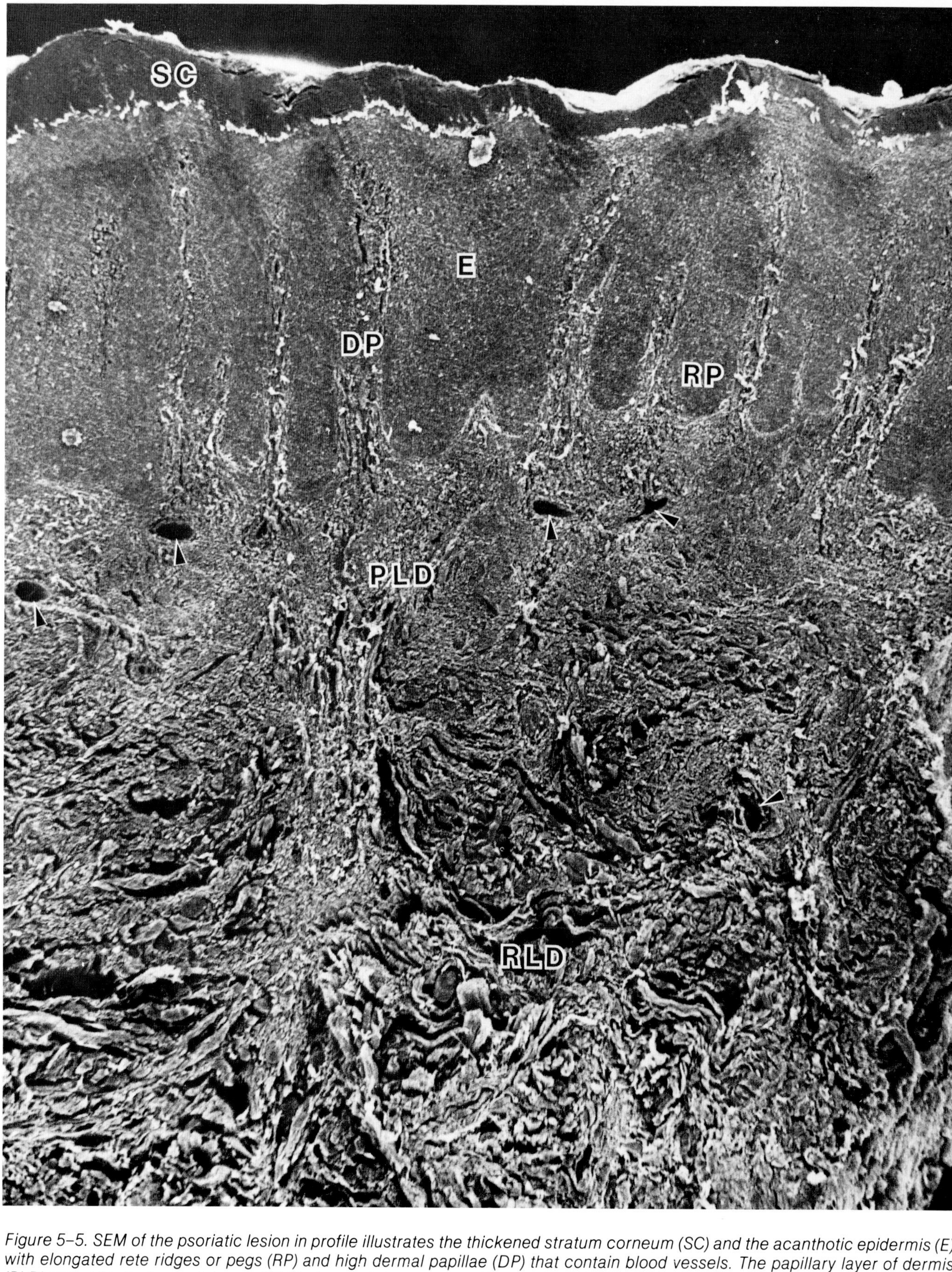

Figure 5–5. SEM of the psoriatic lesion in profile illustrates the thickened stratum corneum (SC) and the acanthotic epidermis (E) with elongated rete ridges or pegs (RP) and high dermal papillae (DP) that contain blood vessels. The papillary layer of dermis (PLD) and reticular layer of dermis (RLD) also contain numerous blood vessels (arrows) located between the bundles of collagen. × 140.

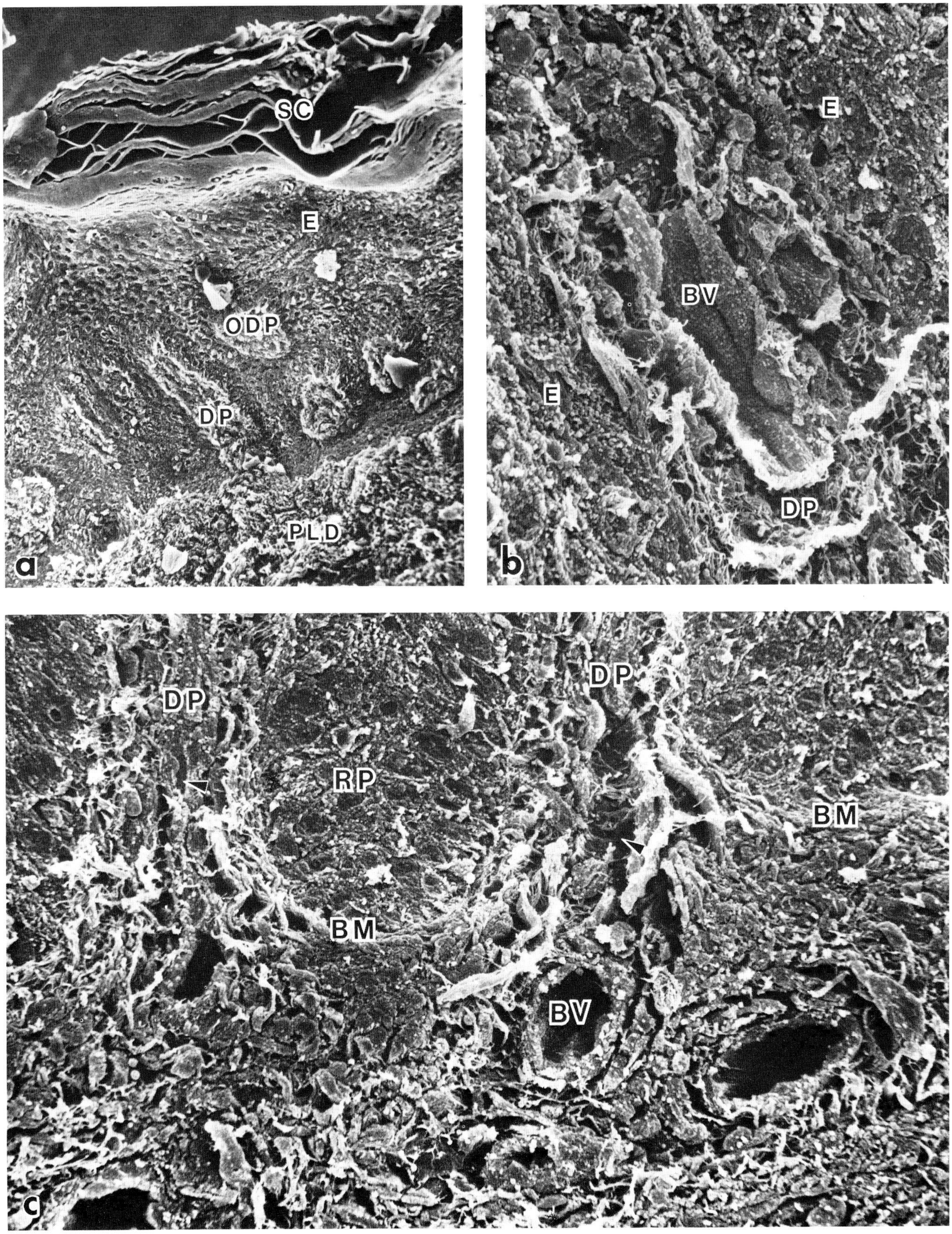

Figure 5–6. a. The central portion of a psoriatic lesion has a thick stratum corneum (SC) with spaces between the lamellae of scales. Extravascular blood tends to accumulate in the spaces. Dermal papillae in oblique section (ODP) seem confined to the epidermis (E), but serial longitudinal sections show that each dermal papilla (DP) connects with the papillary layer of the dermis (PLD). ×180.

b. Higher magnification of a dermal papilla (DP) reveals a blood vessel (BV) close to the epidermis (E). The vessel lumen is lined by elongated endothelial cells. ×1,620.

c. Portions of three epidermal ridges or rete pegs (RP) and two dermal papillae (DP) are shown. A basement membrane (BM) separates the epidermis and dermis. Branches (arrows) from several blood vessels (BV) extend into the highly vascular and cavernous papillae. ×2,375.

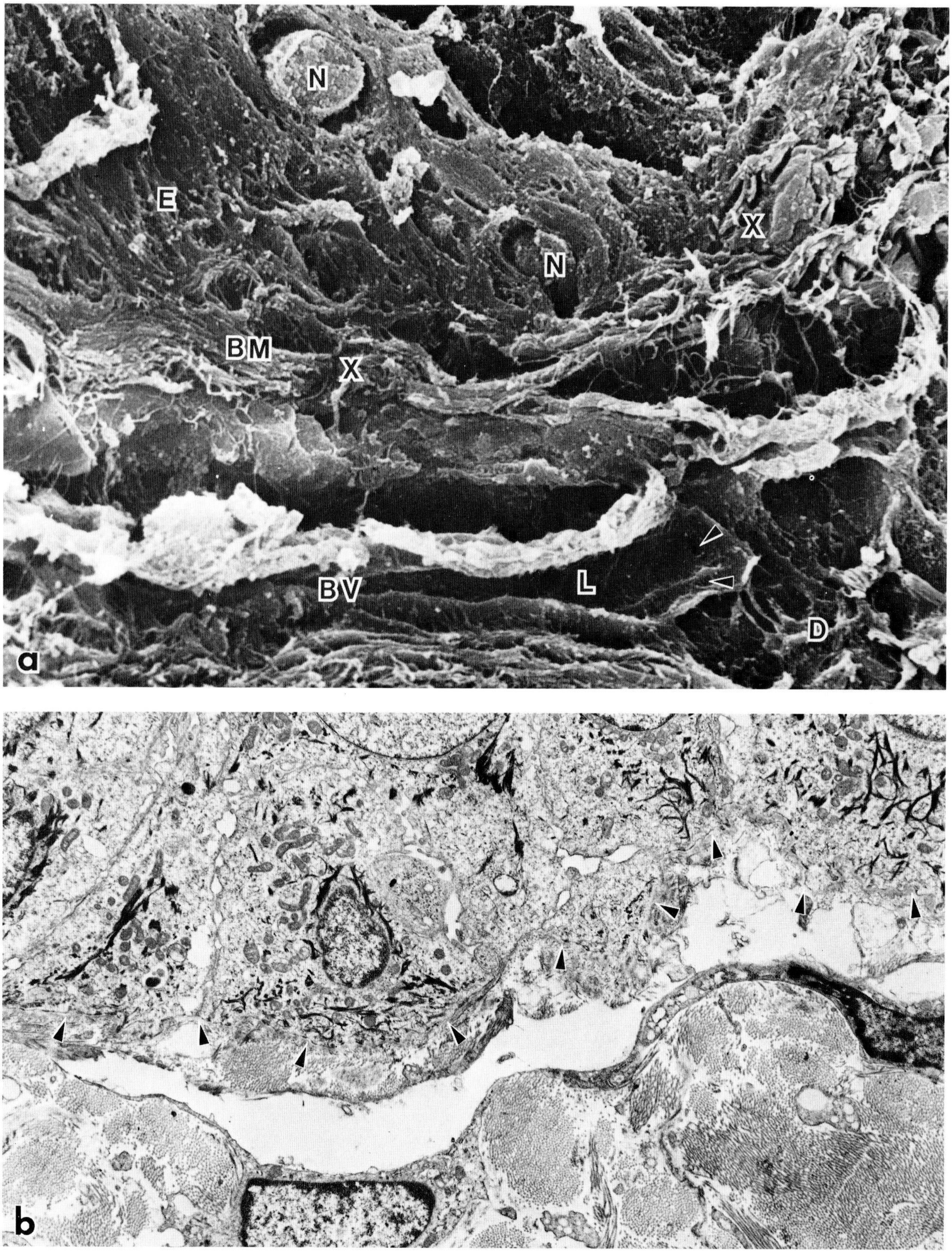

Figure 5–7. a. *A blood vessel (BV) in longitudinal section lies between the epidermis (E) and dermis (D). Nuclei (N) are visible in some keratinocytes. The basement membrane (BM) at some sites may be thin, discontinuous or porous (X), thereby altering the barrier between the epidermis and dermis. Holes (arrows) and gaps are present in the endothelial cells that surround the vessel lumen (L). The importance of discontinuities of the basement membrane and endothelium is that they permit the cellular and non-cellular components of blood to pass into the epidermis where they may have a stimulatory effect on epidermal mitotic activity.* ×3,105.

b. *For correlation with SEM, the dermal-epidermal junction is illustrated by TEM. The basement membrane (arrows) is extremely thin at some sites and is absent at a few sites.* ×5,850.

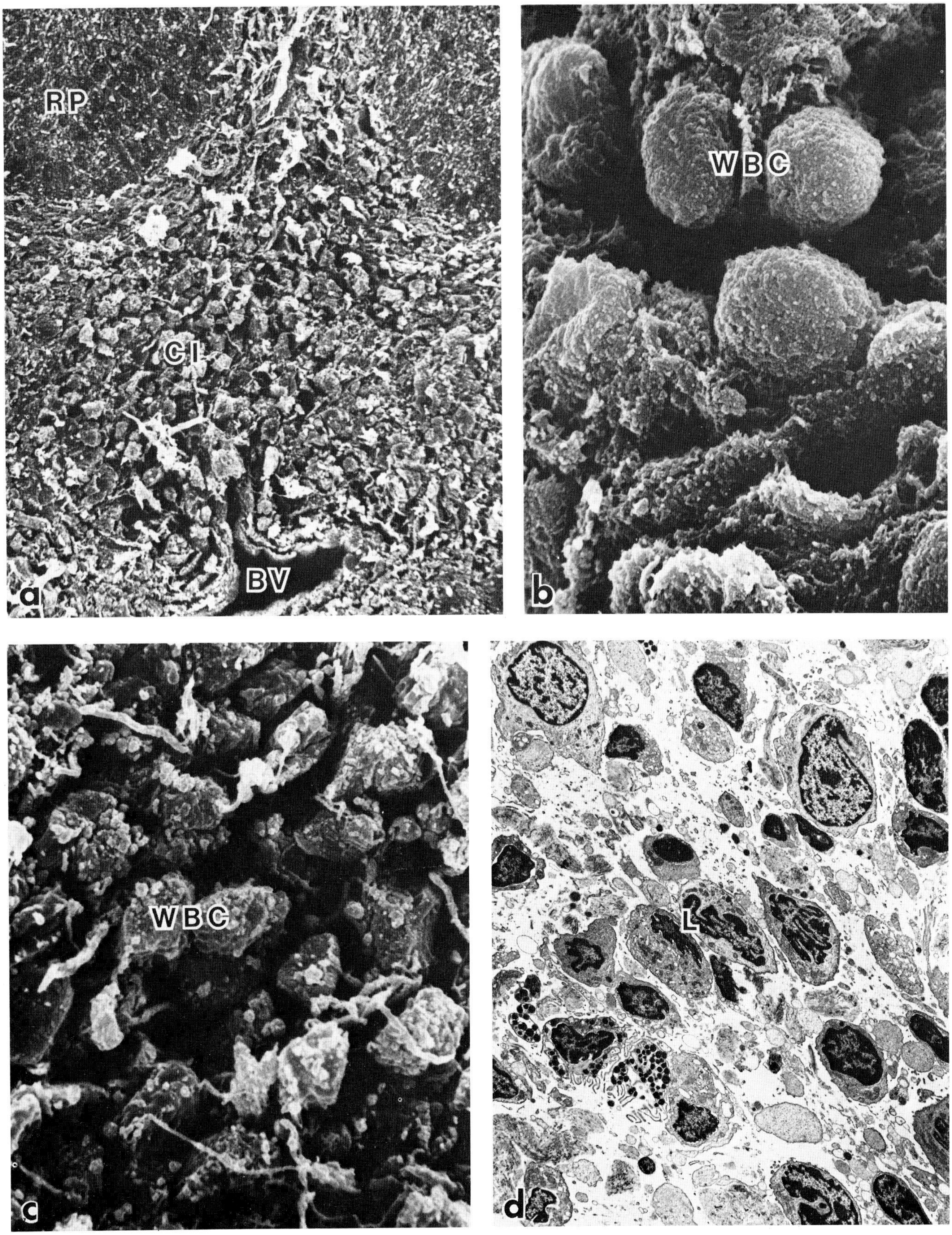

Figure 5–8. a. *The dermis below the rete ridges or pegs (RP) is heavily infiltrated with cells (CI = cellular infiltrate) that have migrated from the dilated blood vessel (BV). × 725.*

b. *Several leukocytes (WBC) from the blood are within a channel of the epidermis. They eventually form Munro-Sabouraud abscesses in the stratum corneum. × 4,425.*

c. *An accumulation of leukocytes (WBC) in a Munro-Sabouraud abscess. × 3,905.*

d. *Correlative TEM of the same psoriatic lesion depicted by SEM shows a rich dermal infiltrate of blood cells composed predominately of lymphocytes (L) × 2,650.*

SEBORRHEIC KERATOSIS 6

Seborrheic keratosis is perhaps the most common tumor of adult skin and is inherited as an autosomal dominant trait. The lesion is sometimes designated by other names, such as seborrheic wart, basal cell papilloma, and senile wart. The tumor has been called the prototype of benign neoplasms. Changes in the skin associated with aging, irritation, or infection may trigger the development of these tumors, and they usually occur in persons aged 40 or older. Tumors are not more labile to malignant changes than is the normal skin adjacent to them.

Lesions are usually multiple, light to dark brown in color, and range in size from several millimeters to several centimeters. They may be flat or rise a variable distance above the level of the normal skin. The lesion's surface may appear smooth, rough, truly verrucous, or even pedunculated. Common sites include the chest, interscapular region, waistline, and face, but the lesion may develop anywhere on the skin with the exception of the palms and soles. Histologically, the tumor contains horn cysts and is often hyperkeratotic, papillomatous, acanthotic, and pigmented.

Most frequently seborrheic keratosis is an asymptomatic growth, but it can become inflamed and cause itching or minor burning. Some believe the inflammation results from bacterial proliferation in the keratinous crypts which are prominent in the more verrucous lesions. Despite the tumor's benign nature, cases have been reported where a basal cell carcinoma has developed in a lesion of seborrheic keratosis. It remains to be demonstrated if such cases represent a malignant transformation of seborrheic keratosis or the confluence of two different adjoining tumors.

Clinical diagnosis of seborrheic keratosis can be accurately made in most instances and the tumor can be removed by a mildly destructive method, such as cryosurgery, fulguration, or topical application of trichloracetic acid. Proper use of these methods leads to complete eradication without major cosmetic defects. In those instances where clinical diagnosis is in doubt, complete surgical excision and histopatholigical examination are required to rule out the malignancies that may mimic seborrheic keratosis, including malignant melanoma, pigmented basal cell carcinoma, lentigo maligna, and melanotic freckle.

The material from which the following micrographs were made consisted of 15 non-irritated seborrheic keratoses removed from 6 male and 9 female Caucasian patients who ranged in age from 40–77 years. Part of each lesion was processed for LM, TEM, and SEM. Each lesion was diagnosed histologically as a definitive seborrheic keratosis.

Horn cysts arose from vellus hair follicles and from keratinocytes that had detached and aggregated within the epidermis. Both methods of horn cyst formation occurred in each lesion with the follicular type outnumbering the extrafollicular type about 7:1. Hyperkeratinization of the free surface was attributed to abnormal scales with pores which branched and interlocked so extensively that the process of desquamation was slowed. Yeasts and bacteria were especially abundant on the free surfaces and in the crevices of some of these common warty growths.

References

Braun-Falco, O., A. Kint, and W. Vogell. Zur Histogenese der Verruca seborrhoica. II. Elektronenmikroskopische Befunde. Arch. klin. exp. Dermatol. 217: 627–651, 1963.

Lachapelle, J. M. Isotopic labelling of cutaneous structures. Br. J. Derm. 81: 299–305, 1969.

Sanderson, K. V. Dynamic aspects of wartiness. Trans. St. John's Hospital Dermatological Soc. 55: 127–140. 1969.

Sanderson, K. V. Tumors of the Skin. *In: Textbook of Dermatology.* A. Rook. D. S. Williamson, and F. J. G. Ebling (eds.), 2nd edition, Oxford, Blackwell Scientific Publications, London, 1972, p. 1911–2007.

Wilborn, W. H., S. G. Carrington, and L. F. Montes. A tridimensional view of seborrheic keratosis. SEM/1980/III, SEM Inc., AMF, O'Hare, IL 60666, p. 485–494.

Wilborn, W. H., D. E. Dismukes, and L. F. Montes, Ultrastructural identification of Langerhans cells in seborrheic keratosis. J. Cut. Path. 5: 368–372, 1978.

Wilborn, W. H., and L. F. Montes. Scanning electron microscopy of yeasts in seborrheic keratoses. J. Cut. Path. 7: 1–7, 1980.

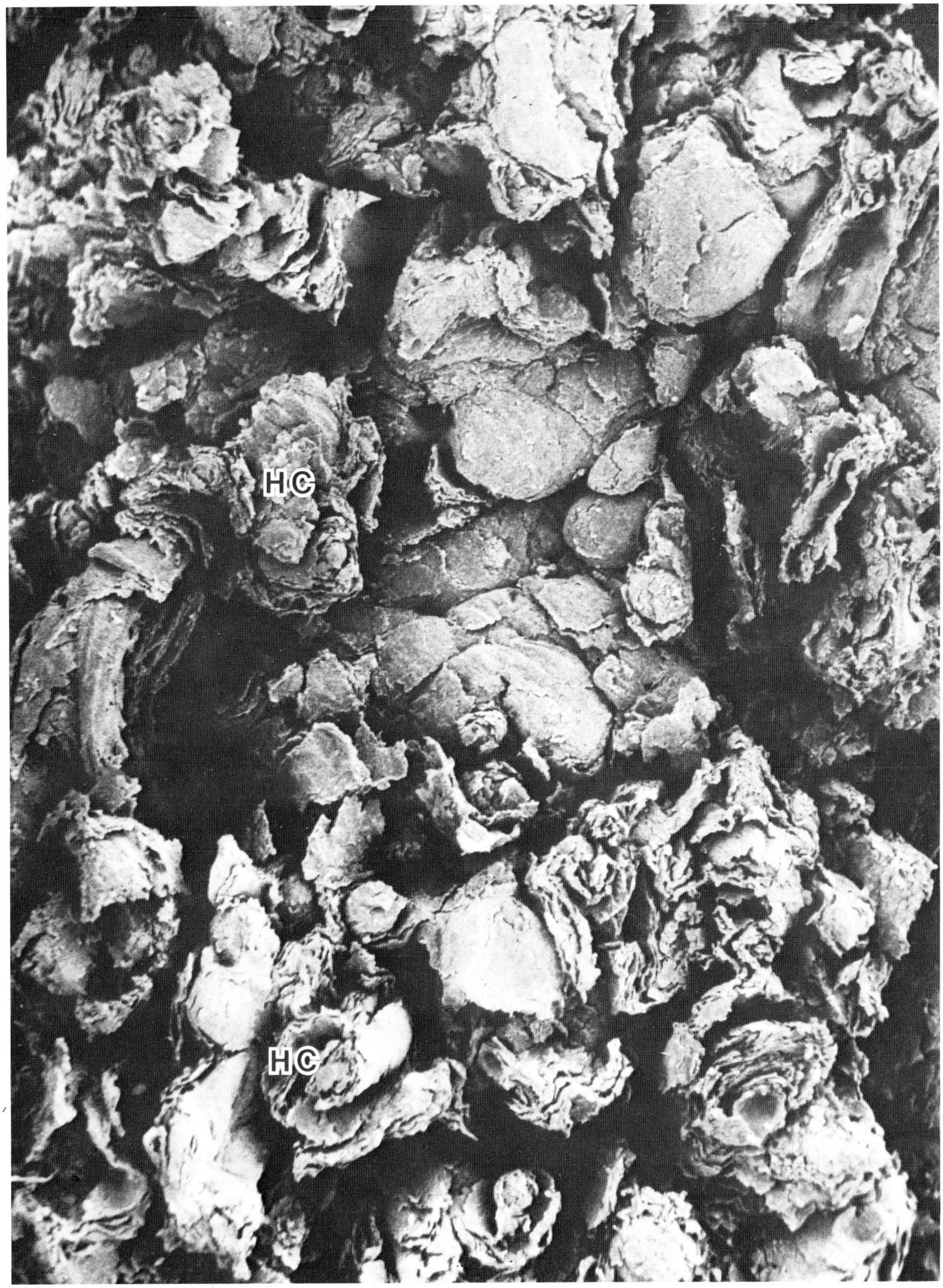

Figure 6–1. The free surface of the lesion viewed at low magnification appears highly irregular and contains numerous horn cysts (HC). A typical horn cyst is composed of several layers of scales arranged in a lamellar pattern and has a "cabbage-like" appearance. Horn cysts detach easily and some of the deep pits represent sites they formerly occupied. ×55.

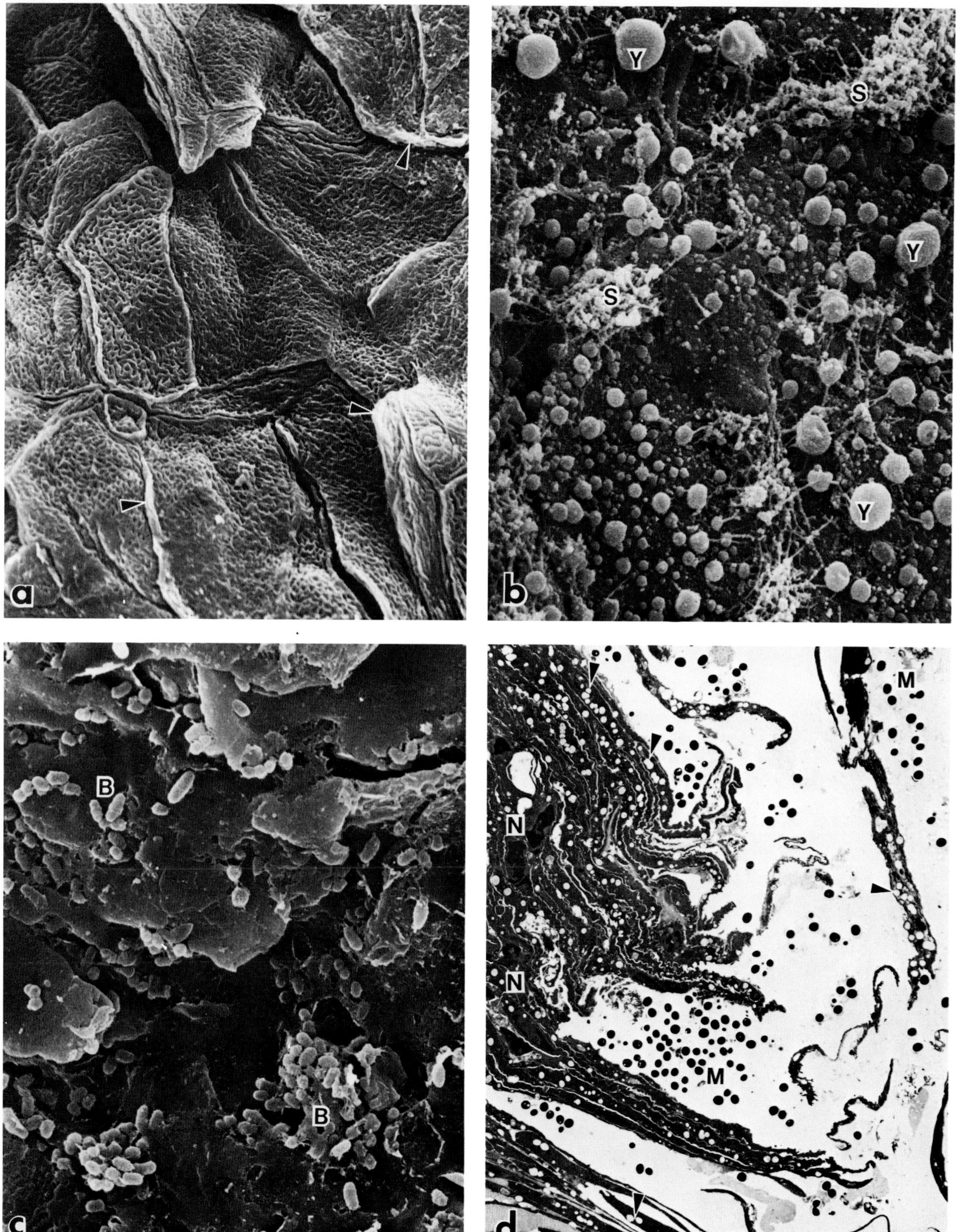
a
Y
S
S
Y
Y
b
B
B
c
M
N
N
M
d

Figure 6–2 a. *Scales of the stratum corneum may have pronounced microridges and microgrooves that occupy their entire surface except their slightly elevated free borders (arrows). Scales of some horn cysts have similar microridges and microgrooves. Such surface patterns are associated with growing lesions and indicate incomplete keratinization typical of mucous membranes of stratified squamous epithelia.* ×*2,600.*

b. *Yeasts (Y) in close association with strands and droplets of sebum (S) are shown on the free surface of a lesion. It is not unusual to find yeasts in crevices and at the free surface. Irritation caused by yeasts often leads to scratching the lesion and further irritation.* ×*4,800.*

c. *Bacteria (B), resembling* P. acnes, *are especially numerous among the scales and sebum droplets of some lesions. They may occur singly or in microcolonies.* ×*3,900.*

d. *Correlative TEM shows an abundance of microorganisms (M) in the spaces between squames at the free surface of the lesion. Scales may contain parakeratotic nuclei (N) and holes (arrows).* ×*1,950.*

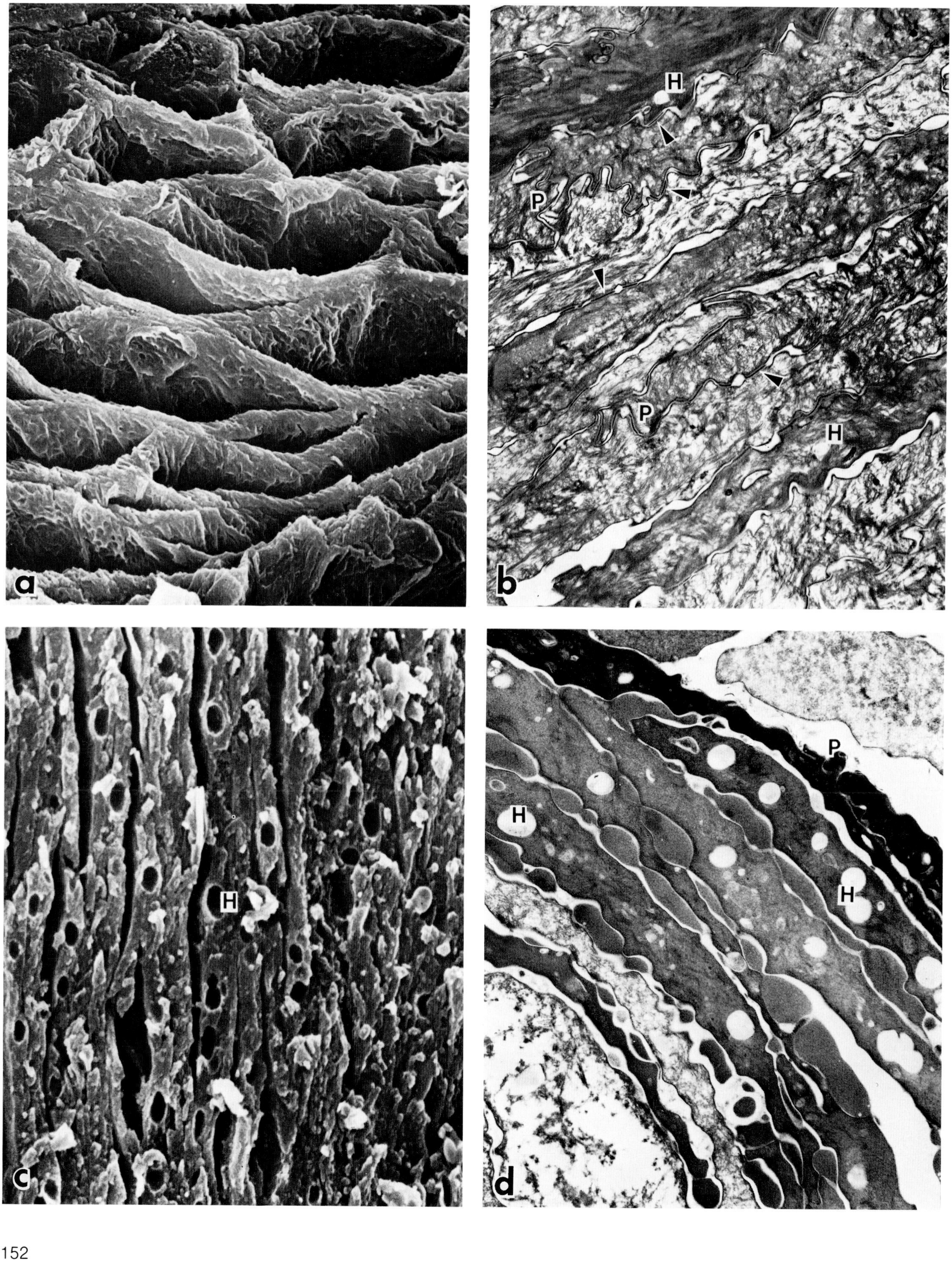
a
b
H
P
P
H
c
H
d
H
H
P

Figure 6–3. a. *Scales of the stratum corneum are shown in profile to illustrate that they branch and appear to anastomose extensively with each other.* × *2,080.*

b. *By TEM, profiles of scales of the stratum corneum have interdigitating processes (P), holes (H), and numerous dense, intercellular plaques (arrows). The plaques represent desmosomes that have not degenerated completely. Many scales in lesions of seborrheic keratosis lack the closely-packed, parallel arrangement of tonofilaments that characterize normal scales. This suggests that the normal process of keratinization is altered to some degree in seborrheic keratosis.* × *13,510.*

c. *Closely packed lamellae of scales at the periphery of a horn cyst branch and contain holes (H) as do scales of the stratum corneum depicted in a.* × *7,800.*

d. *Holes (H) in scales from the central portion of a horn cyst are illustrated by TEM. These scales are older than those at the periphery of the lesion. The fact that they have fewer processes (P) and desmosomes than the younger, peripheral scales may account for the tendency of the central, superficial portion of a horn cyst to be lost when lesions are removed and processed for microscopic study.* × *11,900.*

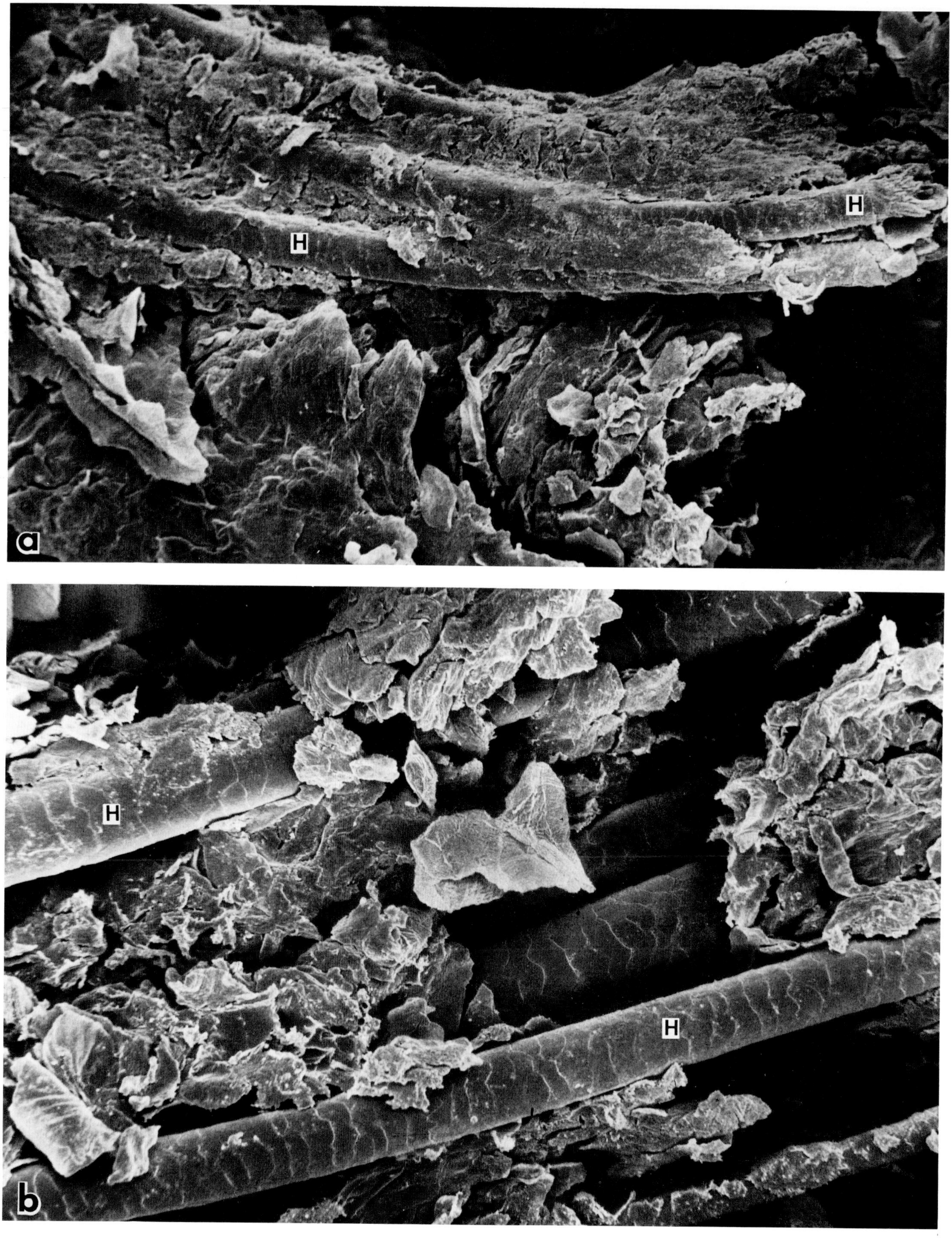

Figure 6–4. a. *Small hairs (H), 8–25 μm in diameter, are partially hidden by an encrustation on scales at the free surface of a lesion. Similar hairs can be found embedded in the scales of most horn cysts.* ×*390.*

b. *At higher magnification, the vellus hairs (H) embedded in the lesion show normal cuticles consisting of a single layer of overlapping cells.* ×*780.*

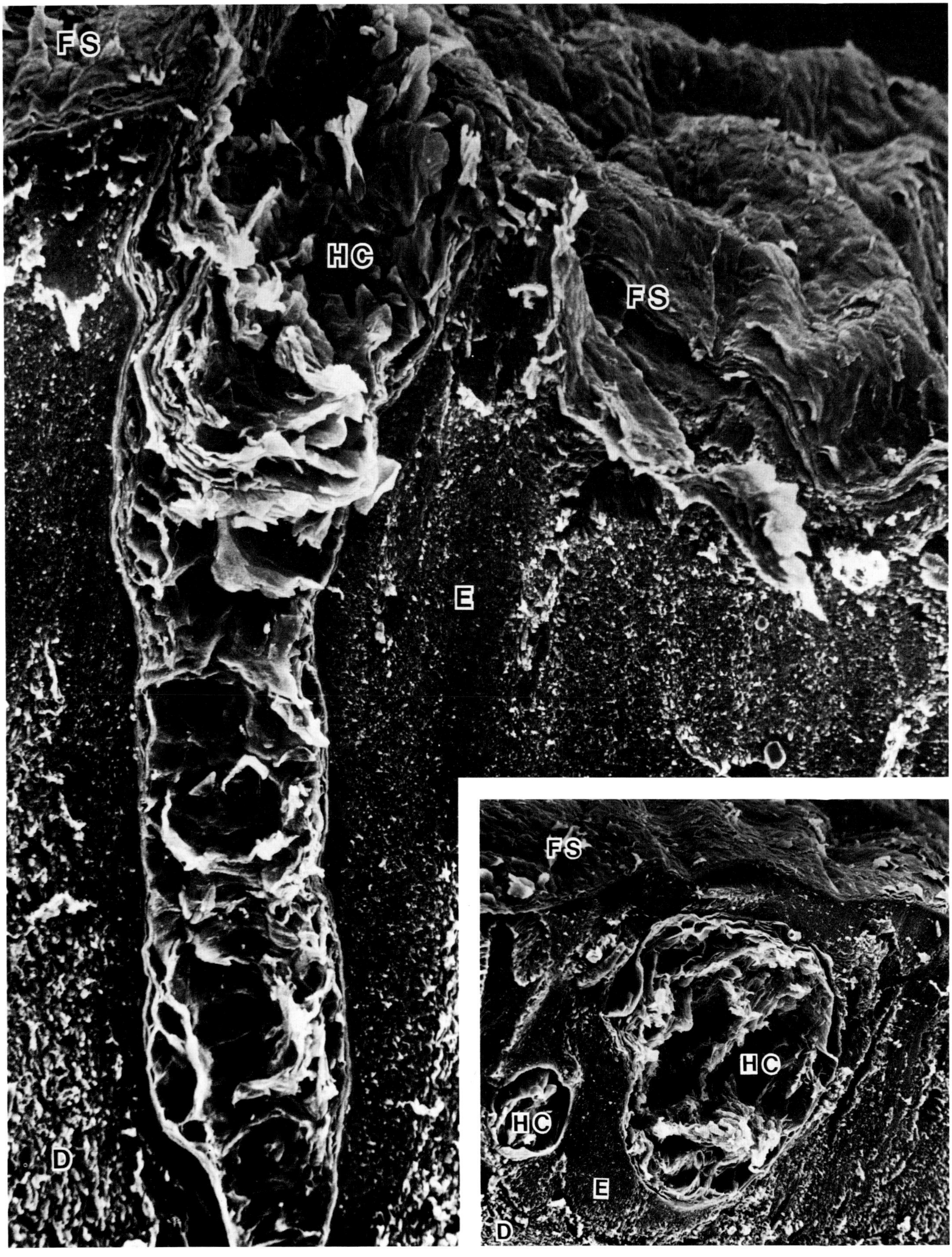

Figure 6–5. A horn cyst (HC) in longitudinal section occupies a hair follicle and extends from deep in the dermis (D) to the free surface (FS). The hair, because of its wiry texture, was probably lost from the follicle during sectioning. E, epidermis. ×285.

The inset shows one large and one small horn cyst (HC) in cross section. D, dermis; E, epidermis; FS, free surface. ×145.

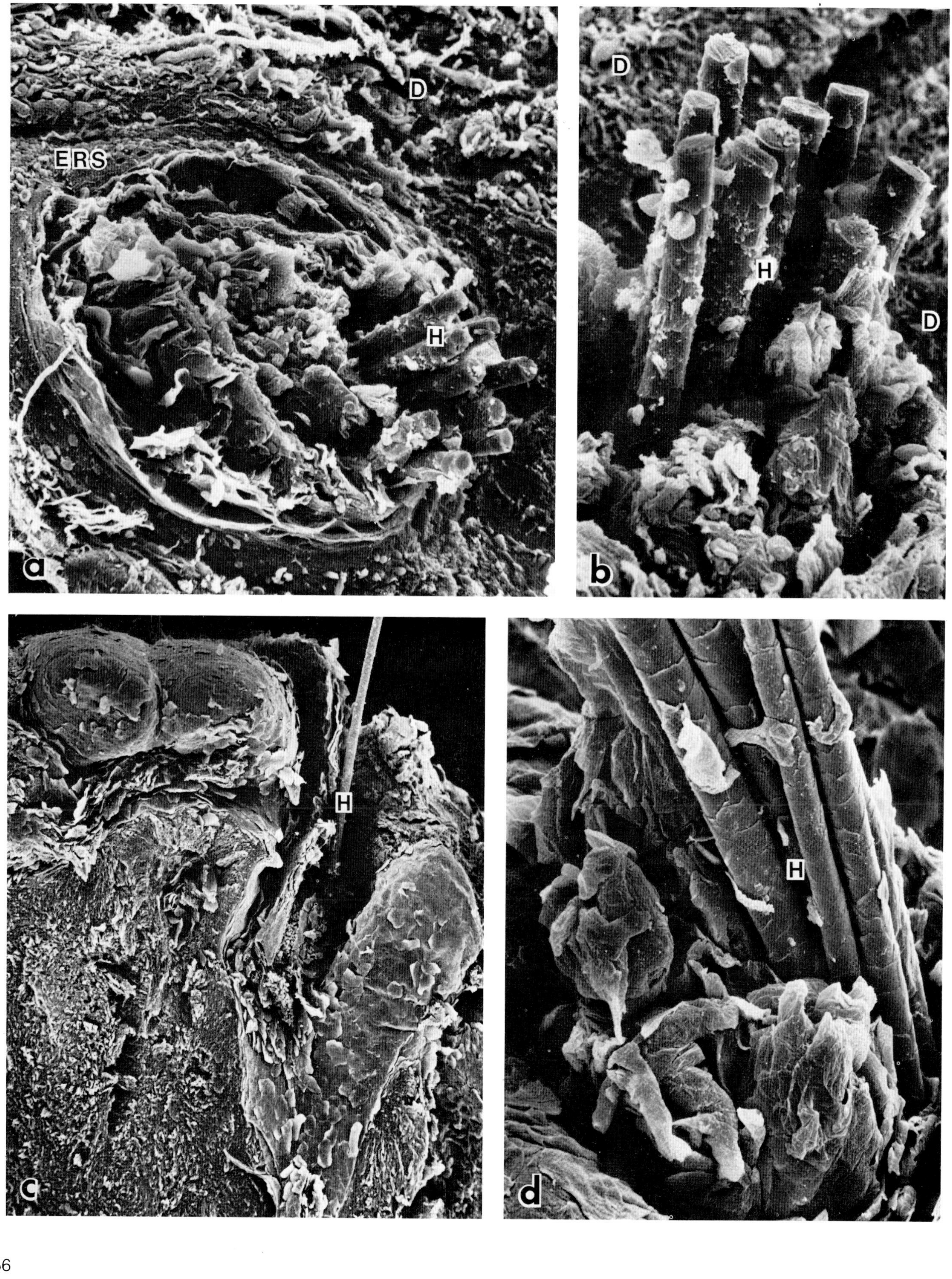

ERS
D
H
a
D
H
D
b
H
c
H
d

Figure 6–6 a. *Several small hairs (H) and loose scales are within a hair follicle of the dermis (D). The epithelial root sheath (ERS) is thickened and the follicular lumen is dilated. The follicle is a developing horn cyst.* ×*390.*

b. *A cluster of vellus hairs (H) is within a dermal follicle. Such hairs are apt to be dislodged when histological sections are prepared. The loose cells in the follicular orifice came from the epithelial root sheath.* ×*730.*

c. *A lesion in profile reveals a hyperkeratotic free surface with a hair (H) in the cavity of a horn cyst.* ×*215.*

d. *A tuft of hairs (H) extends from the center of a small horn cyst to the free surface of the lesion.* ×*780.*

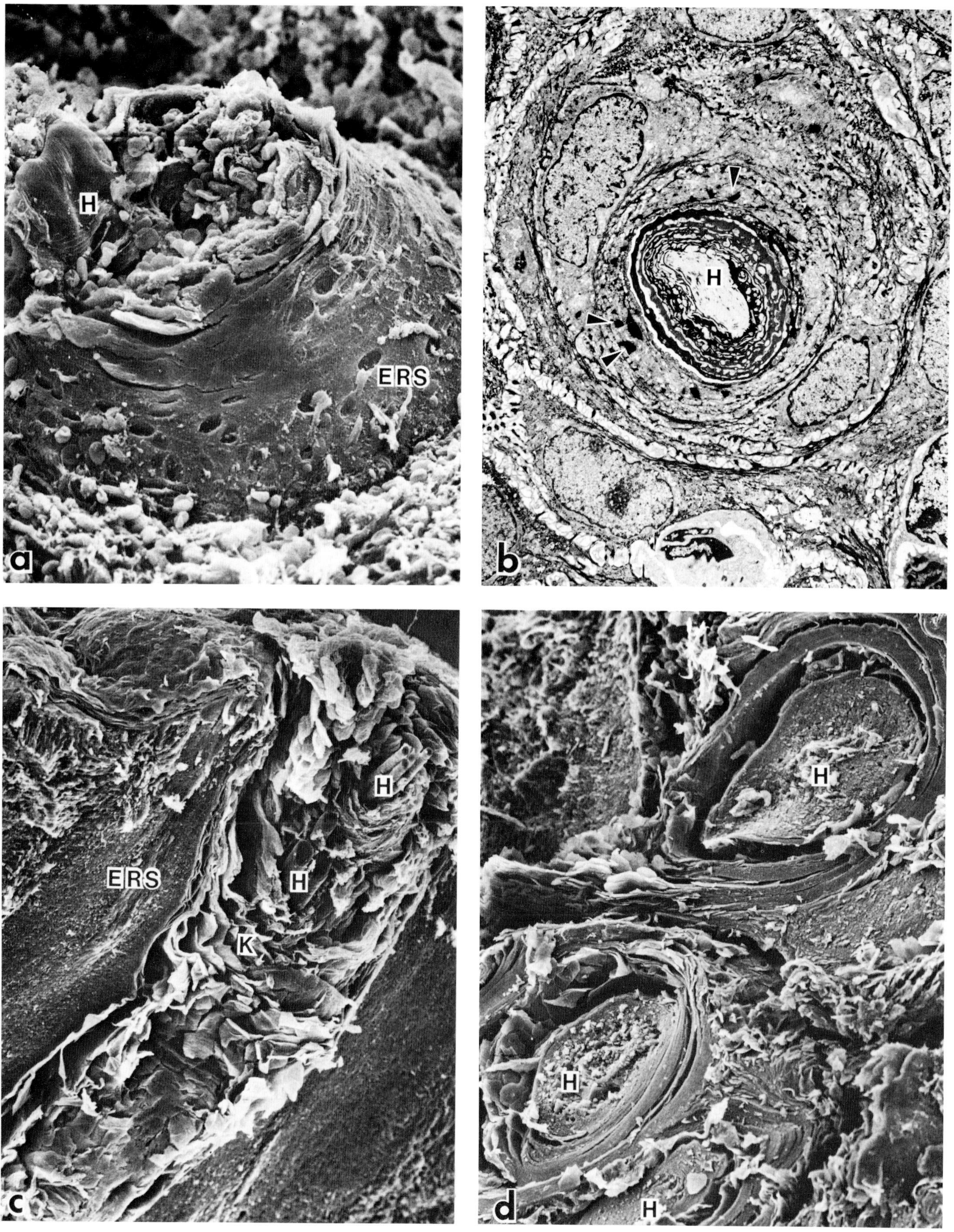
a
H
ERS
b
H
c
H
ERS
H
K
d
H
H
H

Figure 6–7. Follicular origin of horn cysts.

a. *The formation of a follicular horn cyst is initiated in the dermis. Loose cells accumulate in the follicular cavity between the hair (H) and the thick epithelial root sheath (ERS).* $\times 520$.

b. *An early stage in the histogenesis of a follicular horn cyst in the epidermis is shown by TEM. Epidermal cells with giant trichohyaline granules (arrows) surround the small hair (H).* $\times 2{,}470$.

c. *The horn cyst contains two groups of multiple hairs (H) that are enclosed by lamellae of keratinized cells (K). The cyst extends from deep in the dermis to the free surface. ERS, epithelial root sheath.* $\times 255$.

d. *The interior of a horn cyst is shown at the level of the stratum corneum. Hairs (H), surrounded by lamellae of scales, are identifiable in the keratinous mass.* $\times 155$.

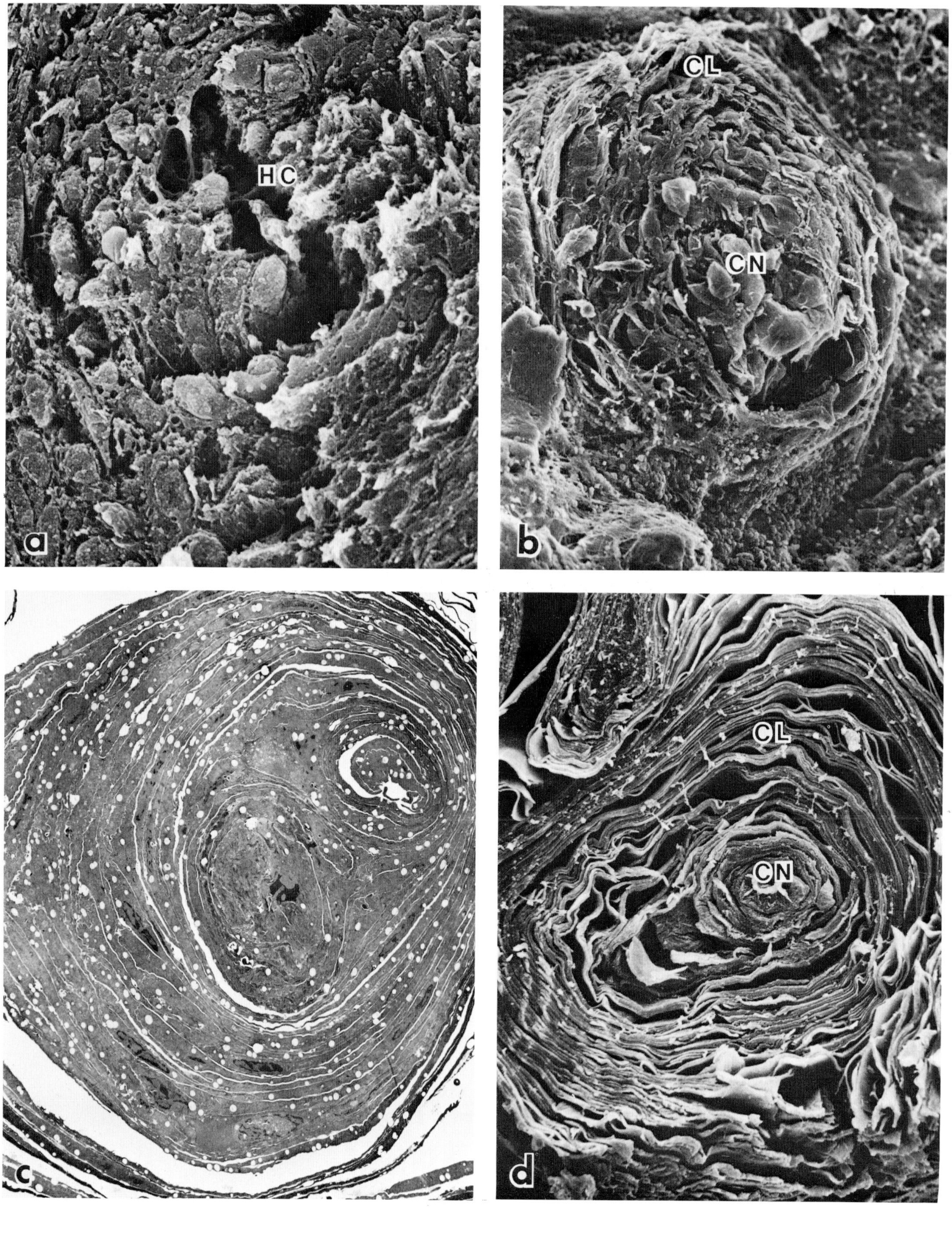
HC
a
CL
CN
b
c
CL
CN
d

Figure 6–8. Extrafollicular origin of horn cysts.

a. *The development of an extrafollicular horn cyst (HC) begins in the lower epidermis when keratinocytes detach from each other, as shown in the center of the micrograph. ×390.*

b. *At a later stage in the development of a horn cyst, detached cells aggregate into a central nidus (CN) which serves as the hub of the lesion while concentric lamellae (CL) of cells are added peripherally. ×210.*

c. *TEM depicts the holes in the central nidus of cells of a developing horn cyst, an indication that the keratinization process is abnormal. ×2,470.*

d. *Loose scales have been removed in this cross section of a mature extrafollicular horn cyst within the stratum corneum to show the central nidus (CN) and concentric lamellae (CL) of scales. ×780.*

CAPILLARY HEMANGIOMA 7

Hemangiomas are benign vascular tumors of the skin formed by excessive proliferation of cutaneous blood vessels. These tumors may be present at birth or they may appear later in life. Hemangiomas range in size from small, localized lesions to very large lesions that involve extensive areas of the skin, or even an internal organ with the impairment of a body function.

There is no general agreement as to how vascular tumors of the skin should be classified. Four types of hemangiomas are often listed as the most common and important: cavernous hemangioma, nevus flammeus, senile hemangioma, and capillary hemangioma.

The *cavernous hemangioma* is formed by large irregular spaces filled with blood. The spaces are limited by a thin endothelium and surrounded by thin or thick fibrous walls. The vascular spaces are deep in the dermis or in the subcutaneous tissue.

The *nevus flammeus* (port-wine nevus or nevus telanglectaticus) consists of greatly dilated spaces that are lined by endothelium and filled with blood. This type of hemangioma involves the upper dermis.

Senile hemangiomas (cherry angiomas, ruby spots, or De Morgan spots) develop in most people who are beyond 30 years of age. Lesions may occur anywhere on the skin and sometimes in large numbers. The upper trunk is the most common site. The young lesion contains numerous capillaries with narrow lumina and large endothelial cells. The mature lesion is composed of moderately dilated capillaries with flat endothelium.

Capillary hemangiomas (strawberry marks) are soft, reddish tumors formed by numerous capillaries. The endothelial cells proliferate during growth of the young lesion. The capillary hemangioma may undergo fibrosis and involution. Dilated capillaries, lined by flattened endothelial cells that rest on a thin connective tissue layer, are present in older lesions.

The capillary hemangioma was selected to illustrate a vascular tumor of the skin. Five capillary hemangiomas were removed from 4 young adult females and from one 39 year old female. Lesions were completely excised, including the margin of uninvolved skin with dermis and subcutaneous tissue. Gross and histological features of a typical lesion are shown in Figure 7–1.

The middle and deep layers of the dermis were nearly filled with non-fenestrated capillaries. SEM provided new information on the cells that lined the capillary walls. The endothelial cells manifest an unusually large number of microplicae and vesicles. These features indicate that the vessels in the hemangioma have a much higher metabolic activity and absorptive rate than normal cutaneous vessels.

References

Geschickter, C. F., and L. E. Keasbey. Tumors of blood vessels. Am. J. Cancer 23: 568–591, 1935.

Hoepfel-Kreiner, I. Histogenesis of hemangiomas — An ultrastructural study on capillary and cavernous hemangiomas. Path. Res. Pract. 170: 70–90, 1980.

Kojimahara, M., K. Yamazaki, and G. Ooneda. Ultrastructural study of hemangiomas. I. Capillary hemangioma of the skin. Acta Pathol. Jpn. 31: 105–115, 1981.

Walsh, T. S., Jr., and V. N. Tompkins. Some observations on the strawberry nevus of infancy. Cancer 9: 869–874, 1956.

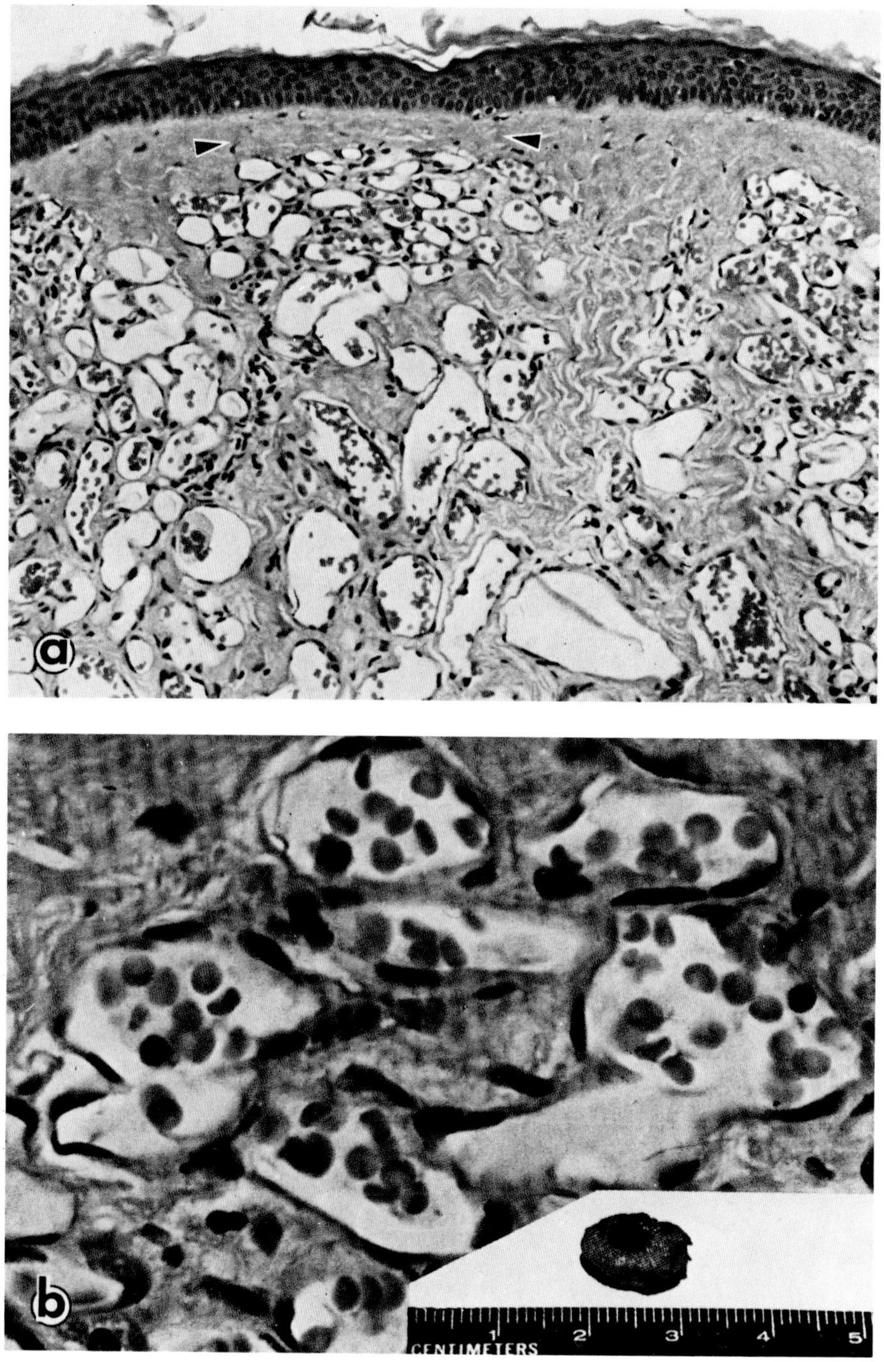

Figure 7–1. Inset *in* b *depicts a capillary hemangioma measuring approximately 5 mm in diameter. The skin surrounding the tumor is also shown. Histologically, as illustrated in* a *and* b, *there are many dilated, erythrocyte-filled blood vessels (BV) in the middle and deep dermis. A "grenz" zone (arrows) separates the upper dermis and epidermis. The epidermis shows mild hyperkeratosis, flattening of the stratum spinosum, and disappearance of the rete ridges.*

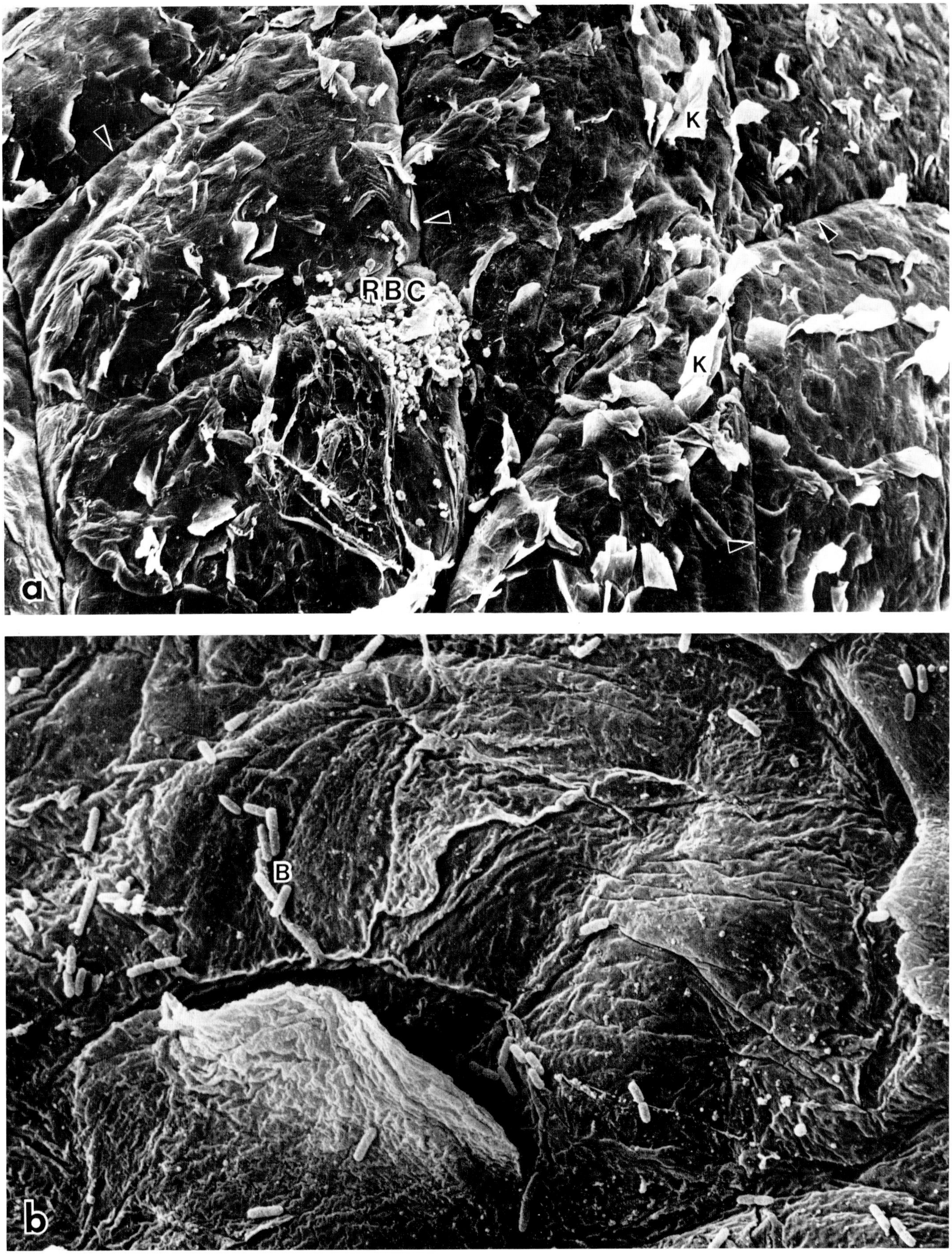

Figure 7–2. a. *The free surface has lobulated protrusions demarcated by creases (arrows). Red blood cells (RBC); exfoliated keratinized cells (K). ×360.*

b. *Bacteria (B) on ruffled scales at free surface of lesion. ×3,750.*

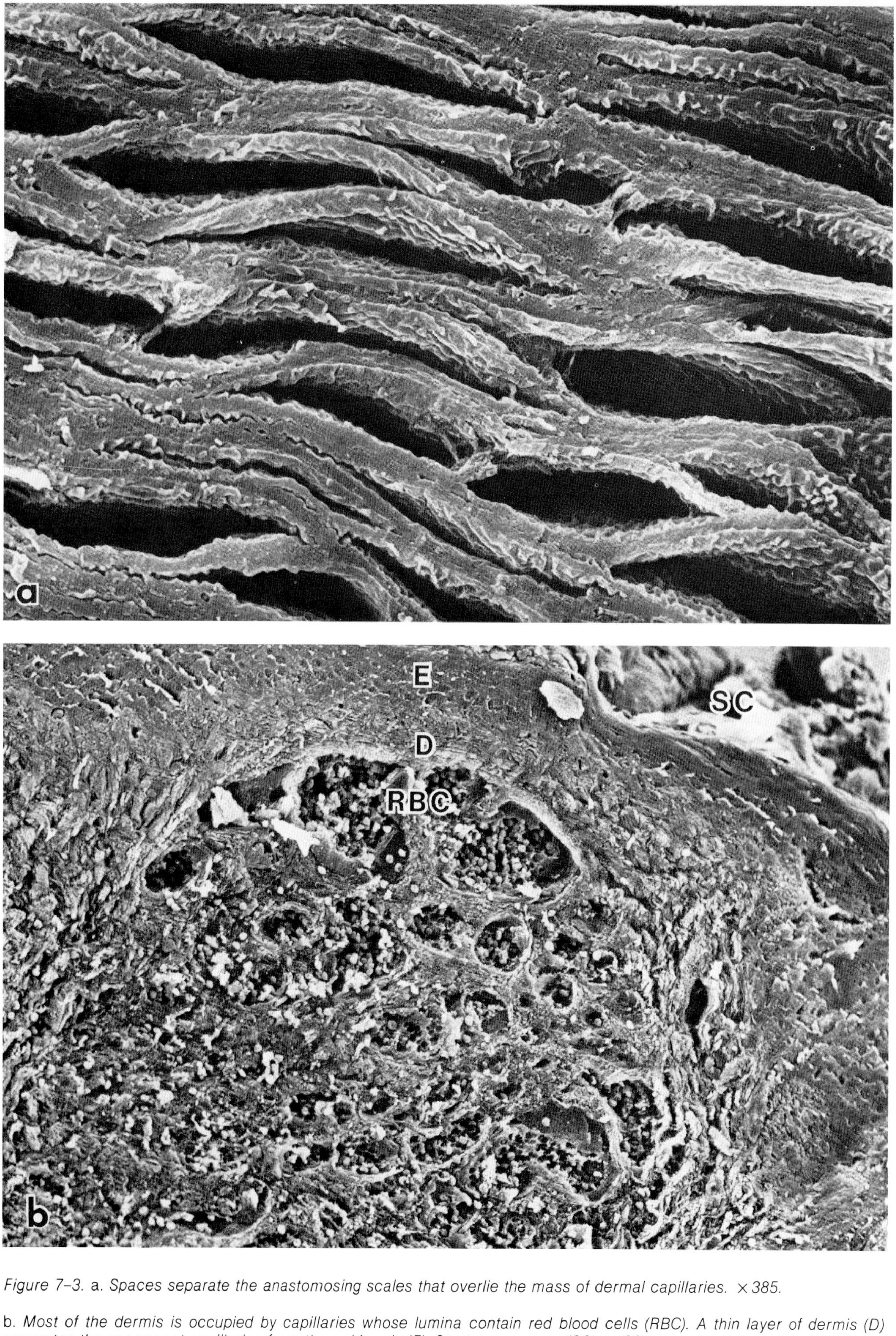

Figure 7–3. a. *Spaces separate the anastomosing scales that overlie the mass of dermal capillaries.* $\times 385$.

b. *Most of the dermis is occupied by capillaries whose lumina contain red blood cells (RBC). A thin layer of dermis (D) separates the uppermost capillaries from the epidermis (E). Stratum corneum (SC).* $\times 965$.

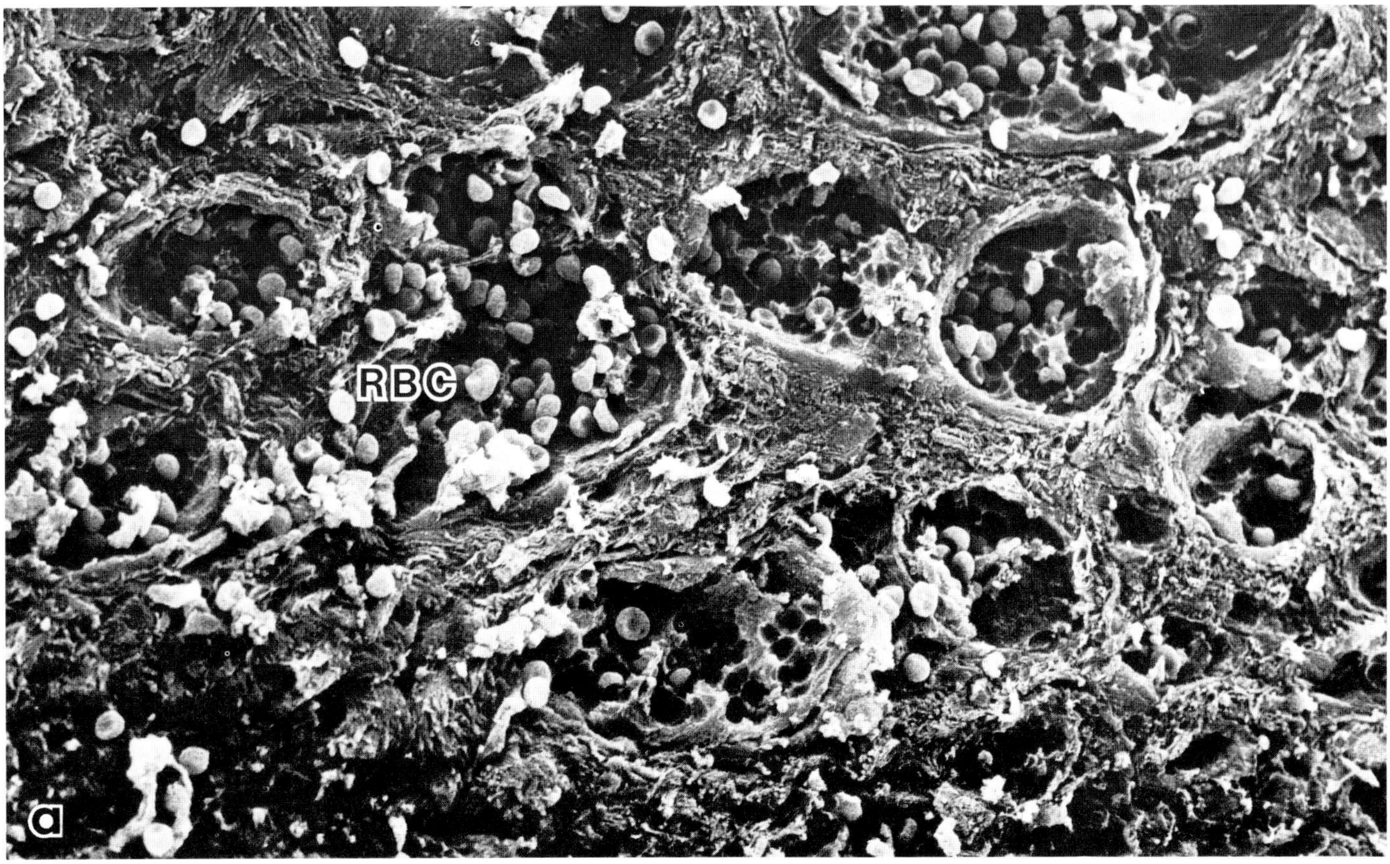

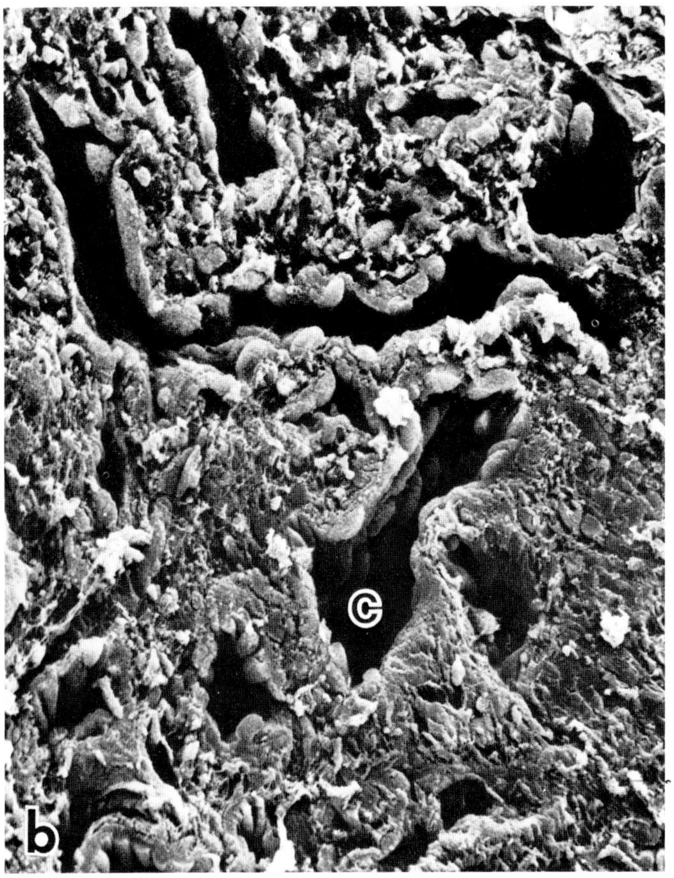

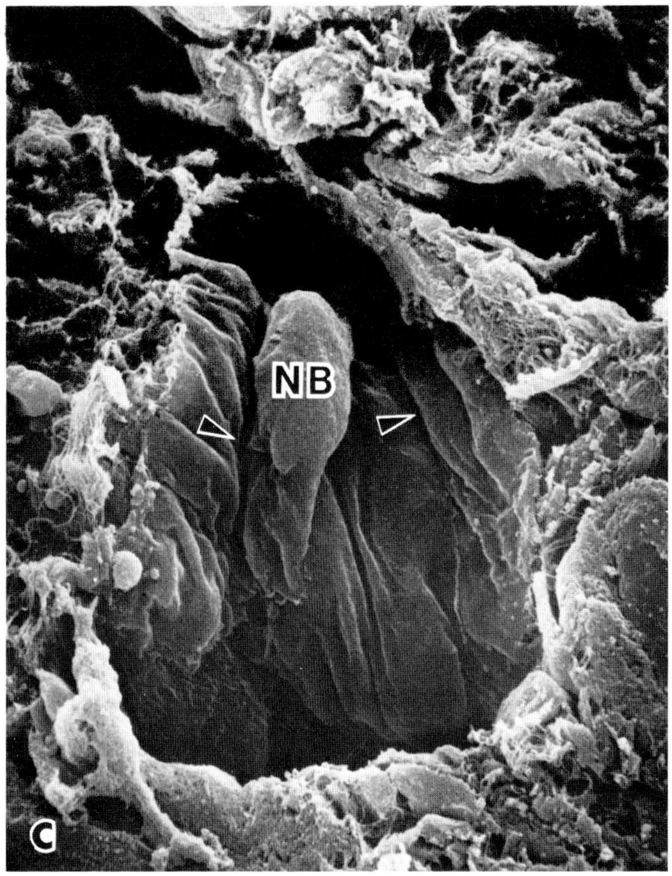

Figure 7–4. a. *Capillaries in dermis. Lumina are distended with red blood cells (RBC). ×965.*

b. *Small, meandrous capillaries (C) in dermis. ×540.*

c. *The capillary lumen is highly irregular. Deep furrows (arrows) separate endothelial cells and are most prominent at sites of nuclei. Protruding nuclei produce nuclear bulges (NB). ×2,250.*

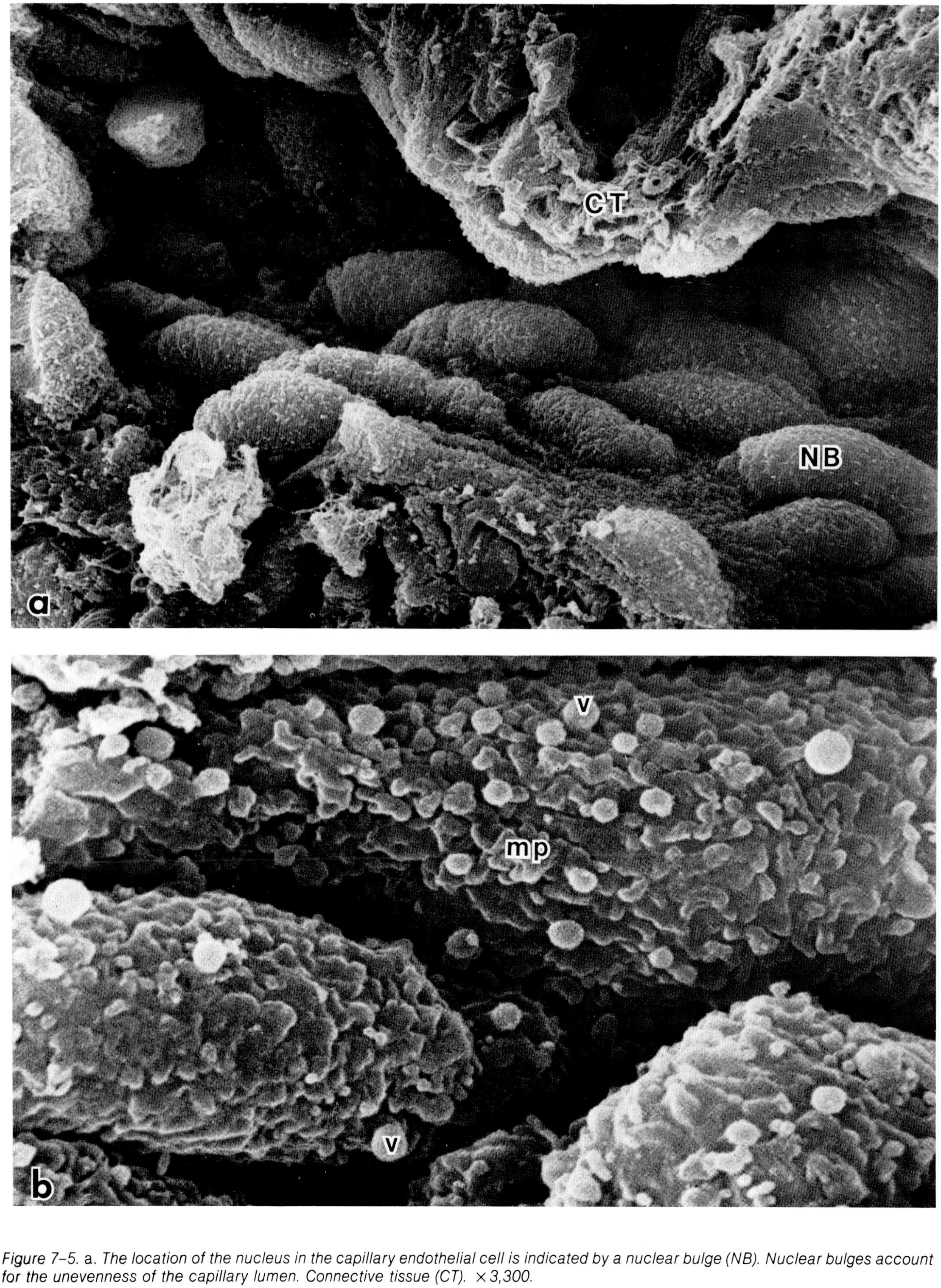

Figure 7–5. a. *The location of the nucleus in the capillary endothelial cell is indicated by a nuclear bulge (NB). Nuclear bulges account for the unevenness of the capillary lumen. Connective tissue (CT). ×3,300.*

b. *Surfaces of endothelial cells viewed at high magnification show vesicles (v) and microplicae (mp). These microprojections indicate a high metabolic activity and absorptive rate. ×13,200.*

BASAL CELL EPITHELIOMA 8

The basal cell epithelioma (BCE) is the most common type of skin cancer. Although opinions differ concerning the exact origin of the BCE, it is generally held that the tumor arises from basal cells of the epidermis, hair follicles, and sweat glands. Some prefer the term basal cell carcinoma for BCE, but most believe the tumor should be designated an epithelioma since it appears to grow by direct extension and rarely metastasizes.

The BCE has a propensity to develop in sun-exposed, anatomically thin epidermis with a high density of sebaceous glands, in irradiated areas, and in old burn scars. It is most frequent on the face (scalp and periorbital region) of elderly persons of fair complexion who live in geographical areas with much sunshine. The tumor seldom occurs on mucous membranes or the palms and soles, the two areas where hair is absent. Rodent ulcer is the term applied to a large, untreated BCE of the nodular type which has destroyed much of the patient's face. Death may result from destruction of vital vessels or structures.

Lever and Shaumburg-Lever (1983) listed five clinical types of basal cell epitheliomas (BCEs): (1) nodular — the most common type (includes nodular-ulcerated and rodent ulcer), (2) pigmented, (3) morphea-like or fibrosing, (4) superficial, and (5) fibroepithelioma. We studied 24 nodular, 5 superficial, and 3 pigmented tumors by SEM. The nodular type, both ulcerated and non-ulcerated, is shown in the following micrographs. Some of the tumors that we examined had differentiated toward hair structures (keratotic BCE), sebaceous glands (cystic BCE), and apocrine or eccrine sweat glands (adenoid BCE). A sharp dividing line could not be drawn when a tumor had more than one type of cutaneous appendage.

It is known that the nodular BCE begins as a circumscribed reddish spot and grows steadily from a few millimeters to several centimeters in size. The growth rate varies in different patients. As the tumor increases in diameter, it rises above the level of the surrounding normal skin and appears as a small, elevated, pale, translucent, firm papule that often shows a few, small telangiectatic vessels on its surface. The tumor slowly becomes button-like with a white, glossy, rolled free edge. The latter is called the "pearly border" which is diagnostic clinically. The center of the lesion may be depressd or ulcerated with ensuing blood and crusting. The usual treatment is surgical excision, electrodessication, or. irradiation.

Tumor cells are sometimes referred to as basiloma cells. They resemble normal basal cells except their nucleus to cytoplasm ratio is larger and the cytoplasm is often poorly defined. The connective tissue about the tumor cells (parenchyma) is called stroma and is arranged in parallel bundles. The stroma is closely associated with the parenchymal cells and grows with them.

We used SEM to define BCEs in a detailed manner and derived the following new information. The free surface is highly irregular with horn cysts and hyperkeratotic follicular openings. Sebum or blood may cover the free surface of the tumor. Extensive exfoliation is associated with BCEs. This finding agrees with previously published cell proliferation studies that show the average cell of the BCE reproduces every nine days which is about 3X the rate of cells in normal epidermis. SEM indicates that the exfoliation rate is comparable to the proliferation rate, a fact that may account for the slow net growth of the tumor observed clinically.

References

Amonette, R., S. Salasche, T. Chesney, C. Clarendon, and R. Dilawara. Metastatic basal-cell carinoma. J. Derm. Surg. 7: 397–400, 1982.

Ishibashi, A., T. Kasuga, and E. Tsuchiya. Electron microscopic study of basal cell carcinoma. J. Invest. Dermatol. 56: 298–304, 1971.

Jacobs, G. H., J. J. Rippey, and M. Altini. Prediction of aggressive behavior in basal cell carcinoma. Cancer 49: 533–537,1982.

Lever, W. F. and G. Schaumburg-Lever. Basal cell epithelioma. *In: Histopathology of the Skin.* J. B. Lippincott Co., Philadelphia, PA, 1983 (6th edition), p. 562–575.

Reidbord, H. E., H. L. Wechsler, and E. R. Fisher. Ultrastructural study of basal cell carcinoma and its variants with comments on histogenesis. Arch. Derm. 104: 132–140, 1971.

Sanderson, K. V. The architecture of basal-cell carcinoma. Br. J. Derm. 75: 455–474. 1961.

Weinstein, G. D., and P. Frost. Cell proliferation in human basal cell carcinoma. Cancer Res. 30: 724–728, 1970.

Zackheim, H. S. Origin of the human basal cell epithelioma. J. Invest. Dermatol. 40: 283–297, 1963.

Zelickson, A. S. An electron microscopic study of the basal cell epithelioma. J. Invest. Dermatol. 39: 183–187, 1962.

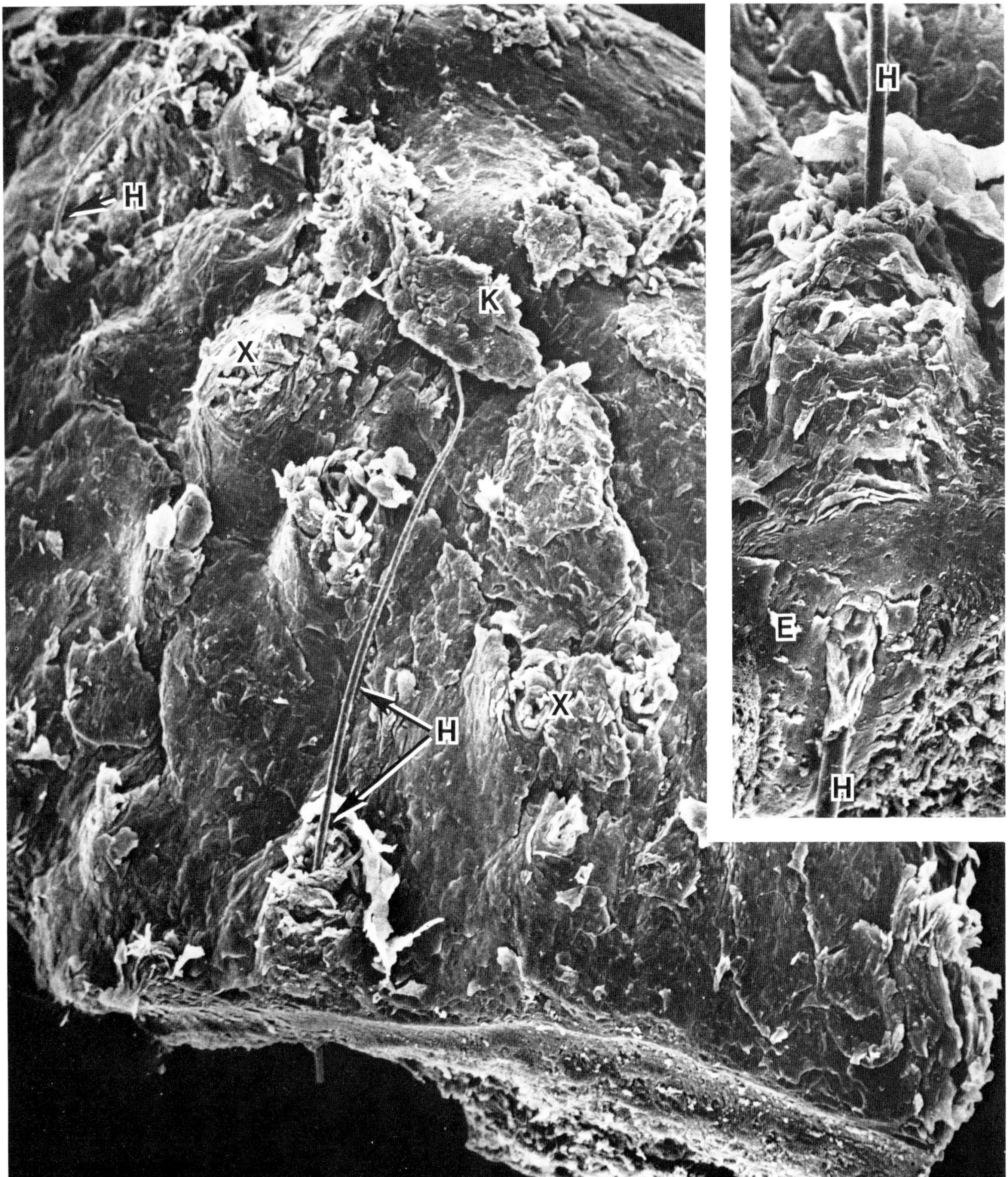

Figure 8–1. Two hairs (H), several elevated follicular orifices without hairs (X), and patches of loosely attached scales (K) undergoing desquamation are illustrated on the free surface of the tumor. The surface of this particular lesion is rough but it is not encrusted. $\times 150$.

Inset. *Profile of hair (H) is shown in follicular orifice at the tumor's free surface and in the epidermis (E).* $\times 300$.

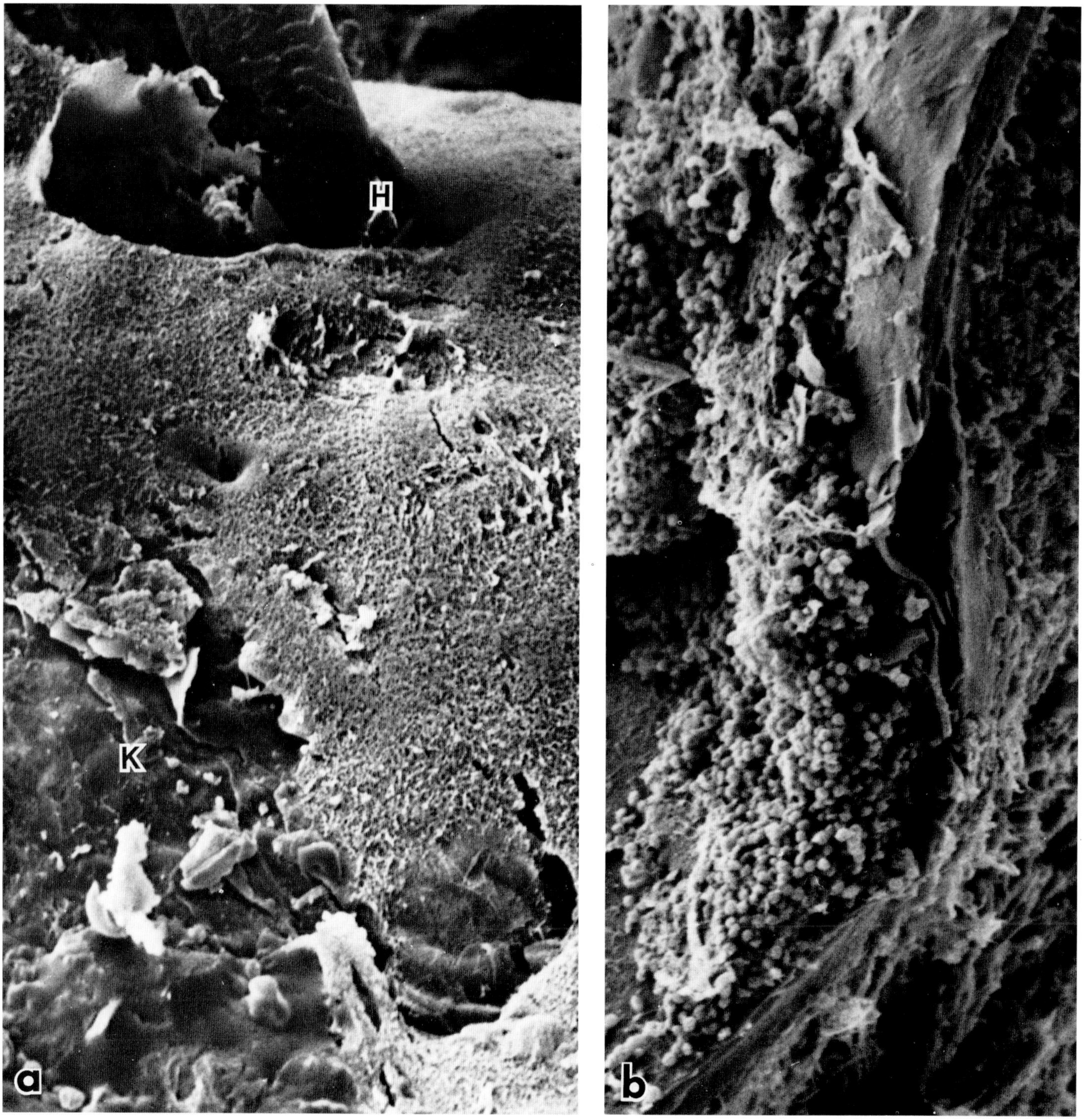

Figure 8–2. Free surface of tumor.

a. *The surface is encrusted by a thin layer of material that also surrounds the hair (H). Scales (K) at lower left are not encrusted.* ×400.

b. *The portion of the encrustation that is depicted in profile is from the central ulcerated area of a basal cell epithelioma. Most of the small structures in the encrustation are lymphocytes.* ×430.

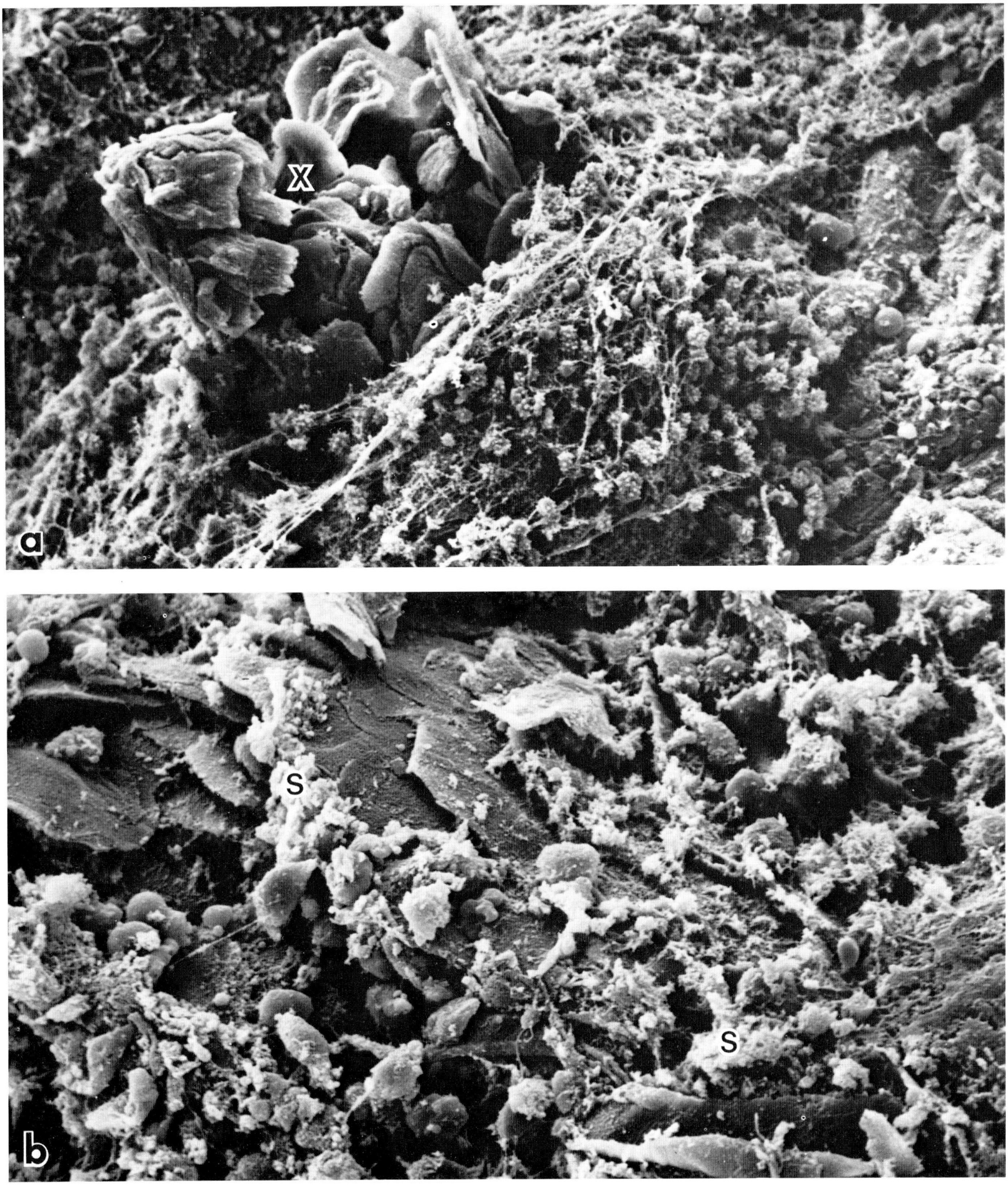

Figure 8–3. Free surface of tumor.

a. *The follicular orifice (X) is filled with keratinized cells and is surrounded by an encrustation of leukocytes, erythrocytes, and fibrin. Encrustations occur in lesions undergoing central ulceration or spontaneous regression. ×640.*

b. *An excess of sebum (S), as shown on the keratinized cells in this micrograph, is a feature of many basal cell epitheliomas. ×830.*

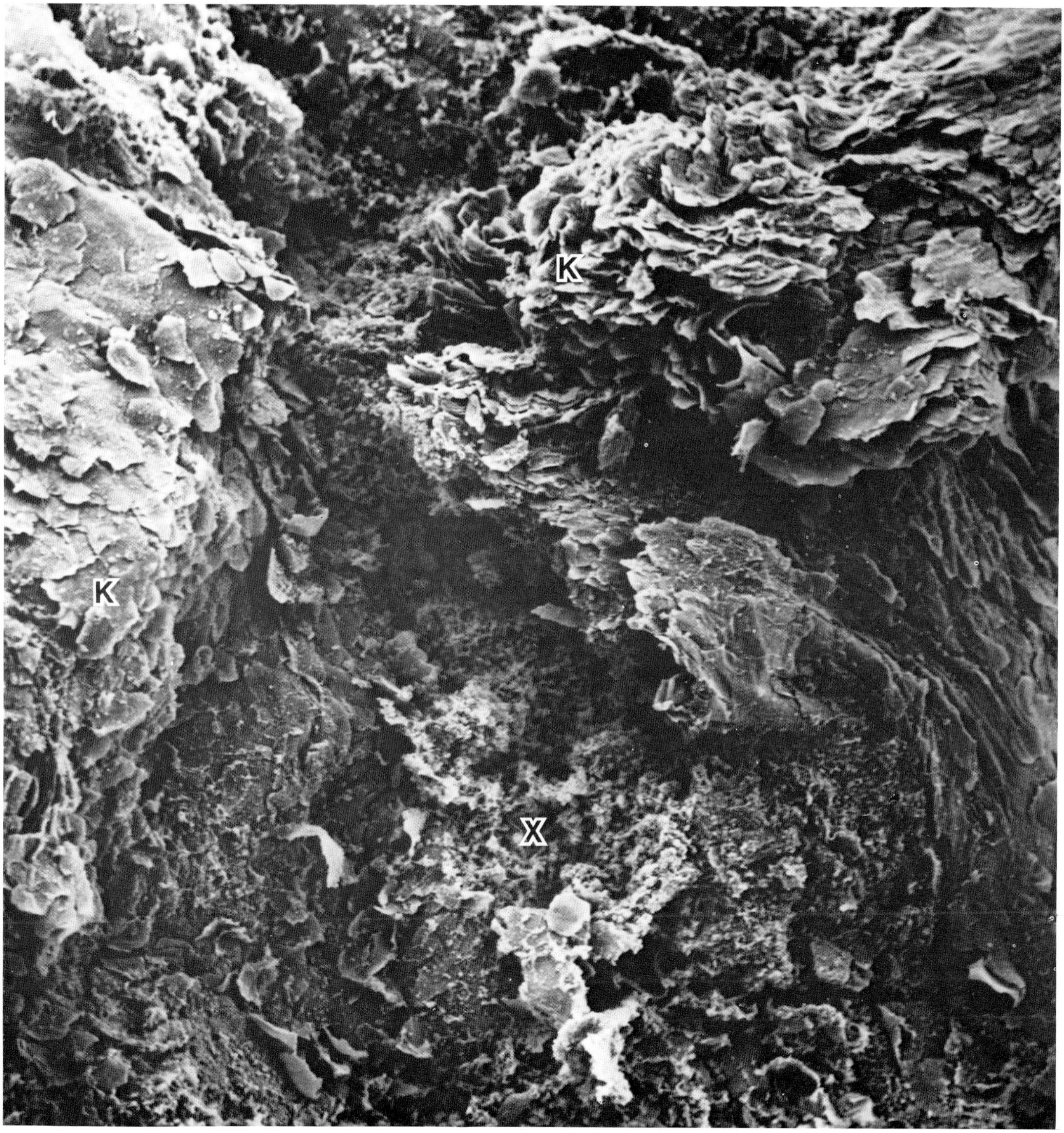

Figure 8–4. Stacks of scales (K) form the periphery of the encrusted, crater-like depression (X). The irregular surface is well suited for the collection of sebum and the growth of microorganisms. Extensive desquamation of scales is a characteristic of the tumor that is readily appreciated by SEM. The loss of cells at the free surface may equal the rather high degree of cell proliferation that other investigators have found in the tumor. ×175.

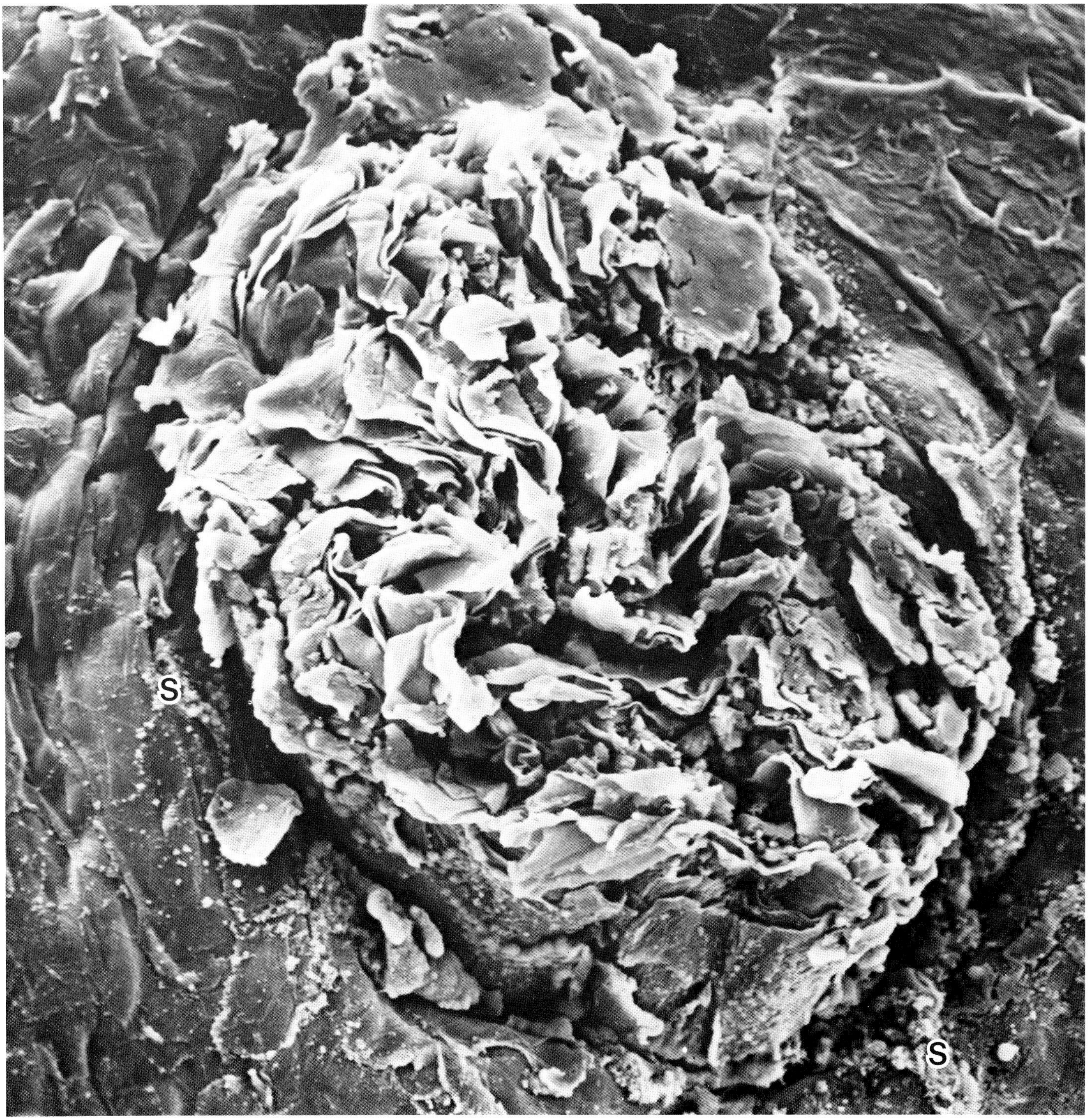

Figure 8–5. The large keratinous cyst in the center of the micrograph has been pushed to the free surface by deeper mitotically-active cells. Sebum (S) is present on the peripheral scales of the cyst. × 705.

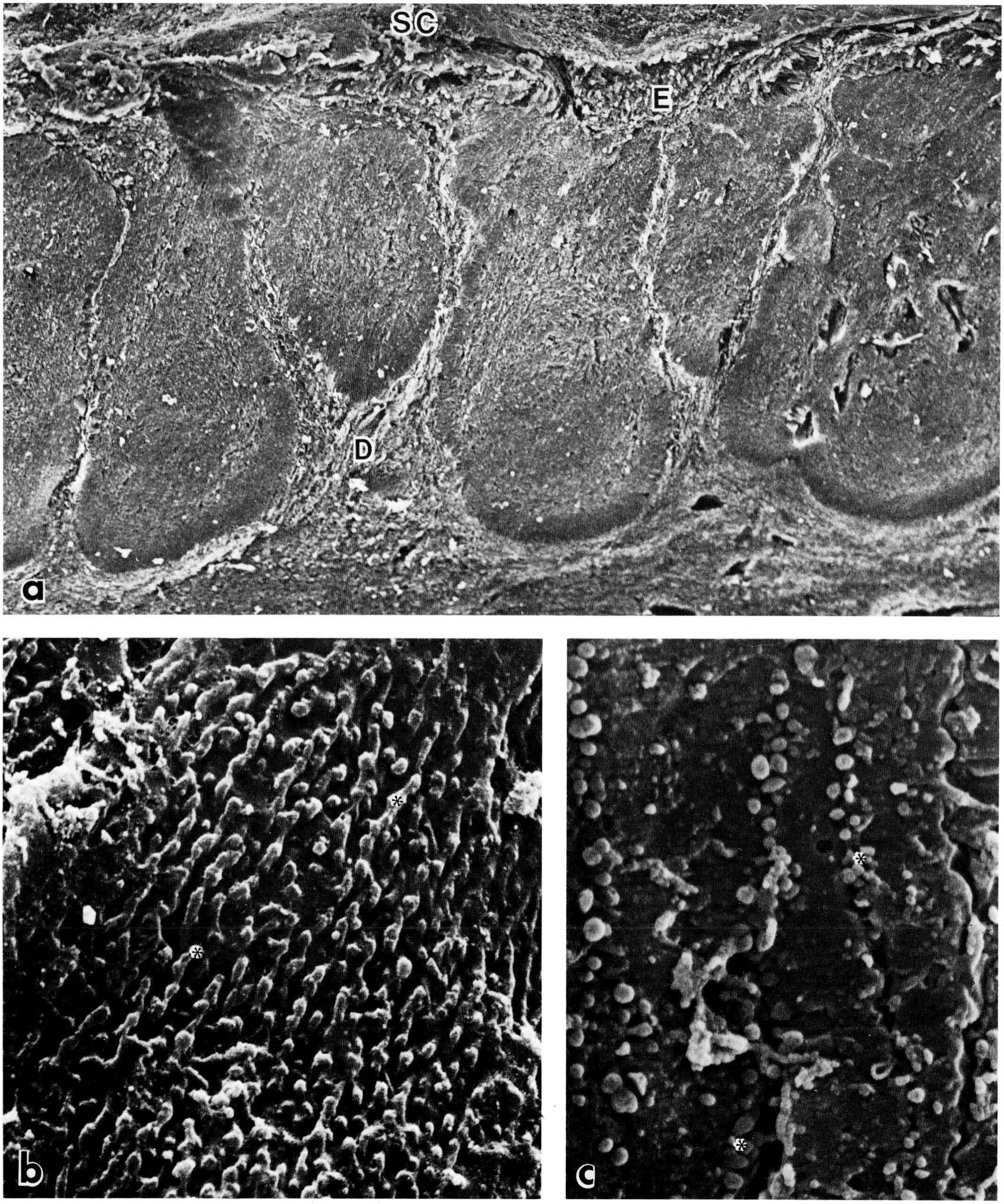

Figure 8–6. a. *Nodular tumor in profile, showing stratum corneum (SC) and masses of tumor cells extending deep into the dermis (D) but still connected to the epidermis (E). The outer dark rim of each nodule is the location of the palisading, columnar basal cells. Tumors are generally separated from the surrounding tissue by a basement membrane. Some cavities are present in the tumor and show signs of keratinization.* × *180.*

b. *Cornified tumor cells are visible on the lesion's free surface at sites devoid of encrustations. The surface topography of these cells is unusual in that they have numerous pointed plicae (*), a feature that is also found on some of the more deeply located non-keratinized cells.* × *9,400.*

c. *Pointed plicae-like projections can be seen on the tumor cells shown in profile in this micrograph. We saw similar projections on epidermal cells of fetal skin.* × *12,550.*

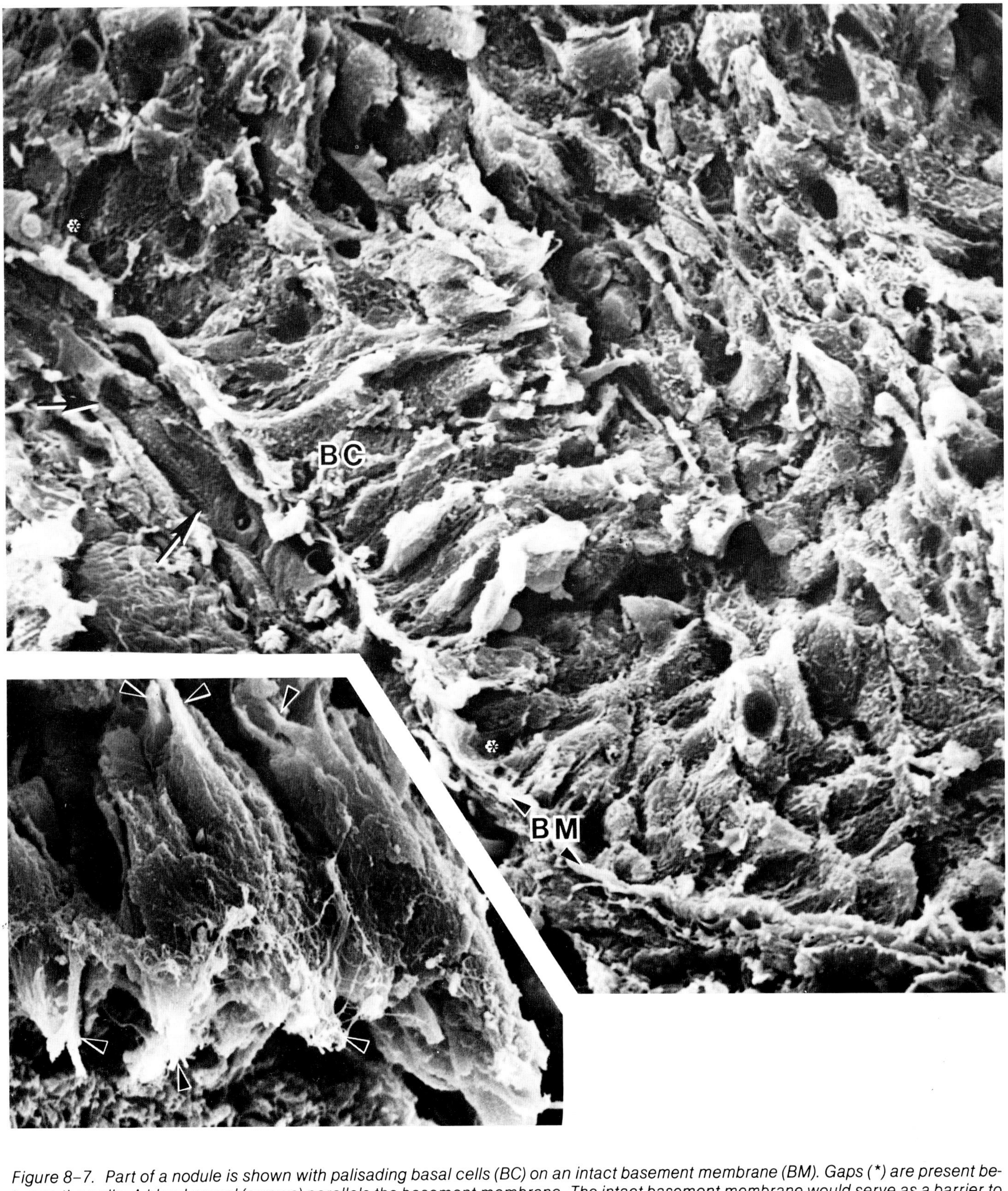

Figure 8–7. Part of a nodule is shown with palisading basal cells (BC) on an intact basement membrane (BM). Gaps (*) are present between the cells. A blood vessel (arrows) parallels the basement membrane. The intact basement membrane would serve as a barrier to metastasis. × 1,410.

Inset. *The outermost basal cells of this nodule have pointed apical and basal processes (arrows). The basal processes are visible because the cells have been dislodged from the basement membrane. TEM has shown desmosomes between the cells, and hemidesmosomes where basal cells attach to the basement membrane. × 2,000.*

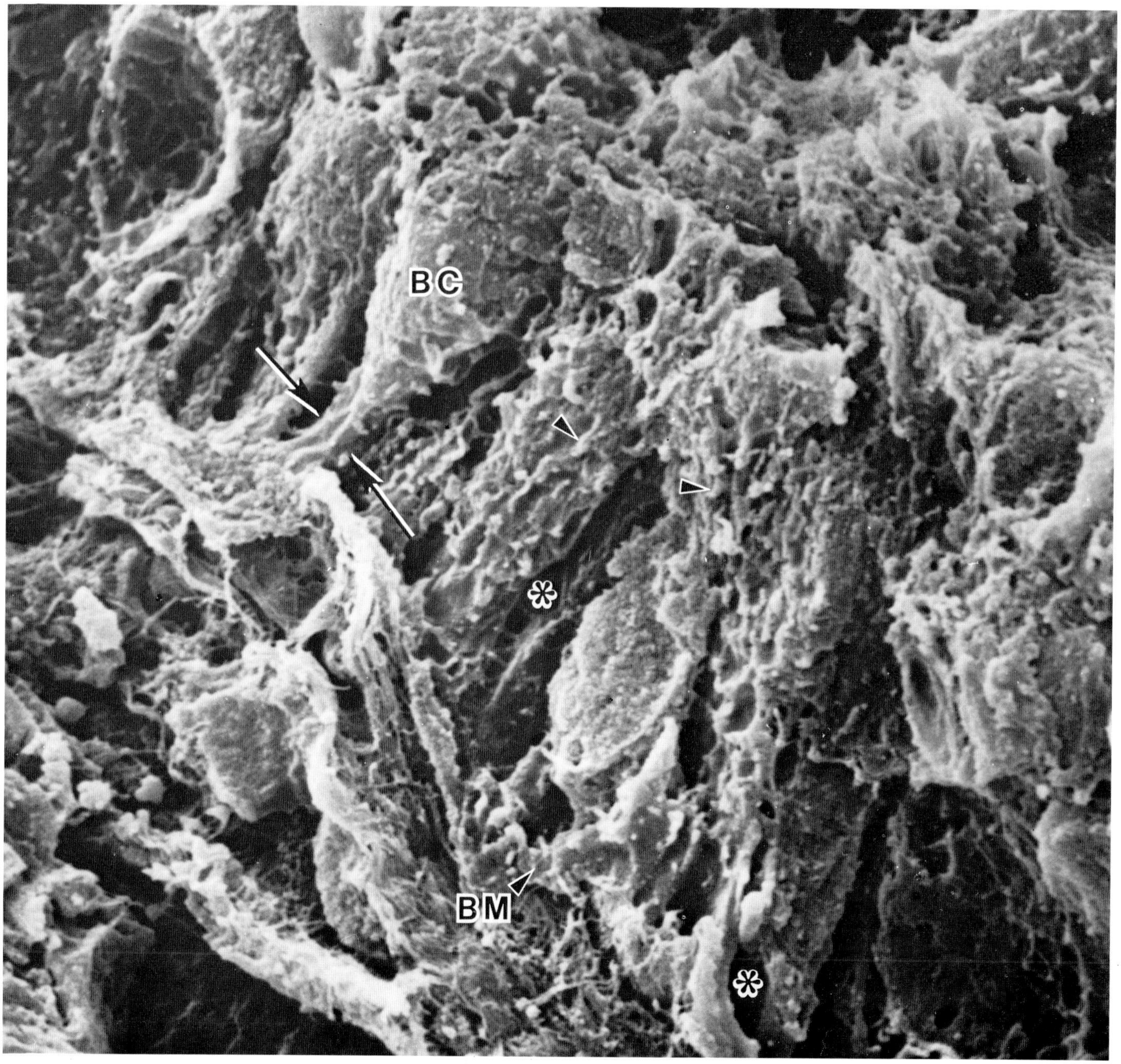

Figure 8–8. Basal cells (BC) and basement membrane (BM) at periphery of nodule. The basal cells are separated by gaps (*) and have a peculiar surface pattern with numerous plicae (small arrows) that give them a ruffled to honeycomb appearance. Cell bases are narrower than cell apices, and form stalk-like attachments (large arrows) to the basement membrane. ×5,500.

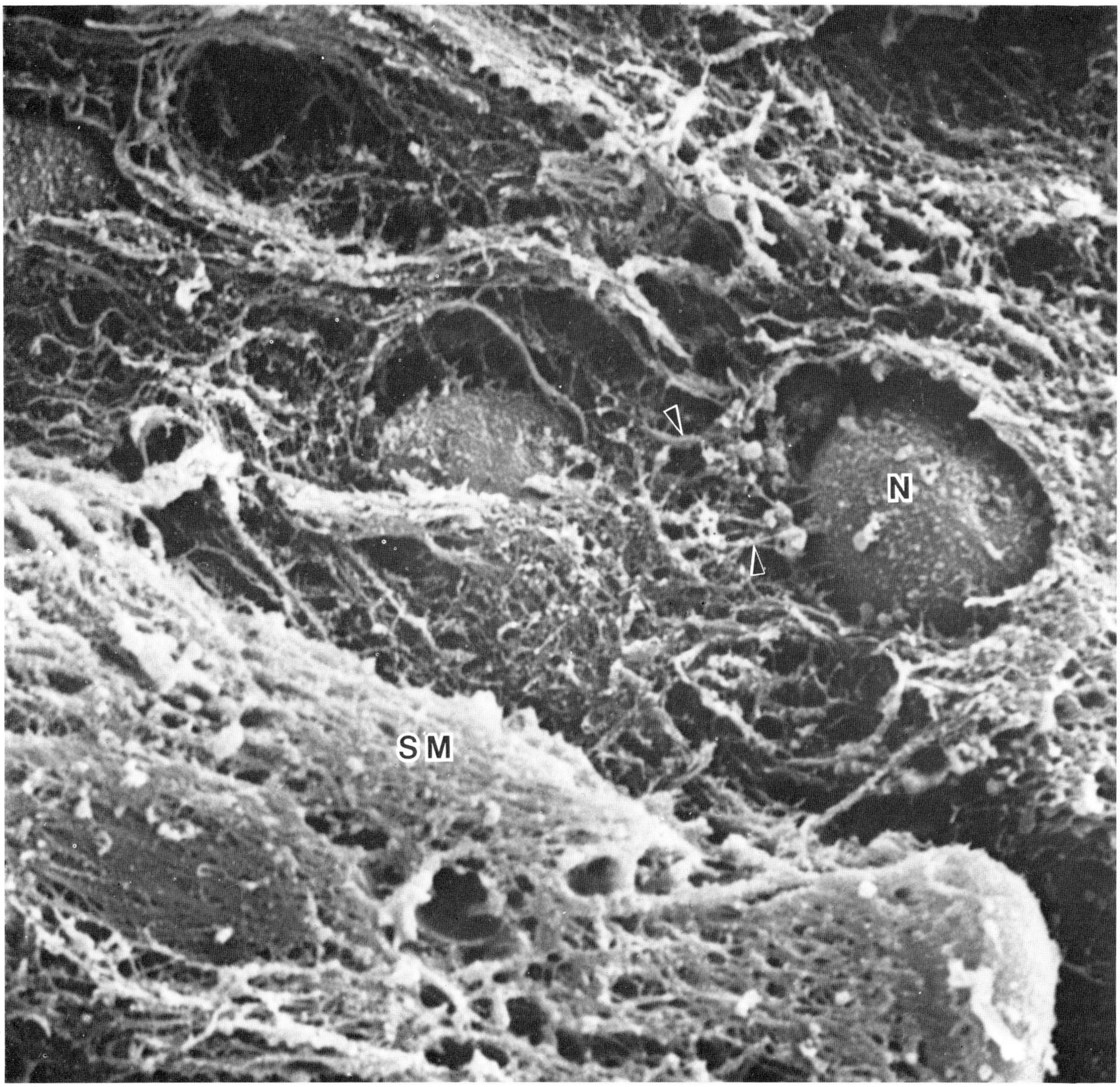

Figure 8–9. High magnification of fractured tumor cells in profile. The cells are located near center of a nodule. A large nucleus (N) is visible in some cells. Note the network of intracellular tonofilaments (arrows). The stringy material (SM) probably represents the mucopolysaccharide that has been reported to accumulate in the tumor. ×5,400.

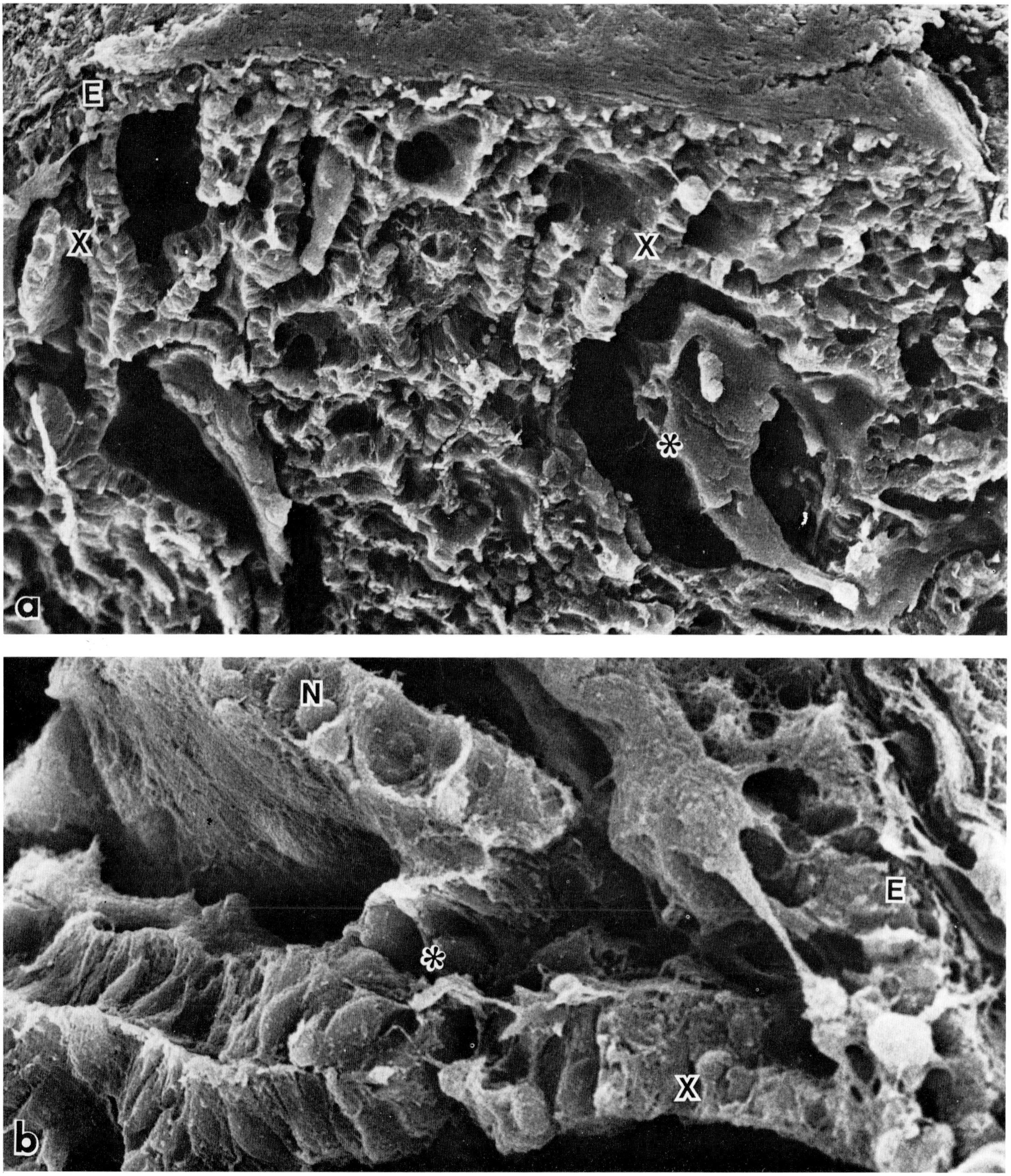

Figure 8–10. Adenoid basal cell epithelioma in profile.

a. *Columns of branching and anastomosing tumor cells (X) extend from the epidermis (E) and almost fill the dermis. Dilated spaces (*) are present between the columns.* ×520.

b. *Higher magnification of a column of tumor cells (X). The column is two cells wide and attached to the epidermis. (E). Note point where column branches (*), and nucleus (N) of tumor cell.* ×1,730.

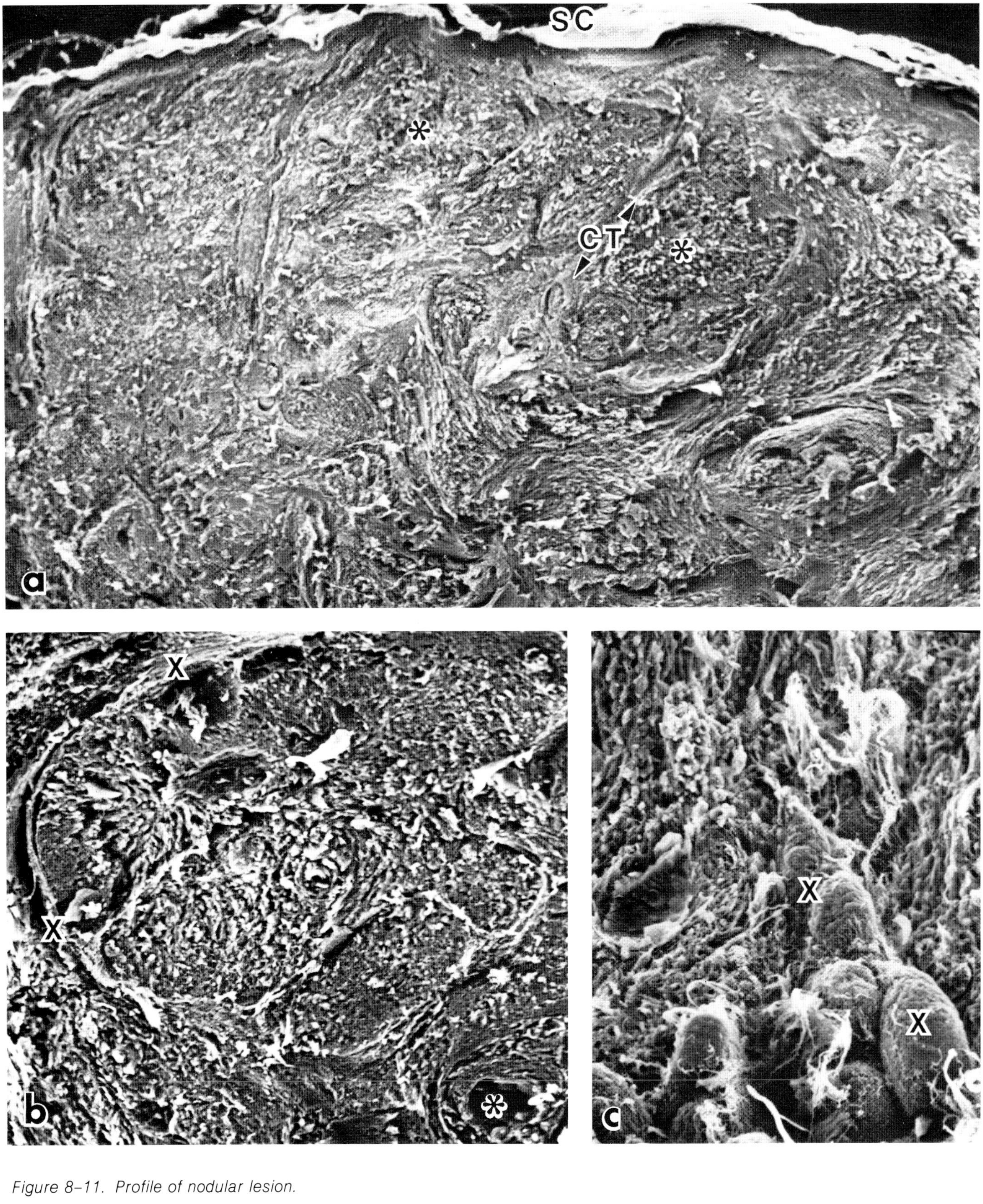

Figure 8–11. Profile of nodular lesion.

a. *Multiple islands of tumor cells (*) are shown in the dermis. The stratum corneum (SC) is represented by the shiny layer at the free surface. Each nodule is known to attach at some point to the epidermis, but the attachment of each nodule cannot be visualized without serial sections. Islands of tumor cells occupy about 60% of the dermis in this section and they are separated by strands of connective tissue (CT). ×80.*

b. *Large island of tumor cells. A basement membrane (X) separates the tumor cells from the dermis with its many blood vessels (*). ×150.*

c. *Small, interconnected islands of tumor cells in dermis. Only the surfaces (X) of the islands are visible. The basement membrane separated from the cells when the specimen was processed for SEM. ×275.*

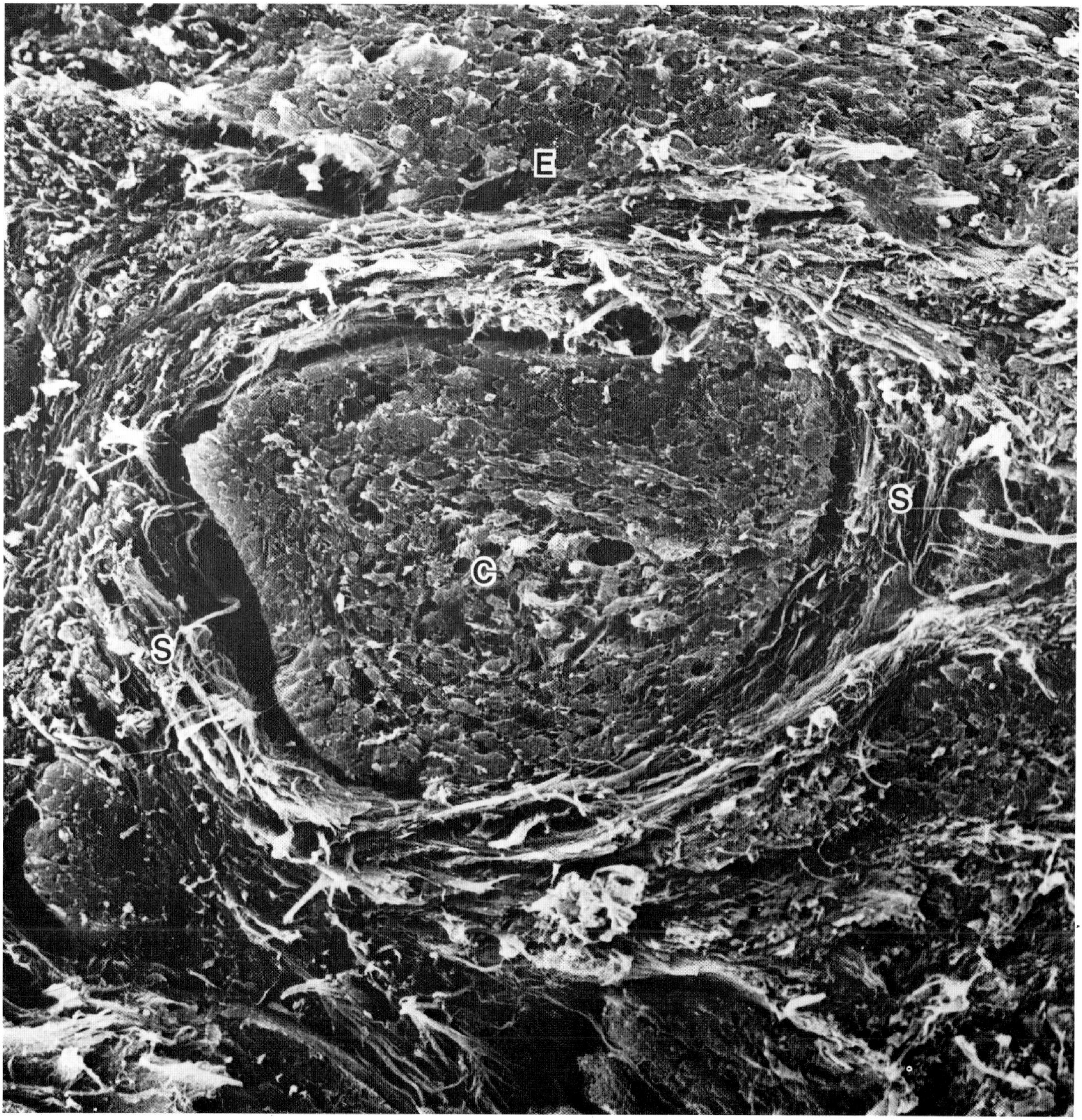

Figure 8–12. Nest of tumor cells near epidermis (E) and surrounded by connective tissue stroma (S). The center (C) of the nest shows signs of keratinization and horn cyst formation, as indicated by the presence of non-cellular debris. Some nests are filled with cells that bear surface projections, other nests contain cells whithout surface projections, and a few nests have a mixture of both cell types. ×690.

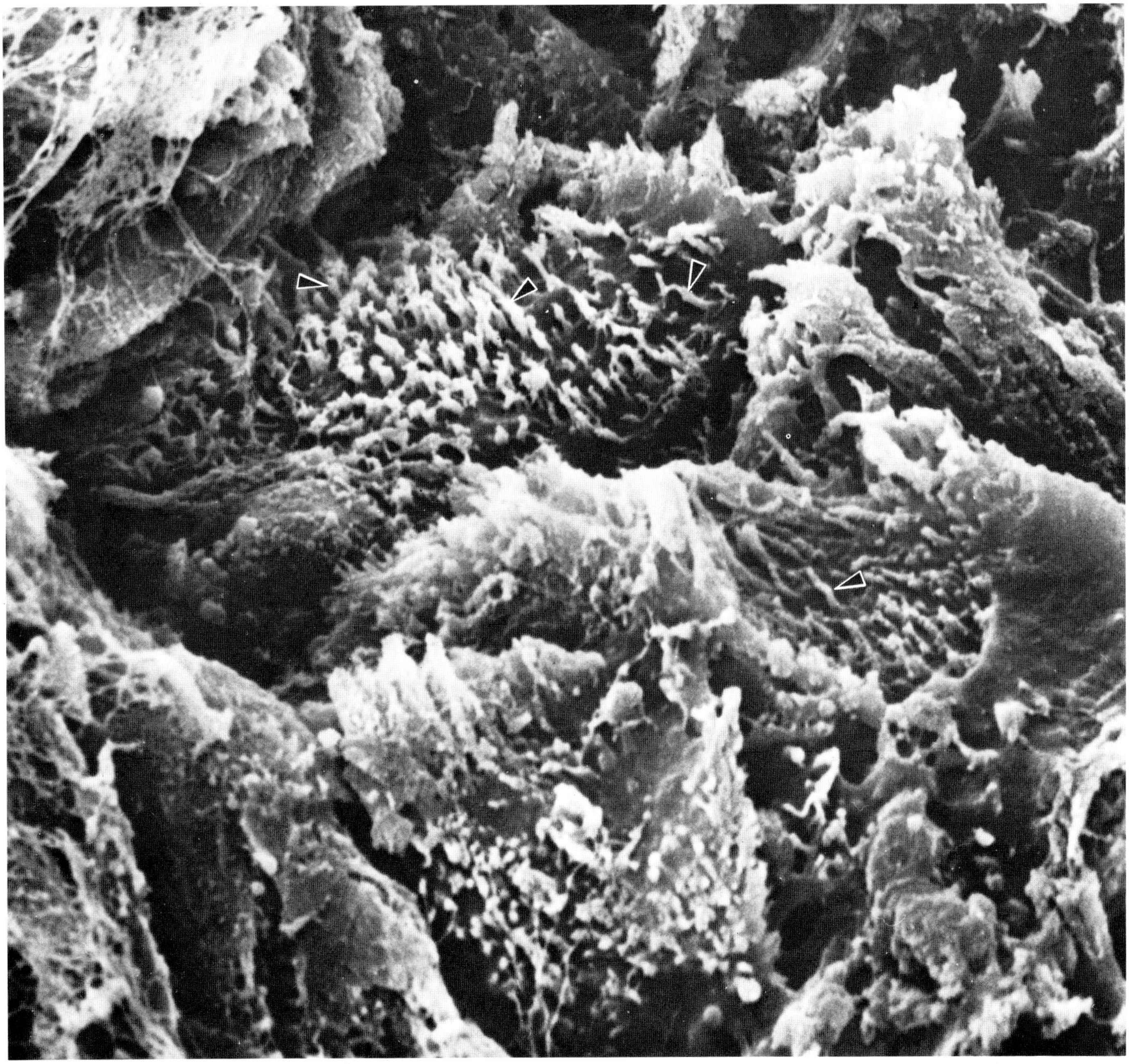

Figure 8–13. Tumor cells in a nest with villous-like projections (arrows). The small processes are not associated with desmosomes. They result from the plicated nature of the cell surface. ×6,600.

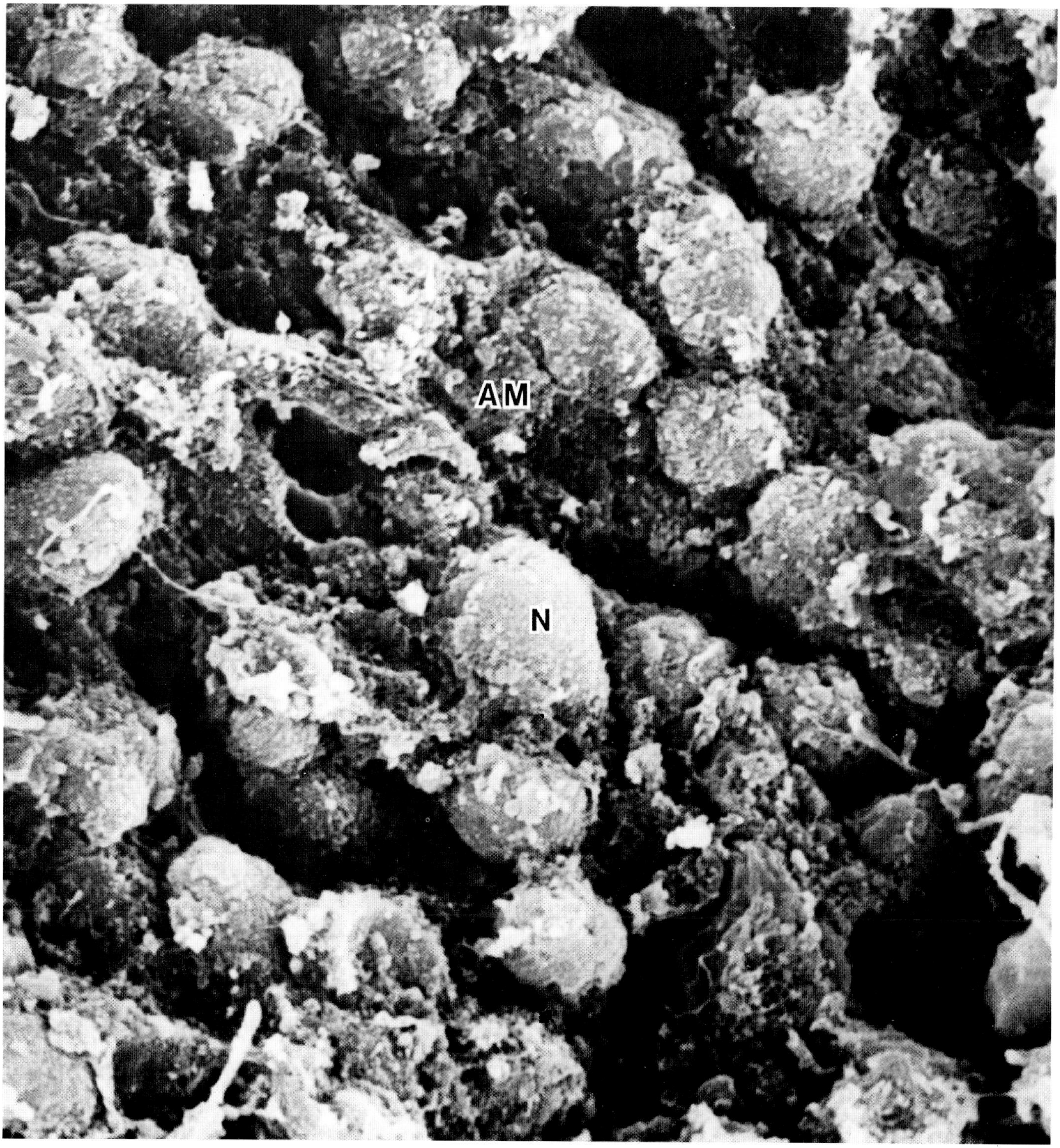

Figure 8–14. Tumor cells without surface projections. Each bulge indicates the location of a nucleus (N). Globules of amorphous material (AM) coat the cells. ×5,500.

SQUAMOUS CELL CARCINOMA 9

The squamous cell carcinoma (SCC) is a malignant tumor that may occur anywhere on the skin or on the mucous membranes. Squamous cells of the epidermis, cutaneous appendages, and mucous membranes that give rise to the tumor have the capability to differentiate and produce keratin. Other synonomous terms for SCC include epidermoid carcinoma, spinocellular carcinoma, prickle cell cancer, and spinalioma. The tumor develops mainly in later life (after 55 years of age), and affects males almost twice as frequently as females.

The SCC occurs most often on sun-exposed areas above the level of the shoulders and on the hands and forearms. Although sun-damage is by far the most common cause of SCC, any skin carcinogen may be responsible (e.g., arsenic, X-rays, coal tar, creosote, and industrial oils). It usually requires years for a SCC to develop following injury to the skin by a carcinogen. Other conditions that may promote the development of SCC include certain premalignant states (e.g., Bowen's disease, actinic keratoses, and leukoplakia) and some of the chronic dermatoses (e.g., discoid lupus erythematosus, lupus vulgaris, syphilis, psoriasis, and lepromatous leprosy).

The clinical features of squamous cell carcinomas (SCCs) are not always as clear as those of the basal cell epithelioma. An early SCC may appear as a scaly, erythematous lesion with ill-defined borders that may be somewhat tender and bleed following removal of the overlying scales. The malignant nature of the tumor requires that it be managed far more aggresively than the basal cell epithelioma. Wide surgical incisions should be made, regional lymph nodes should be examined for possible metastasis, and X-ray therapy along with topical and systemic chemotherapy should be considered.

Broders (see references) described SCCs as having four histological grades of severity. He called the tumor grade 1 if more than 75% of the cells were differentiated, grade 2 if 50% to 75% of the cells were differentiated, grade 3 if 25% to 50% of the cells were differentiated, or grade 4 if 0% to 25% of the cells were differentiated. His method of grading the degrees of malignancy on a histological basis can be applied to any neoplasm. It should be emphasized that differentiation of the SCC is in the direction of keratinization, and that the degree of keratinization is the essential feature of Broders' classification. Therefore, grade 1 tumors are the most benign and the most differentiated (keratinized or mature); grade 4 tumors are the most malignant and keratinization is almost absent.

In addition to the amount of keratinization, it is recognized that the degree of atypicality of the tumor cells and the depth of the lesion should be considered in grading the tumor. Lever and Shaumburg-Lever (1983) have pointed out that grade 1 SCCs have not penetrated below the level of the sweat glands, and most of the tumor cells have intercellular bridges and horn pearls. The latter are composed of concentric layers of wholly or partially keratinized squamous cells. Grade 2 SCCs also contain a few horn pearls, but they are absent in grades 3 and 4 SCCs. Only in grade 4 SCCs are keratinized cells completely absent and the vast majority of tumor cells are atypical and devoid of intercellular bridges.

Histologically, the main hallmark of the SCC is invasion of the dermis by tumor cells through breaks or disruptions of the basement membrane. Irregular masses of normal squamous cells and atypical (anaplastic) squamous cells undergo proliferation in the dermis. The malignancy of the tumor is directly proportional to the number of atypical squamous cells as manifested, e.g., by variation in cell size and shape, the presence of atypical mitotic figures, absence of intercellular bridges, and nuclear hyperplasia and hyperchromasia.

The material for this study consisted of 12 SCCs that were excised from the lips, hands, and forearms of 8 male and 4 female patients who ranged in age from 50 to 71 years. Part of each specimen was used for histology, SEM, and TEM. The clinical diagnosis of each lesion was confirmed in histological sections. All grades of the tumor were represented in the 12 specimens.

By SEM, many scales in the process of exfoliation were present on the free surface of the lesion. Grade 1 tumors were often encrusted with leukocytes. Scales at the free surface were immature as indicated by their anastomotic ridges and grooves. TEM showed that desmosomes were infrequent or absent. Keratinized centers of horn pearls were surrounded by tumor cells. Certain tumor cells had long cytoplasmic processes that gave them a "bearded" appearance. This feature made it possible to distinguish by SEM well differentiated SCCs from keratoacanthomas. Until now the ability to clearly distinguish between these two tumors by conventional microscopy has been difficult.

References

Battifora, H. Spindle cell carcinoma. Ultrastructural evidence of squamous origin and collagen production by the tumor cells. Cancer 37: 2275–2282, 1976.

Broders, A. C. Practical points on the microscopic grading of carcinoma. New York J. Med. 32: 667–671, 1932.

Caro, W. A. Tumors of the skin. Squamous cell carcinoma. *In: Dermatology,* S. L. Moschella, D. M. Pillsburry, and H. J. Hurley (eds). W. B. Saunders Co., Philadelphia, PA, 1975, Vol. 2, p. 1342–1344.

Edmundson, W. F. Microscopic grading of cancer and its practical implication. Arch. Dermatol. Syph. 57: 141–150, 1948.

Evans, H. L., and J. L. Smith. Spindle cell squamous carcinomas and sarcoma-like tumors of the skin. Cancer 45: 2687–2697, 1980.

Kobayas, T. Dermo-epidermal junction in invasive squamous cell carcinoma. Acta Derm.-Venerol. 49: 445–457, 1969.

Lever, W. F., and G. Schaumburg-Lever. Squamous cell carcinoma. *In: Histopathology of the Skin.* J. B. Lippincott Co., Philadelphia, PA, 1983 (6th edition), p. 499–506.

Lund, H. Z. Squamous cell Carcinoma. *In: Tumors of the Skin.* Armed Forces Institute of Pathology, Washington, D.C., 1957, p. 235–258.

Moller, R. M., R. Flemming, and K. Hou-Jensen. Metastases in dermatological patients with squamous cell carcinoma. Arch. Dermatol. 115: 703–705, 1979.

Muller, S. A., C. M. Wilhelm, Jr., E. G. Harrison, Jr., and R. K. Winkelmann. Adenoid squamous cell carcinoma (adenoacanthoma of Lever). Arch. Dermatol. 89: 589–597, 1964.

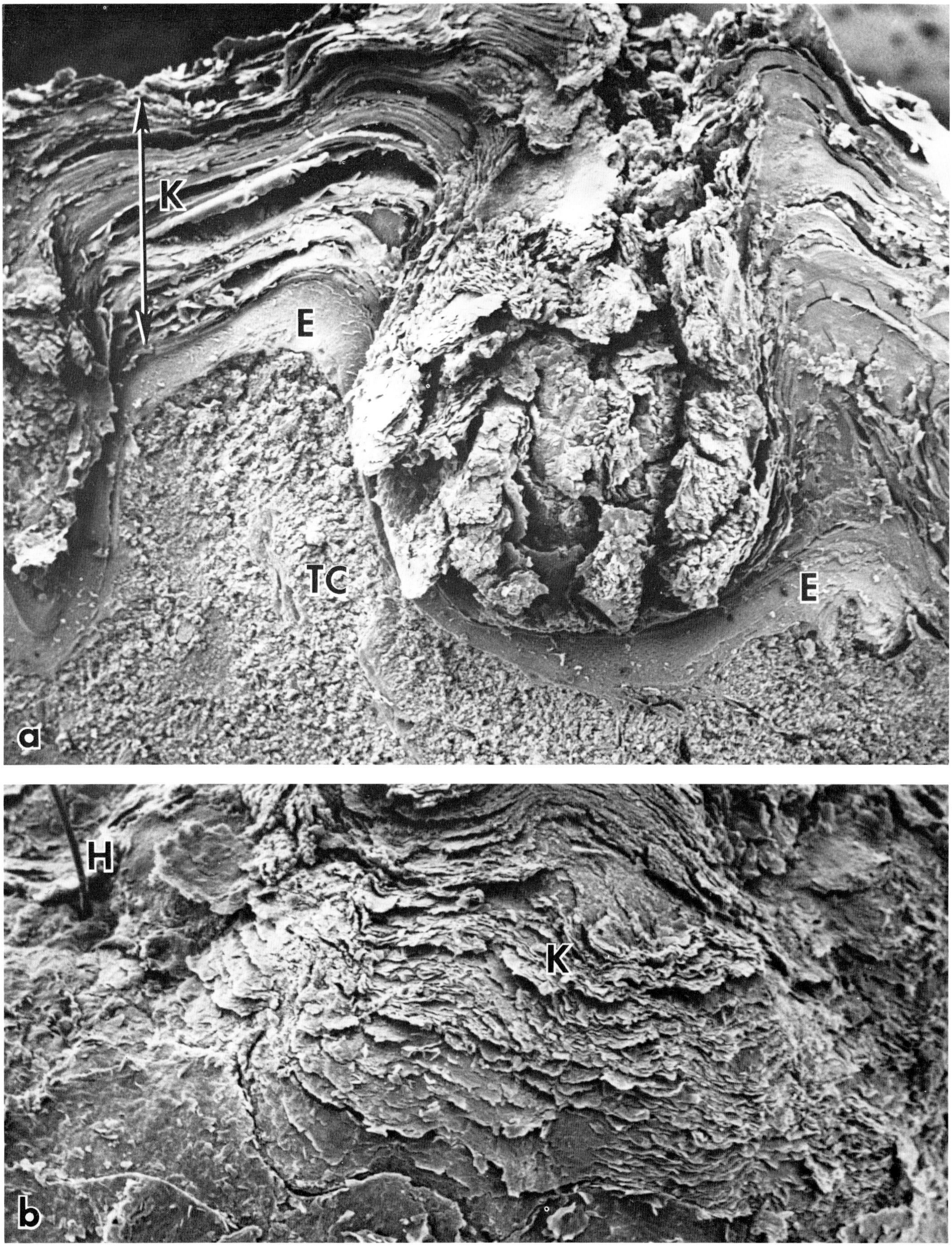

Figure 9–1. Free surface of squamous cell carcinoma.

a. *Lesion in profile. The free surface is hyperkeratotic with multiple layers of keratinized cells (K) whose thickness is indicated by arrows. A plug of scales is in the furrow above the band of non-keratinized epidermal cells (E). Tumor cells (TC) are below the band. ×35.*

b. *A small hair (H) projects through the lamellae of scales (K) at the free surface of the lesion. ×80.*

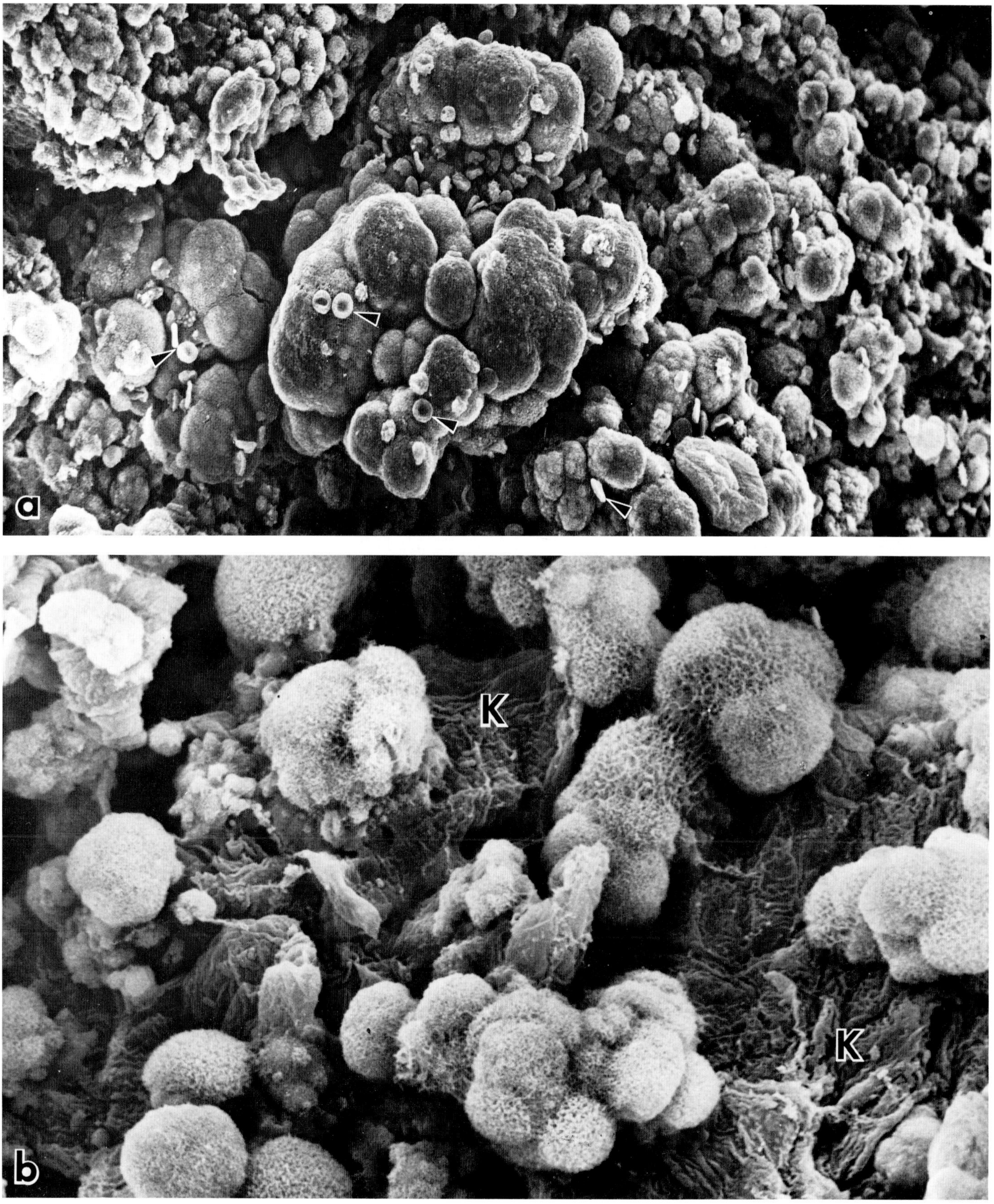
a
b
K
K

Figure 9–2. Encrustation on free surface.

a. *Red blood cells (arrows) are among the aggregates of leukocytes on the uneven free surface of the lesion. × 700.*

b. *Higher magnification of cellular encrustation on the free surface of a lesion. Aggregates of leukocytes matted with fibrillar material overlie the keratinized cells (K). The inflammatory reaction shown here is the type that occurs most frequently in grade 1 squamous cell carcinoma. Leukocytes are believed to reach the free surface following an immune reaction against the underlying malignant cells. × 3,350.*

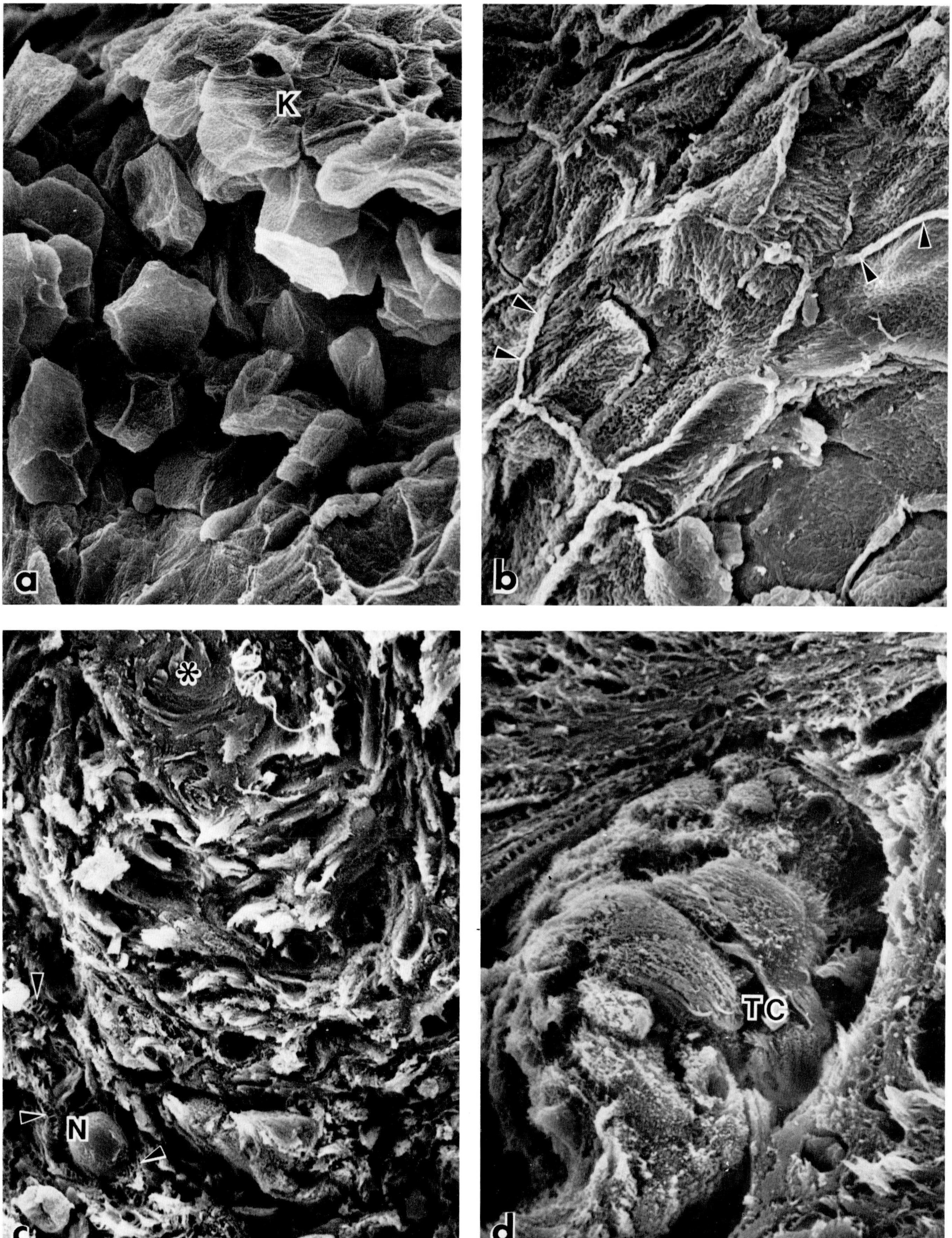
K
a
b
*
N
c
TC
d

Figure 9–3. a. *Loosely arranged keratinized cells (K) in the process of exfoliating are shown at the free surface of the lesion. By TEM, desmosomes are infrequent or even absent between some cells, a fact that may account for the high rate of exfoliation in squamous cell carcinomas.* × *8,400.*

b. *Higher magnification of kertinized cells at surface of lesion. The cells differ from normal scales in that they have anastomotic ridges and grooves and are incompletely keratinized. Boundaries (arrows) overlap between individual cells.* × *1,625.*

c. *Horn pearl with keratinized center (*) surrounded by tumor cells, each of which tends to have a large nucleus (N) and processes (arrows).* × *830.*

d. *Epidermal pocket with cluster of tumor cells (TC) that possibly represent the center of a developing horn pearl.* × *1,090.*

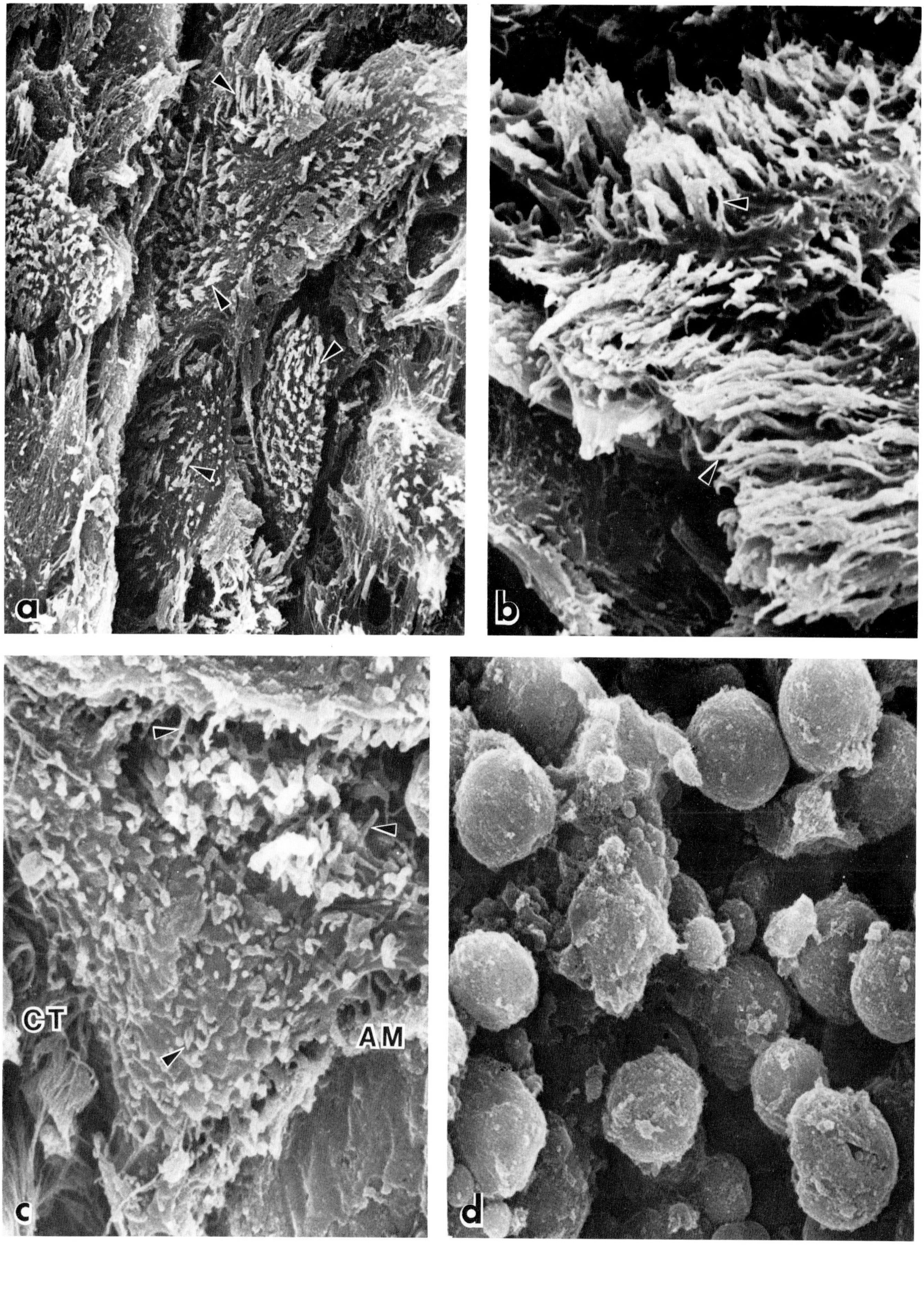
a
b
CT
AM
c
d

Figure 9–4. Special features of tumor cells.

a. *The tumor cells in this micrograph are irregularly-shaped and have cytoplasmic processes (arrows). ×2,100.*

b. *Higher magnification of tumor cell processes (arrows). Long, thin processes of this type have not been observed on tumor cells of the keratoacanthoma, a tumor that is difficult to distinguish from some squamous cell carcinomas by conventional microscopy. The cytoplasmic processes give the cell surface a "bearded" appearance, a feature that permits the SCC to be easily identified by SEM. ×4,000.*

c. *Observe the plicae and processes (arrows) from the tumor cell surface and the two products of the tumor cells — connective tissue fibers (CT) and amorphous intercellular material (AM). ×8,400.*

d. *Round tumor cells. These cells lack cytoplasmic processes and are especially numerous in the higher grades (more undifferentiated) squamous cell carcinomas. ×4,200.*

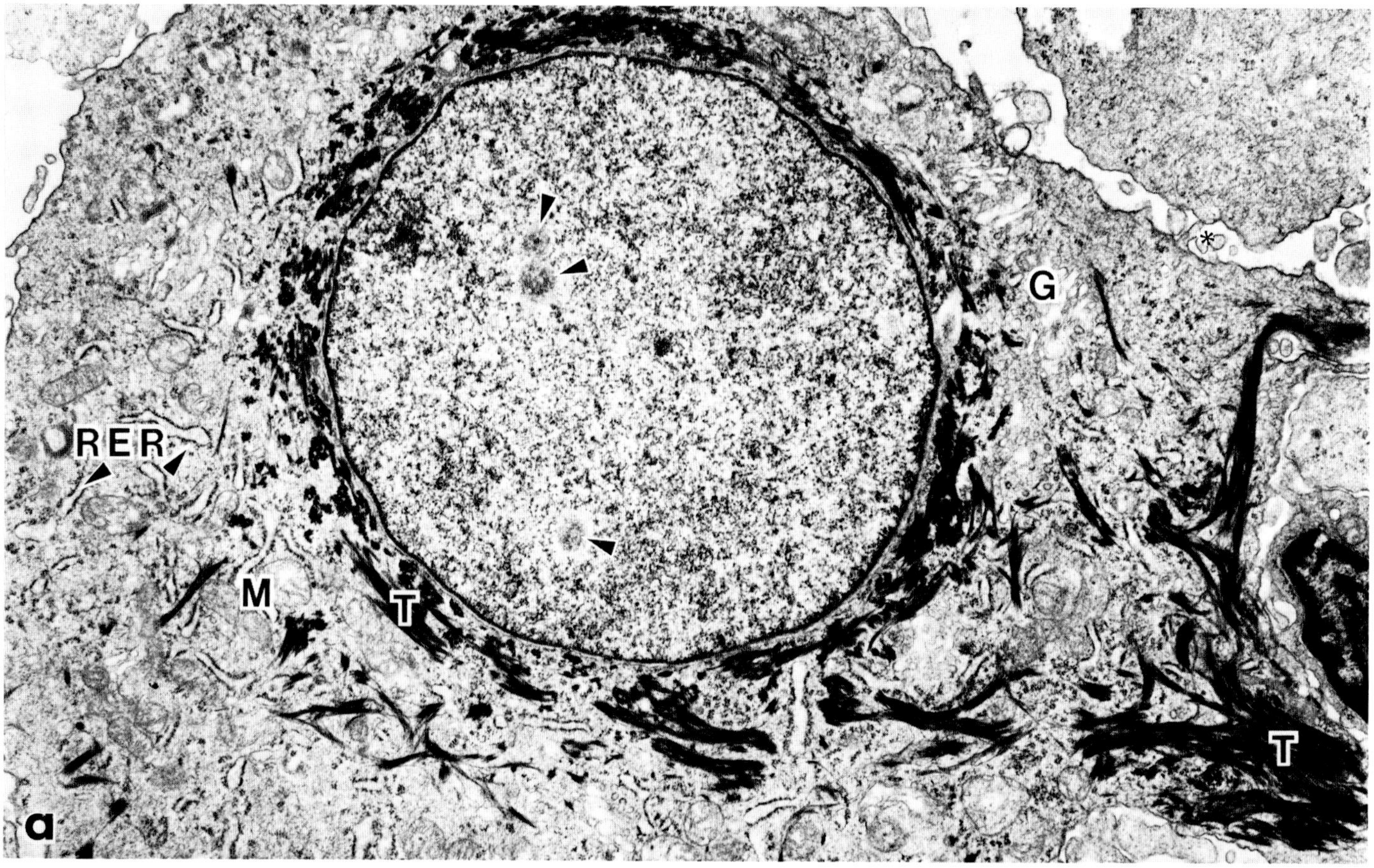

G
RER
M
T
T
a

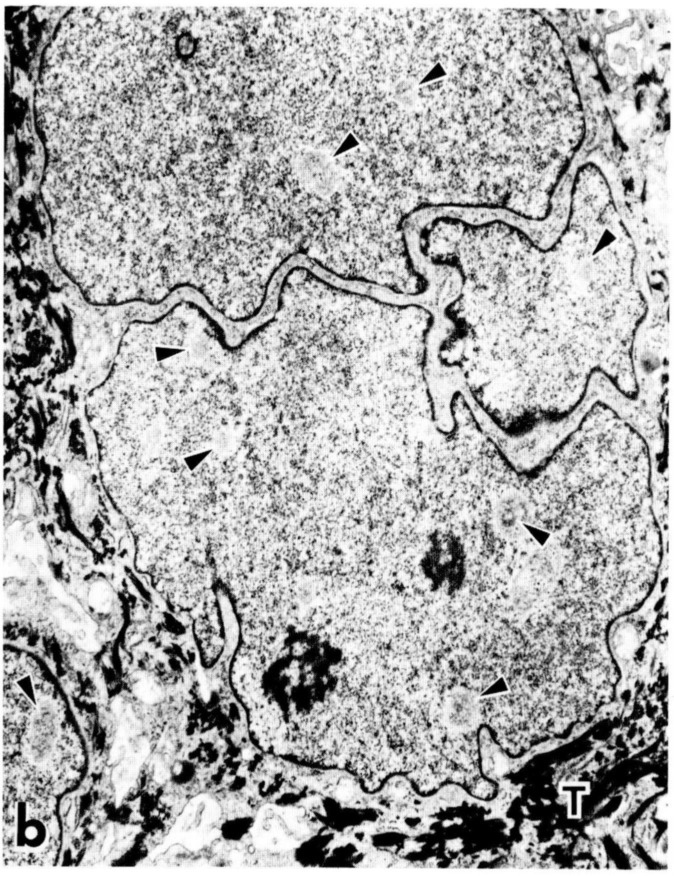

T
b

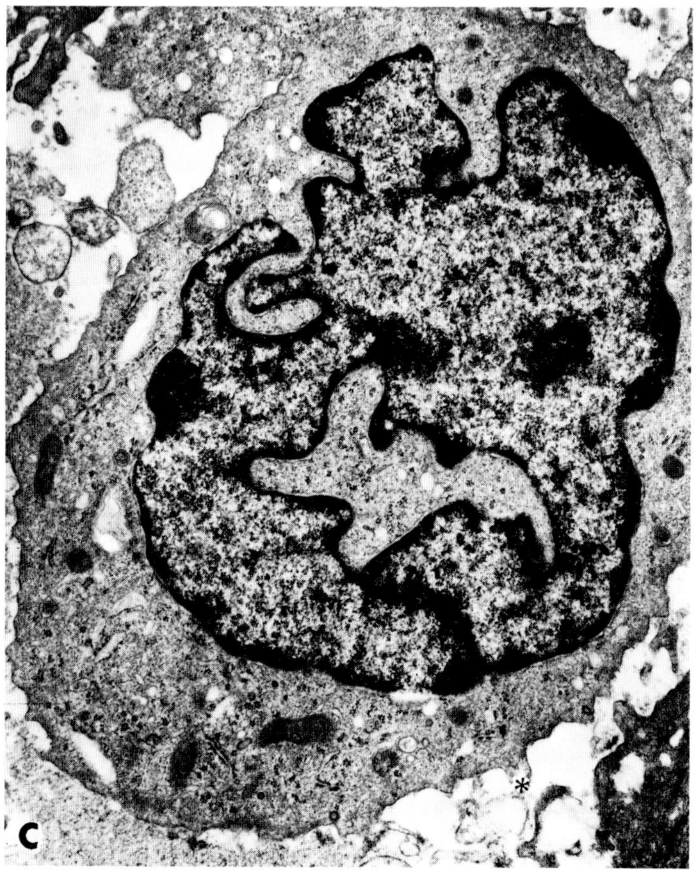

c

Figure 9–5. TEM, tumor cells.

a. *The nucleus is large and contains nuclear bodies (arrows). Bundles of tonofilaments (T) are fewer in number than in normal keratinocytes. They are more concentrated in the vicinity of the nucleus than elsewhere in the cytoplasm. Cytoplasmic processes (*) are present; desmosomes are absent; mitochondria (M), Golgi membranes (G), and segments of rough endoplasmic reticulum (RER) are abundant; intercellular spaces are wide.* × *11,580.*

b. *Bizarre nucleus of tumor cell with nuclear bodies (arrows) and deep invaginations. The nucleus is surrounded by bundles of tonofilaments (T). Nuclear bodies indicate altered metabolism.* × *7,725.*

c. *Undifferentiated tumor cell with highly irregular nucleus. Bundles of tonofilaments and desmosomes are absent. Cytoplasmic processes (*) project into the intercellular space.* × *10,000.*

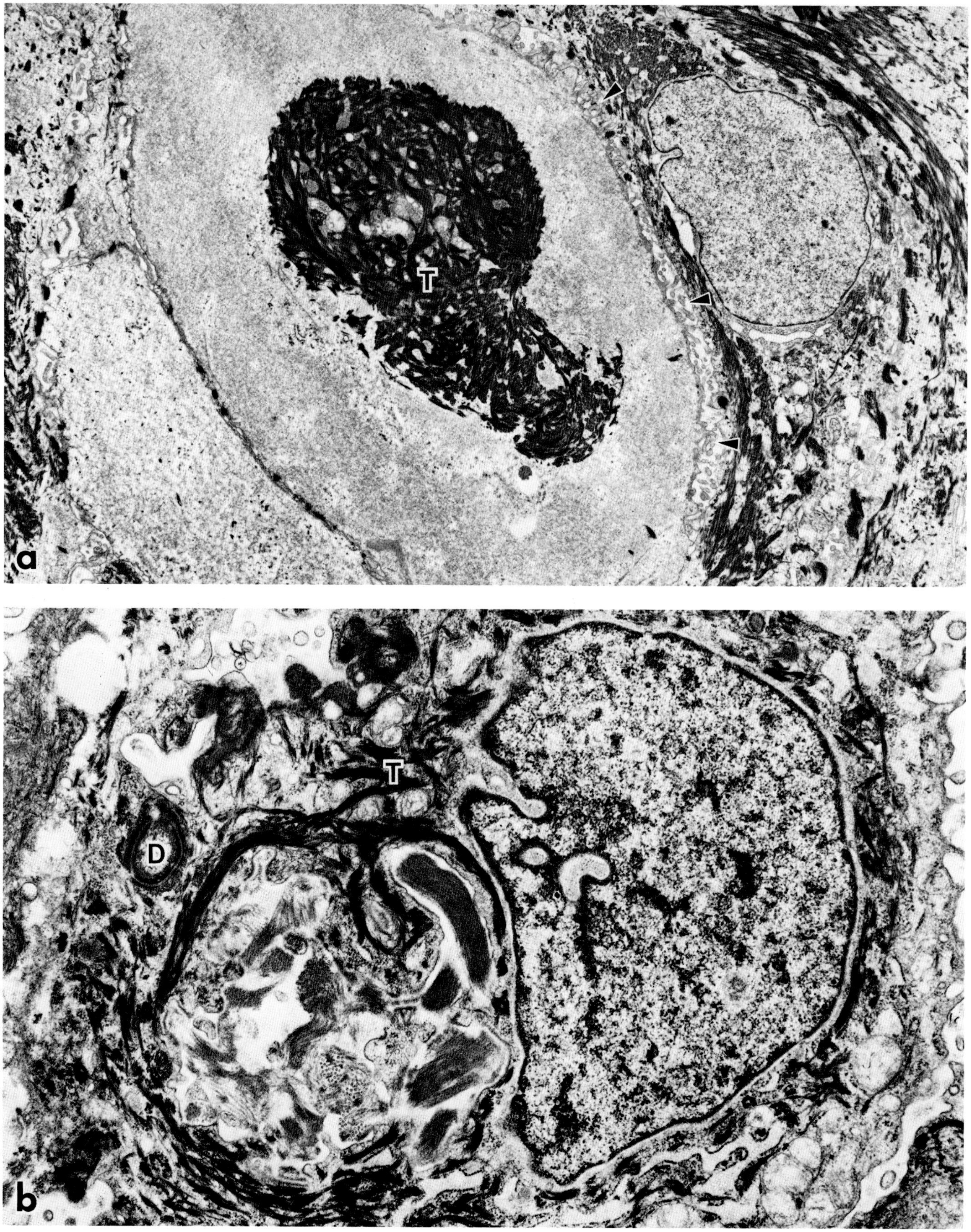

Figure 9–6. TEM, degenerating tumor cells.

a. *Only part of a large tumor cell is shown. The squamous cell at right of tumor cell is of normal size. Note the aggregates of tonofilaments (T) and multitude of cytoplasmic processes (arrows) associated with the tumor cell. × 5,280.*

b. *Bundles of tonofilaments (T) of different diameters surround the irregular nucleus. The intracellular desmosome (D) may have resulted from phagocytosis or from invagination and detachment of the cell membrane. Similar intracellular desmosomes are associated with certain other skin abnormalities, such as the keratoacanthoma. Thus, they are not specific for squamous cell carcinomas. × 16,400.*

KERATOACANTHOMA 10

The human keratoacanthoma (KA) is a benign, hyperkeratotic skin tumor that appears rather suddenly. The KA has been described as a rapidly growing, heavily keratinized lesion of invasive squamous cells which is definitely destructive. If left untreated, it stops growing spontaneously and will eventually subside, often leaving a scar.

Keratoacanthomas (KAs) may occur on any hairy surface of the skin. They have not been reported on the palms, soles, or mucous membranes where hairs are absent. The tumor is uncommon in dark-skinned races and in the Japanese. Males are affected about three times more frequently than females. The incidence of KA increases at middle age, but does not become significantly more frequent in the aged.

The cause of human KA has not been completely resolved. Virus-like bodies have been observed in the tumor and it has been suggested that the tumor has a viral etiology. Proliferation of cells in the infundibula of hair follicles and in the ducts of sweat glands has also been implicated in the pathogenesis of the tumor. Lesions with the histological appearance of human KAs have been produced in rabbits and certain other experimental animals by topical application of dimethylbenzanthracene. The idea is widely held that KAs arise from hair follicles in both man and experimental animals.

Clinically, KAs are rapidly growing, hard tumors that can be accurately diagnosed. Histopathologically, KAs can be confused with squamous cell carcinomas. KAs show considerable irregular hyperplasia of the stratum spinosum which spreads laterally below the epidermis. Careful study of the basement membrane at the epidermal-dermal junction fails to show any serious disruption as seen in squamous cell carcinomas. The center of a KA is a keratin-filled crater. Foci of concentrically arranged scales, the "horned pearls" or keratin plugs, are present in the keratin crater. The dermis surrounding the crater contains a chronic inflammatory infiltrate. The tendency of KAs to recur following excision can be reduced by topical application of retinoic acid and 5-fluorouracil after healing of the surgical wound.

Material for this study consisted of 18 KAs obtained by surgical excision under xylocaine anesthesia. The 17 patients from which the lesions were removed ranged in age from 37 years to 75 years. Thirteen KAs were mature lesions; 5 were young lesions. Each specimen was bisected and one-half used for histopathology and the remainder for correlative SEM and TEM.

Tumor cells of KAs are modified keratinocytes that are larger than normal. They contain vacuoles and intracellular desmosomes. Keratinized tumor cells have a "honeycomb" appearance due to prominent microridges and microgrooves which interdigitate to produce a "tongue and groove" effect.

Keratin plugs arise from hair follicles and from extrafollicular tumor cells. The latter may be derived from hair follicles. Each plug has a central nidus surrounded by concentric lamellae of tumor cells. Viruses were not observed, and there was no evidence that sweat ducts, sebaceous glands, or Langerhans cells were involved in the pathogenesis of the lesion. SEM provides further confirmation that hair follicles give rise to human KAs.

References

Freeman, R. G. On the pathogenesis of pseudoepitheliomatous hyperplasia. J. Cut. Path. 1: 213–237, 1974.

Carrington, S. G., and W. H. Wilborn. A tridimensional view of keratoacanthoma. Scanning Electron Microscopy, Vol. III, 1980, SEM Inc., Chicago, IL, pp. 495–504.

Ghadially, F. N. Role of hair follicles in origin and evolution of some cutaneous neoplasms of man and experimental animals. Cancer 14: 801–816, 1961.

Kern, W. H., and M. K. McCray. The histopathologic differentiation of keratoacanthoma and squamous cell carcinoma of the skin. J. Cut. Path. 7: 318–325, 1980.

Pinkus, H., and A. H. Mehregan. *A Guide to Dermatopathology,* Appleton-Century-Crofts, New York, 1981 pp. 413–414.

Prutkin, L. Antitumor activity of vitamin A acid and fluorouracil used in combination of the skin tumor, keratoacanthoma. Cancer Res. 33: 128–133, 1973.

Reed, R. J. Actinic keratoacanthoma. Arch. Dermol. 106: 858–864, 1972.

Rook, A. J., and R. H. Champion. Keratoacanthoma. *In: Biology of Cutaneous Cancer,* Monograph No. 10, National Cancer Institute, Bethesda, MD, pp. 257–273, 1963.

Sanderson, K. V. Tumors of the skin. *In: Textbook of Dermatology.* Rook, Williamson, and Ebling, eds., 2nd edition, Oxford, Blackwell Scientific Publications, London, 1972, pp. 1911–2007.

Zelickson, A. S., and F. W. Lynch. Electron microscopy of virus-like particles in the keratoacanthoma. J. Invest. Dermatol. 37: 79–83, 1961.

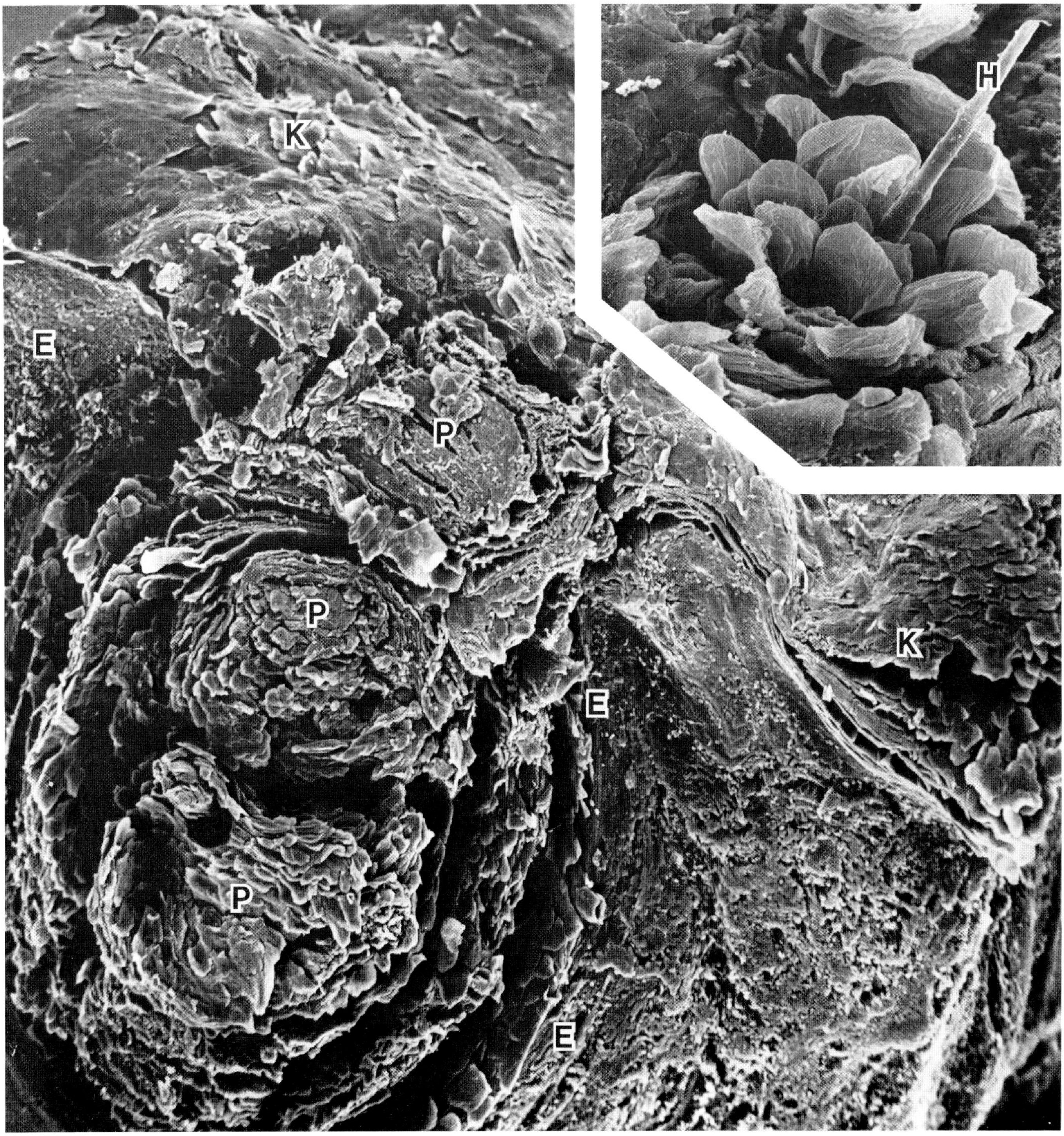

Figure 10–1. KA at low magnification, depicting the lesion's characteristic keratin-filled crater. The crater contains foci of concentrically arranged scales, the "horn pearls" or keratin plugs (P). Exfoliating keratinized cells (K) at free surface of lesion; epidermis (E) at sides and bottom of crater. × 155.

In the inset, a vellus hair (H) projects from an elevated, hyperkeratotic follicular orifice that is filled with scales. Follicular orifices are present at the free surface of the KA, but few contain hairs. × 705.

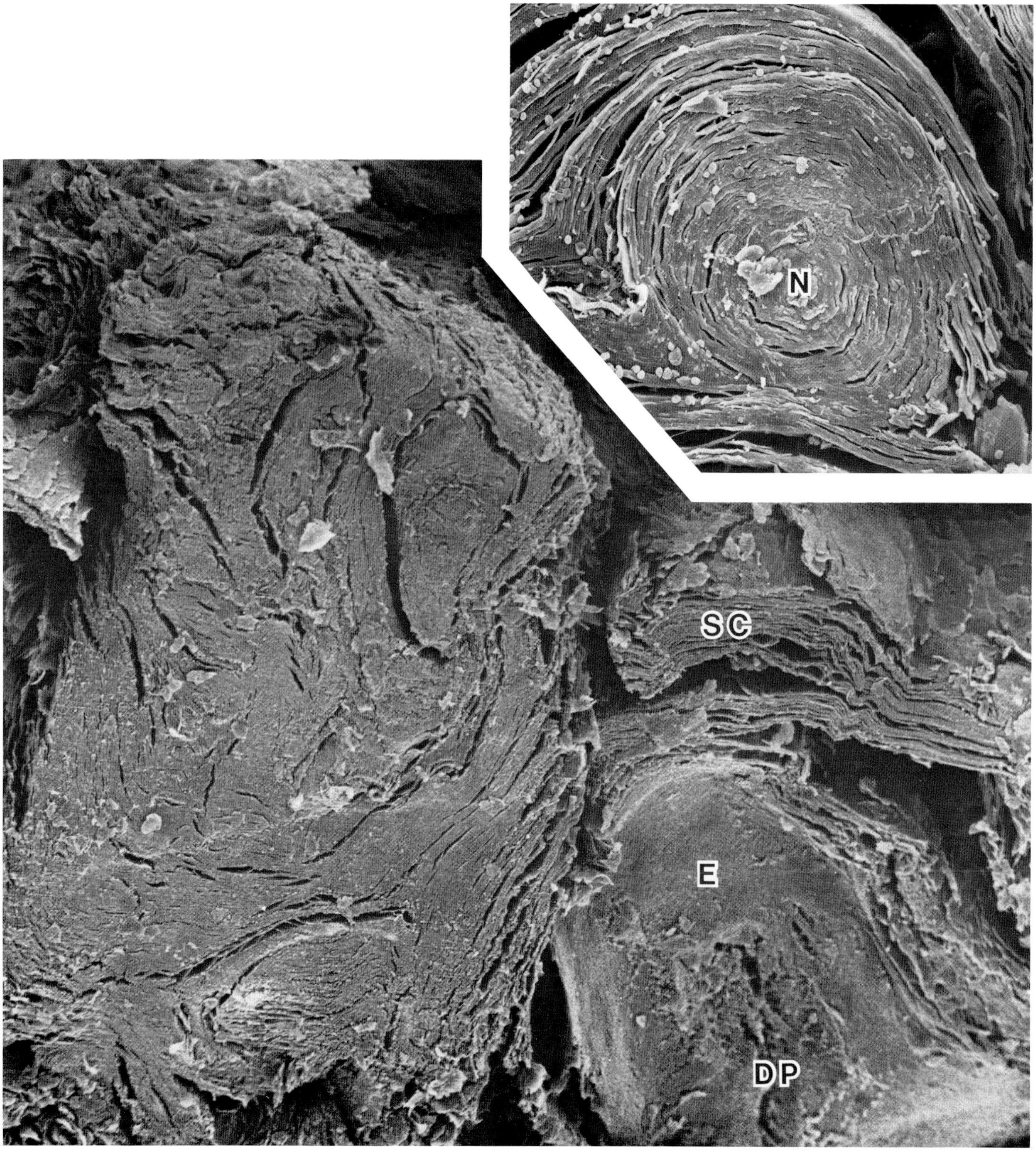

Figure 10–2. Profile of massive keratin crater in mature KA. To the right of the tightly packed scales of the crater, note dermal papilla (DP), acanthotic epidermis (E), and thick stratum corneum (SC). × 80.

Inset *shows the concentrically arranged scales of a keratin plug which has a central core or nidus (N). × 330.*

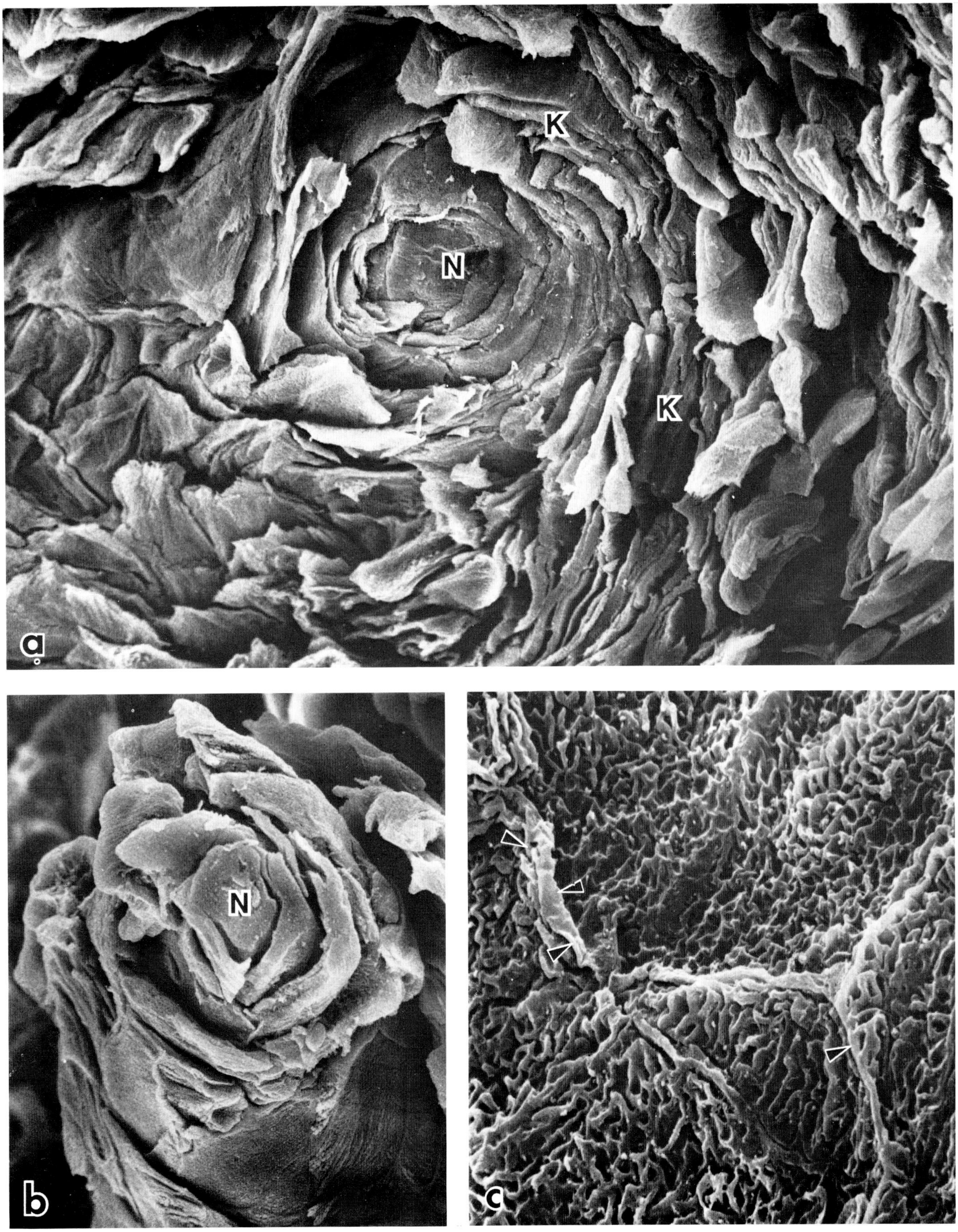

Figure 10–3. Outer, free surface of a keratin plug viewed from above to illustrate the lamellae of keratinized cells (K) that surround central nidus (N) of scales. × 660.

b. *Peripheral scales have been removed from the keratin plug, exposing the keratinized cells of the nidus (N). × 1,150.*

c. *Scales of keratin plugs have a "honeycomb" appearance produced by anastomosing microridges separated by deep depressions. Scales vary in size and have elevated free edges (arrows). × 7,200.*

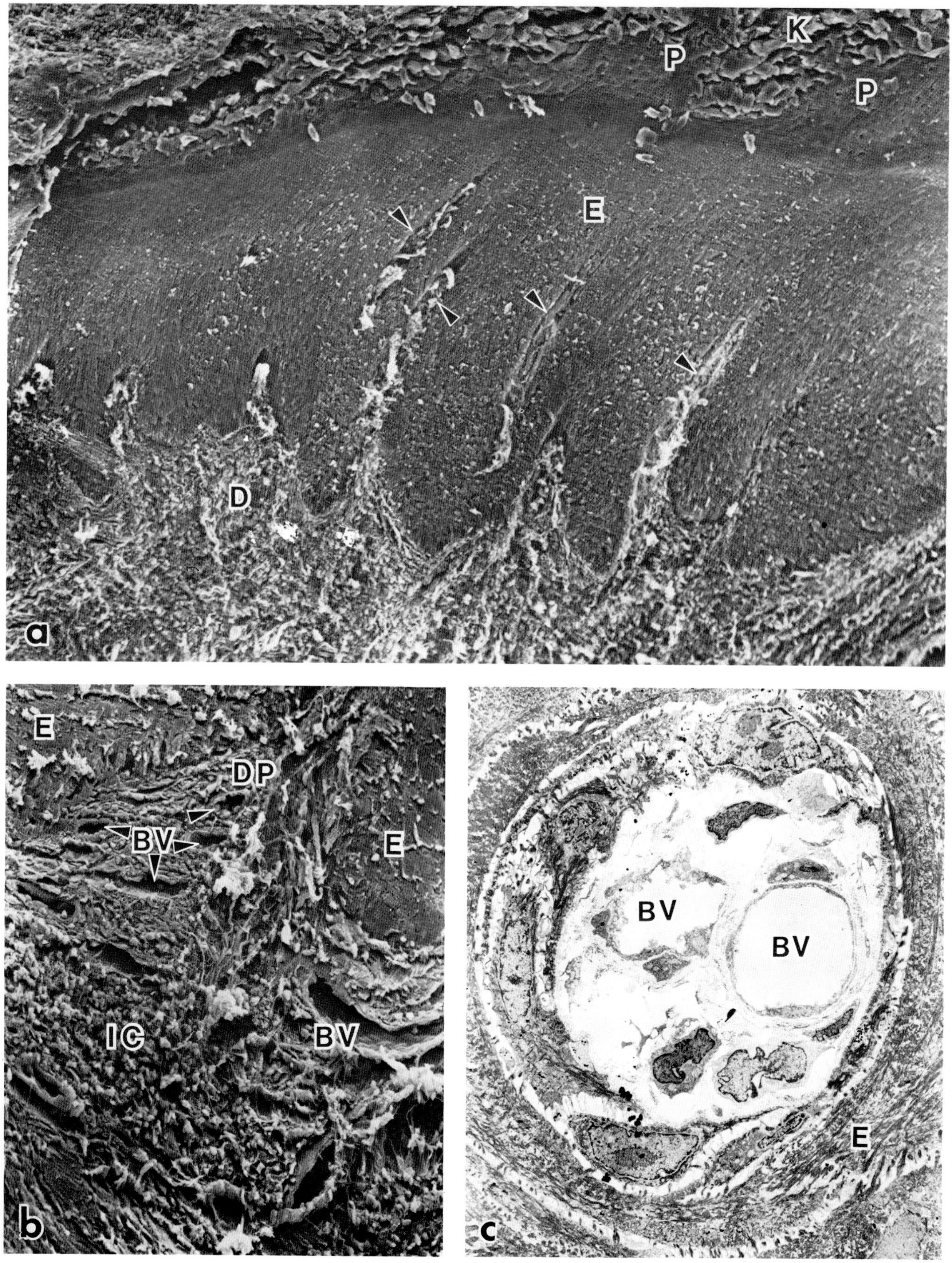

Figure 10–4. a. *Profile of KA, revealing acanthosis and epidermal projections (P) extending into lower border of keratin crater (K). Narrow papillae (arrows) from the dermis (D) deeply indent epidermis (E).* ×150.

b. *Blood vessels (BV) are especially abundant in upper dermis and are shown continuing into a dermal papilla, delineated on either side by lower epidermis (E). Focal infiltrates of inflammatory cells (IC) are common.* ×2,075.

c. *TEM, small dermal papilla surrounded by keratinocytes of upper epidermis (E) and containing two, thin-walled blood vessels (BV). Tissue spaces between keratinocytes permit passage of extravascular blood elements through the epidermis.* ×2,060.

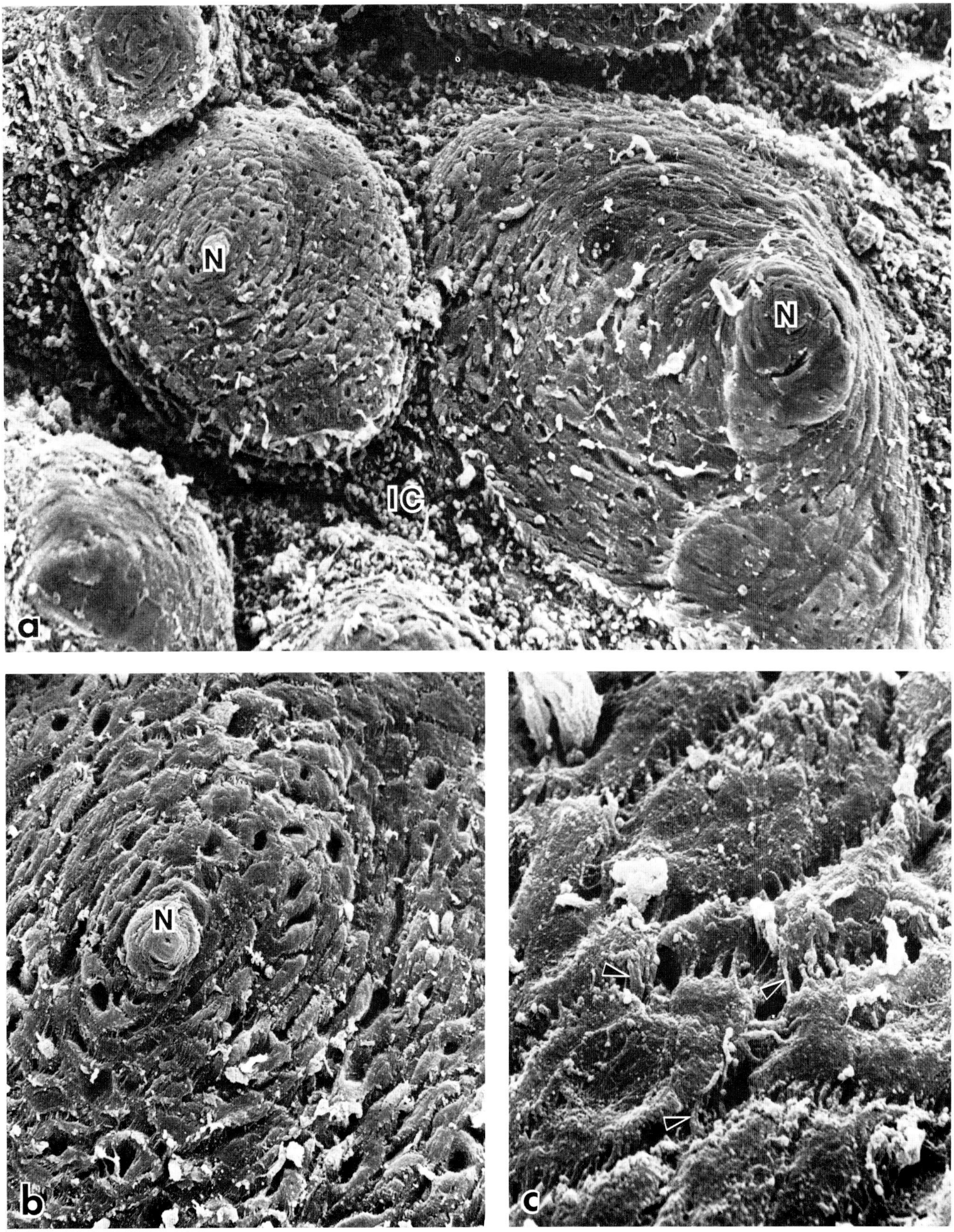

Figure 10–5. a. *Malpighian layer of epidermis viewed from above after removal of keratin crater. Several "cell islands" are illustrated. Each is composed of tumor cells concentrically arranged about a nidus (N) of closely packed cells. A type of cell island that is more frequently encountered has a much larger nidus and is associated with a hair follicle. Its center is hollow if the hair has been lost. Both types of cell islands are surrounded by inflammatory cells (IC), and keratin plugs appear to originate from both types. ×290.*

b. *Higher magnification of a cell island in Figure 10–5a. Tumor cells surround a nipple-like nidus (N). ×815.*

c. *Higher magnification of tumor cells in Figure 10–5b, illustrating spinous process (arrows) between adjacent cells. TEM shows that desmosomes join the processes. ×3,400.*

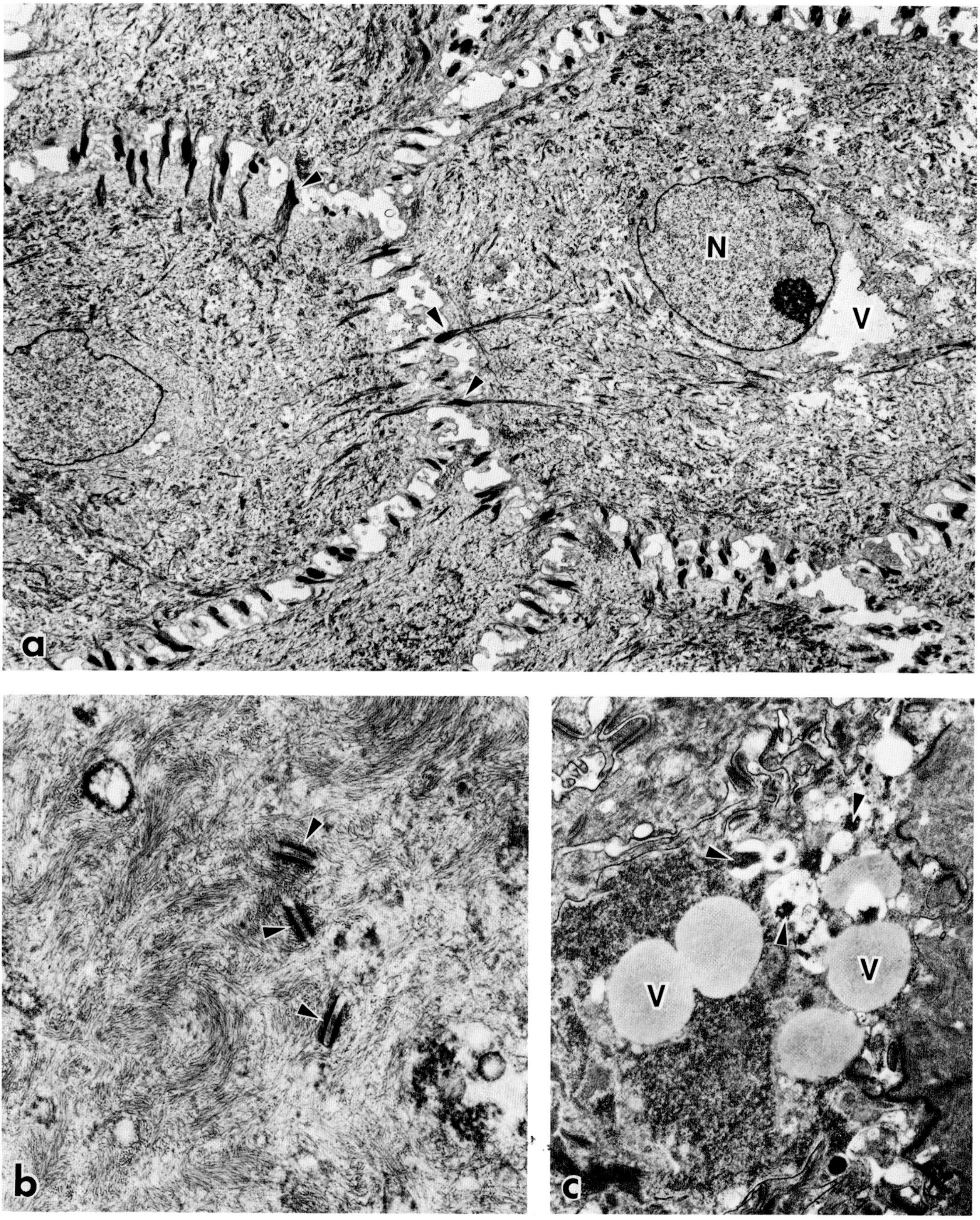
a
N
V
b
c
V
V

Figure 10–6. a. *TEM, tumor cells in cell island. The modified keratinocytes are larger than normal keratinocytes and may reach giant size. The nucleus (N) is often indented and the cytoplasm contains vacuoles (V) of various sizes. Tonofibrils are concentrated in the peripheral cytoplasm and many course toward the numerous desmosomes (arrows) associated with the spinous processes observed by SEM. ×3,800.*

b. *Intracytoplasmic desmosomes (arrows) are an interesting feature of tumor cells. They indicate the ability of tumor cells to incorporate free desmosomes from the intercellular spaces. ×36,000.*

c. *TEM, vacuoles (V) in adjacent tumor cells. Vacuoles form in areas of tumor cell cytoplasm rich in tonofilaments and tonofibrils. Vacuoles contain tonofilaments in their early formative stages, but tonofilaments (arrows) become difficult to recognize as the vacuoles mature. ×15,700.*

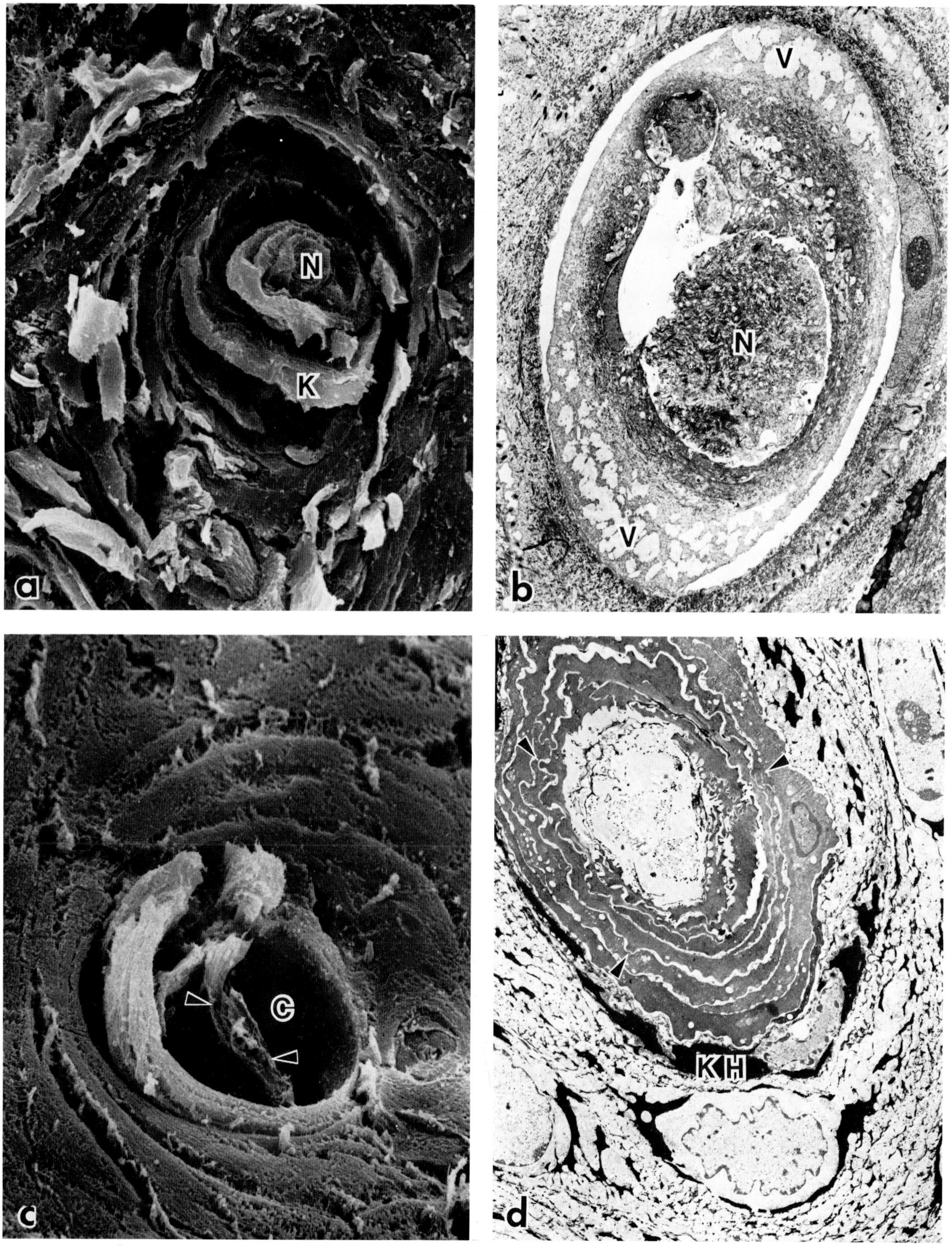
a
N
K
b
V
N
V
c
C
d
KH

Figure 10–7. a. *Some keratin plugs originate from cell islands unassociated with hairs while others arise from cell islands in which hairs or their remnants serve as focal points for plug formation. The histogenesis of an extrafollicular keratin plug is shown here. It involves the addition of concentric layers of cells about a nidus (N). Cells (K) nearest the plug's center are the first to cornify. Growth continues laterally and upward as lamellae of tumor cells are added and keratinize. × 1,440.*

b. *TEM, early extrafollicular plug formation. The nidus (N) conists of degenerating tumor cells with vacuoles (V). × 2,470.*

c. *Follicular plug formation with remnants of former hair (arrows) in center (C) of cell island. Keratin plugs of the follicular type outnumber those of the extrafollicular type about 7:1. × 1,800.*

d. *TEM, hollow center of plug in* c. *The center contains remnants of hair and is surrounded by keratinized cells with interdigitating microridges and microgrooves (arrows). Keratohyalin granules (KH) are large and typical of those associated with hairs. × 2,850.*

PIGMENTED NEVUS 11

The pigmented nevus or common mole is a malformation of the skin that usually affects everyone. Nevi may occur anywhere on the skin and they may involve large cutaneous areas.

Clinically, most pigmented nevi can be grouped into three broad categories: (1) dark, flat, macular; (2) slightly elevated, and (3) dome-shaped, pedunculated. Most of the flat types are junctional (intraepidermal) nevi. Most raised ones are compound nevi, and nearly all dome-shaped nevi are intradermal (dermal) nevi. Therefore, as their names imply, nevus cells (melanocytes) can be located in the epidermis (junctional nevus), in both the epidermis and dermis (compound nevus), or only in the dermis (intradermal nevus).

Pigmented nevi, espicially those of the junctional type, have the potential for transformation into malignant melanomas. This change can be anticipated when a nevus shows a sudden increase in size, darkening, inflammation, bleeding, or tenderness. The recommended treatment for pigmented nevi is complete surgical excision followed by thorough microscopic study in order to permit an accurate diagnosis and prognosis. Special management is required for pigmented nevi associated with mucous membranes, such as the vulva, oral mucosa, and conjunctiva.

Three types of nevus cells can be recognized in pigmented nevi: (1) Type A, epithelioid cells in the upper dermis and epidermis; (2) Type B, round cells in the middle dermis; (3) Type C, elongated cells in the lower dermis. Melanin is present in Types A and B cells, but it is absent in Type C cells. Type A cells are cuboidal to ovoid, Type B cells approximate lymphocytes in size and shape, and Type C cells resemble fibroblasts or Schwann cells. Nevus cells in the epidermis are usually of the Type A variety. Most nevus cells in the epidermis and dermis are located in nests; the remaining occur as bands, strands, or as single cells. Individual cells and aggregates of nevus cells enter the dermis from the epidermis by the so-called "dropping-off" process ("Abtropfung" or more correctly, "abtropfen").

The following text and micrographs are based on the study of 10 junctional nevi, 20 intradermal nevi, and 12 compound nevi. These lesions were excised from 8 male and 16 female patients who ranged in age from 26 to 64 years. Each specimen was bisected and one part was processed for correlative SEM and TEM, and the other portion for histopathology.

SEM has unveiled previously unrecognized features of the lesion, such as its deep invaginations of the keratinized free surface, criss-crossing creases, and a preponderance of follicular openings with multiple hairs. SEM shows that each type of nevus cell (A, B, and C) has distinctive features. These features can be used to diagnose nevus cell lesions and to gain a better understanding of their histogenesis.

References

Bhawan, J. Melanocytic nevi. A review. J. Cut. Path. 6: 153–169, 1979.

Jurecka, W., H. Lassman, and W. Gebhart. The relation of nervous elements to intradermal nevi. An electron microscopic study. Arch. Dermatol. 261: 219–230, 1978.

Kopf, A. W., and R. Andrade. A histological study of the dermo-epidermal junction in clinically "intradermal" nevi, employing serial sections. I. Junctional theques. Ann. N.Y. Acad. Sci. 100: 200–222, 1963.

Masson, P. My conception of cellular nevi. Cancer 4: 9–38, 1951.

Mishima, Y. Macromolecular changes in pigmentary disorders. Arch. Dermatol. 91: 519–557, 1965.

References con't.

Mishima, Y. Melanotic Tumors. *In: Ultrastructure of Normal and Abnormal Skin.* A. Zelickson, ed., Lea & Febiger, Philadelphia, 1967, p. 388–424.

Shelley, W. B., and R. P. Arthur. Nerve fibers, a neglected component of intradermal cellular nevi. J. Invest. Dermatol. 34: 59–69, 1960.

Stegmaier, O. C. Natural regression of the melanocytic nevus. J. Invest. Dermatol. 32: 413–421, 1959.

Traub, E. F. The "common mole." Its clinicopathologic relations and the question of malignant degeneration. Arch. Dermatol. & Syph. 41: 214–252, 1940.

Unna, P. G. *The Histopathology of the Diseases of the Skin.* Translated by N. Walker. MacMillan & Co., N.Y., 1896, p. 1129–1140.

Wilborn, W. H., and L. F. Montes. A tridimensional view of intradermal nevi as revealed by scanning electron microscopy. J. Cut. Path. 6: 170–179, 1979.

Winkelmann, R. K. Cholinesterase nevus: Cholinesterases in pigmented tumors of the skin. Arch. Dermatol. 82: 17–23, 1960.

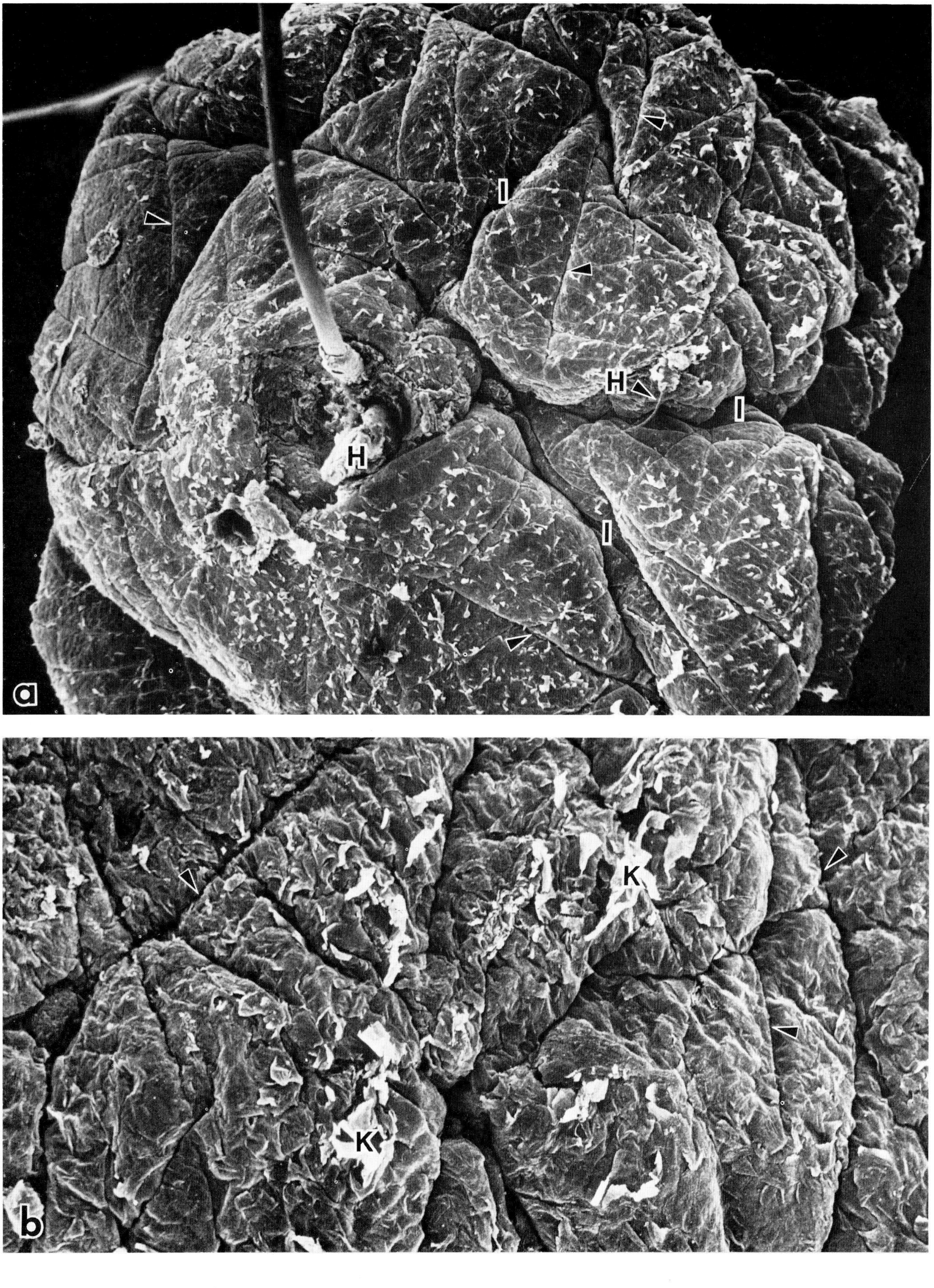

Figure 11–1. a. *The free surface has deep invaginations and criss-crossing creases (arrows). Keratinized cells have detached, resulting in a depression where the two hairs emerge. One hair (H) is broken and the other is intact. A tiny hair (H) is present in another part of the lesion (right of center).* ×65.

b. *Higher magnification of free surface of nevus, depicting loose, keratinized cells (K) and creases (arrows).* ×270.

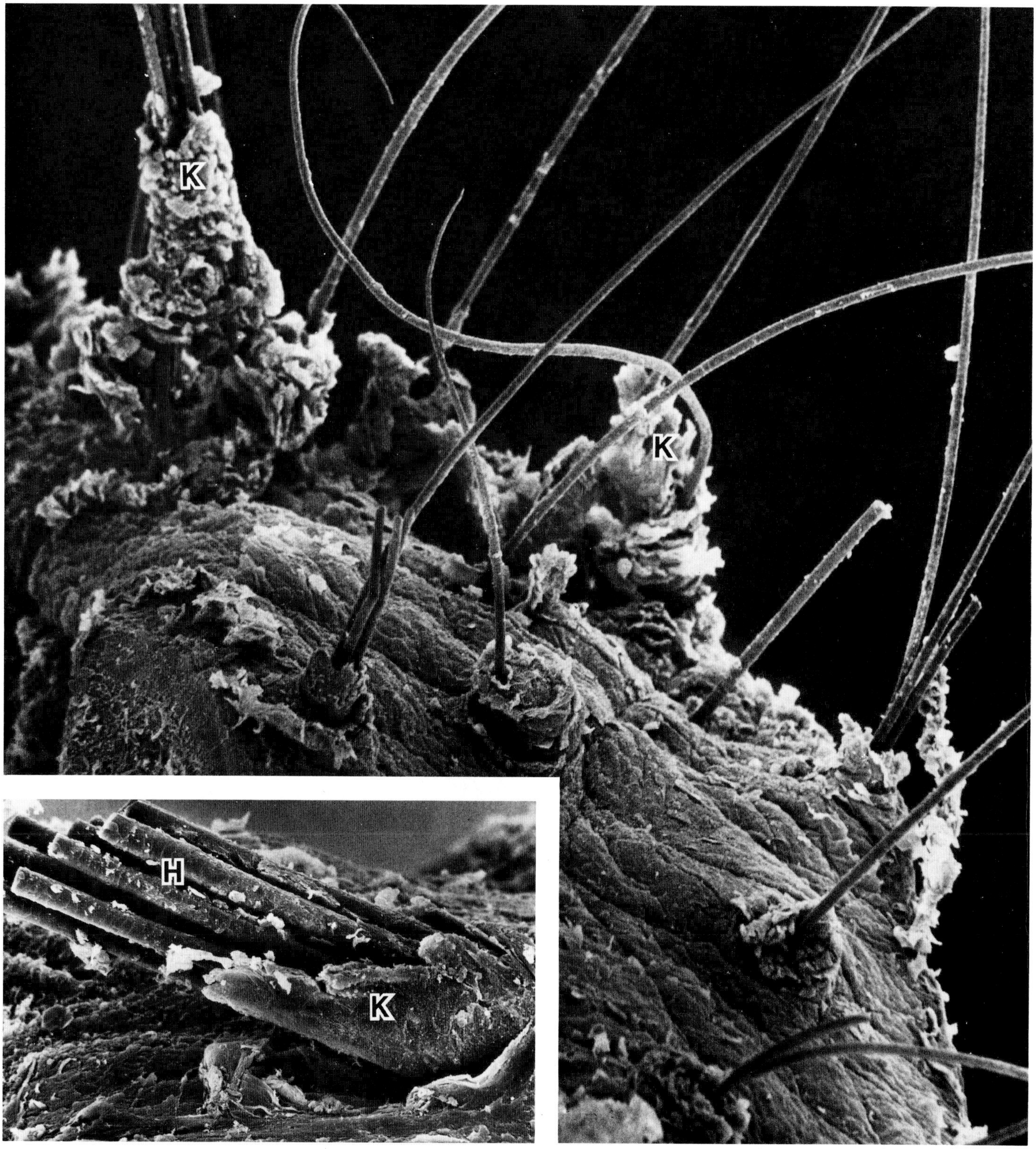

Figure 11–2. Multiple hairs, 14–19 μm in diameter, in a single follicular opening. Shafts of many hairs are encrusted with scales (K). ×165.

Inset *illustrates a follicular orifice with multiple hairs (H) surrounded by keratinized cells (K). Follicles with multiple hairs are characteristic of the pigmented nevus. ×350.*

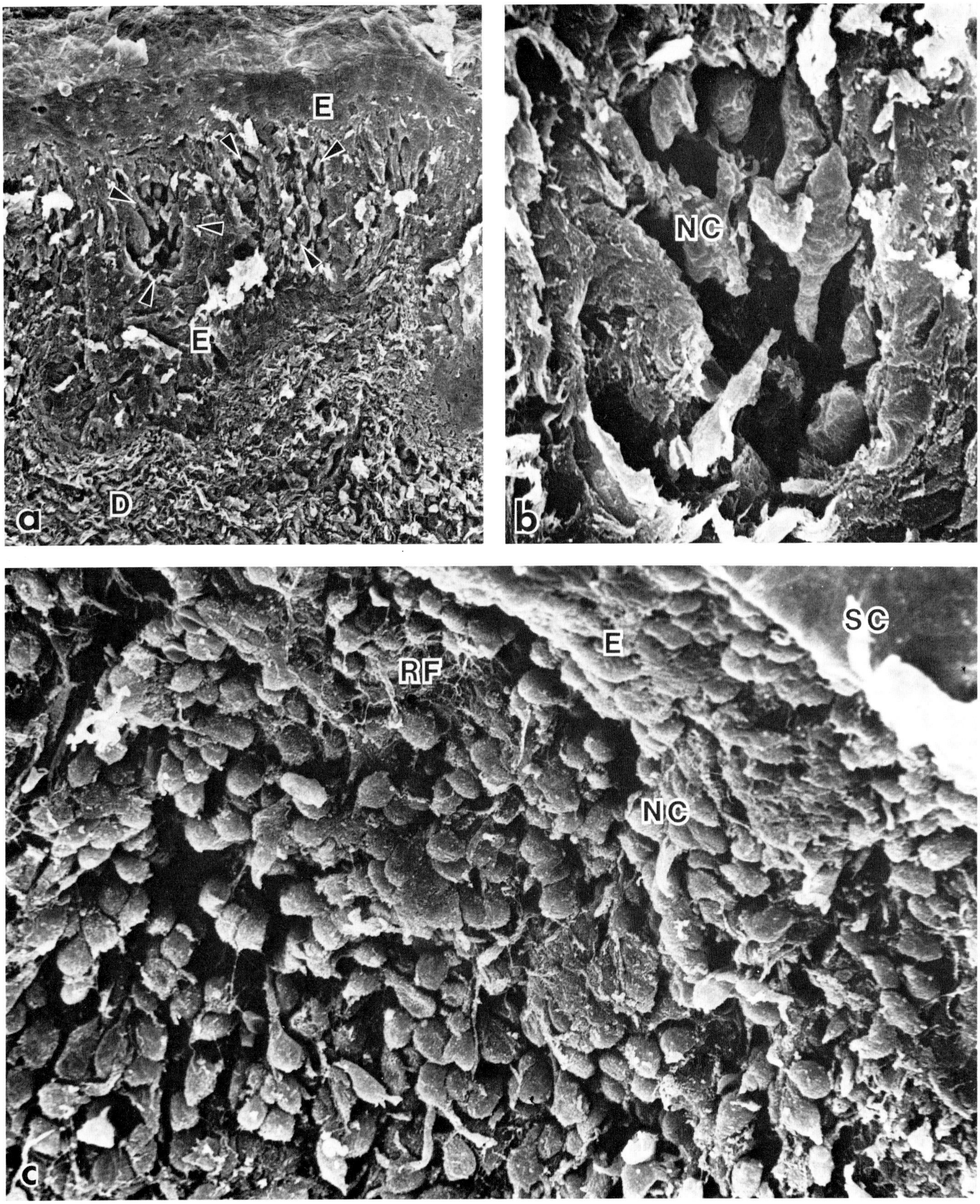

Figure 11–3. a. *Junctional nevus in profile: epidermis (E), dermis (D), and nests of nevus cells (arrows) within the epidermis.* $\times 350$.

b. *Higher magnification of a, showing nest of nevus cells. Nevus cells (NC) are large Type A, epithelioid cells which lack desmosomal attachments and are separated by wide intercellular spaces.* $\times 3{,}600$.

c. *Compound nevus in profile. Type A nevus cells at one site (NC) appear to be in the process of "dropping-off" from the epidermis (E) into the upper dermis. Nevus cells nearly fill the dermis in which a few reticular fibers (RF) can be identified. Stratum corneum (SC).* $\times 1{,}320$.

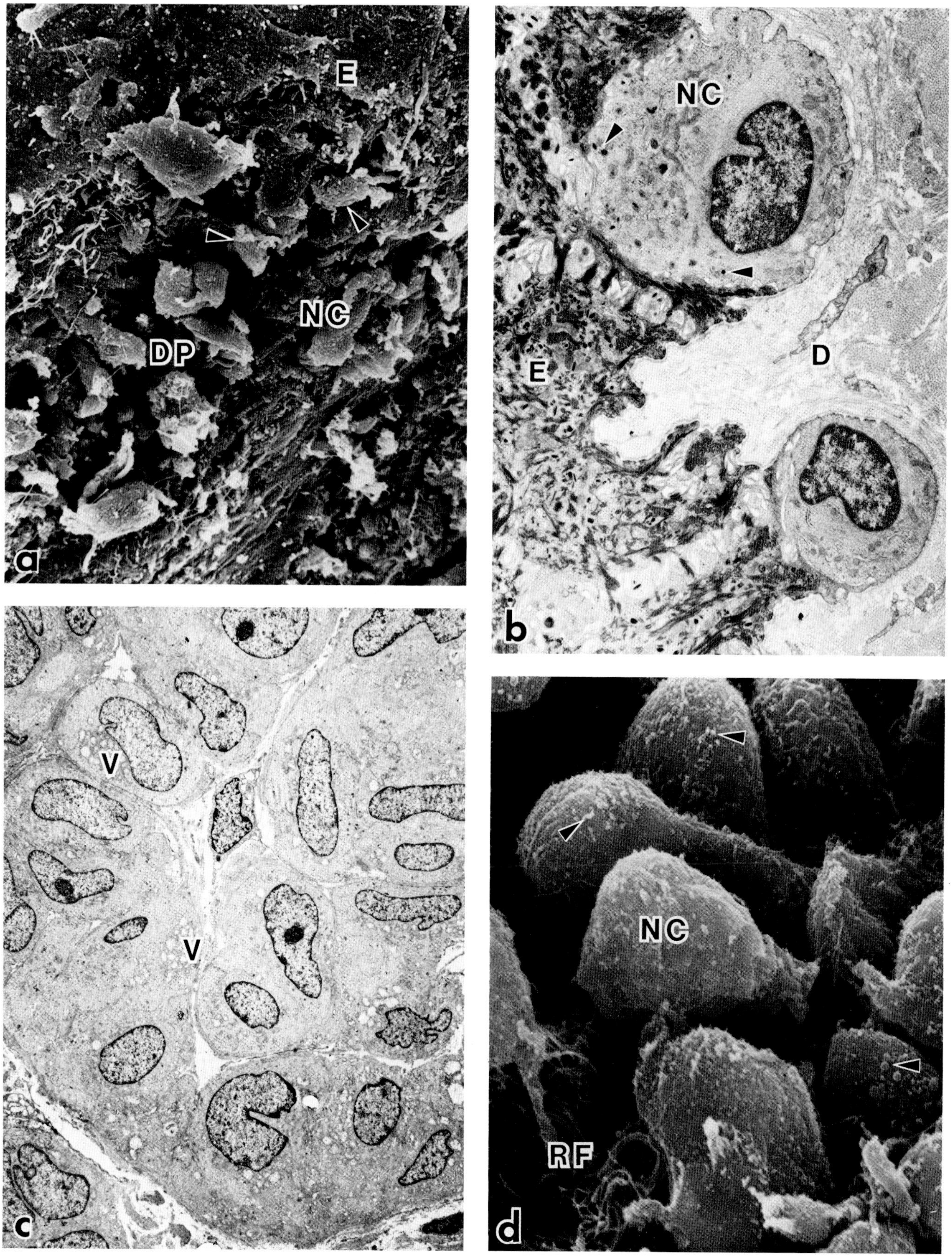
E
NC
DP
a
NC
E
D
b
V
V
c
NC
RF
d

Figure 11-4. a. *Dermal papilla (DP) in compound nevus. Type I nevus cells (NC) are in dermal papilla and some cells (arrows) appear to be migrating into the papilla from the epidermis (E). × 1,500.*

b. *TEM, epidermal-dermal junction of compound nevus with two, pale nevus cells. Each nevus cell (NC) is in the process of "dropping-off" (abtropfen) from the epidermis (E) into the dermis (D). Nuclei of nevus cells are characteristically indented. The cytoplasm lacks tonofibrils and desmosomes, but often contains melanin pigment (arrows). × 5,780.*

c. *TEM, compound nevus, nest of Type A nevus cells in upper dermis. Nevus cells have accumulated in upper dermis after passing through the basement membrane. Many cells are in close contact, but lack attachment plaques. As the lesion ages, mitochondria lose their cristae and become vacuoles (V). Little melanin pigment is present, but the amount is related to the age of the cell. × 1,900.*

d. *Type A nevus cells (NC) in upper dermis. The cells vary in shape and have small cytoplasmic protuberances (arrows). Microplicae and vesiculations of the cell surface indicate that the cells are not in a quiescent physiological state. Reticular fibers (RF). × 4,080.*

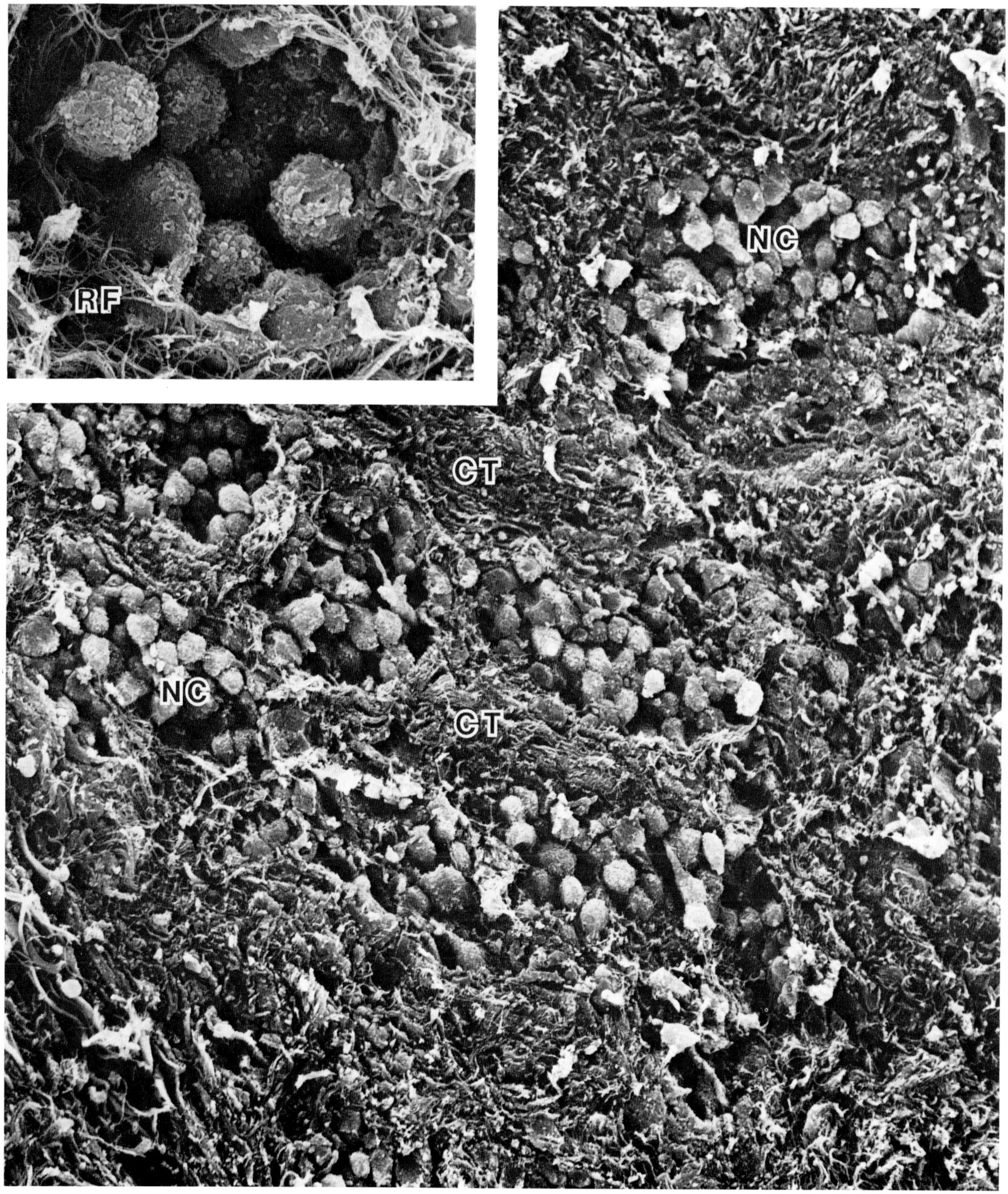

Figure 11–5. Several nests of nevus cells (NC) in middle dermis of intradermal nevus. Most nests contain a mixture of elongated Type A cells and round Type B cells. Round cells resemble lymphocytes. Connective tissue (CT) separates the nests. ×865.

Inset *is a higher magnification of a nest of small, round Type B cells. Cell surfaces are more ruffled and plicated than surfaces of Type A nevus cells. Reticular fibers (RF) surround nest. ×3,200.*

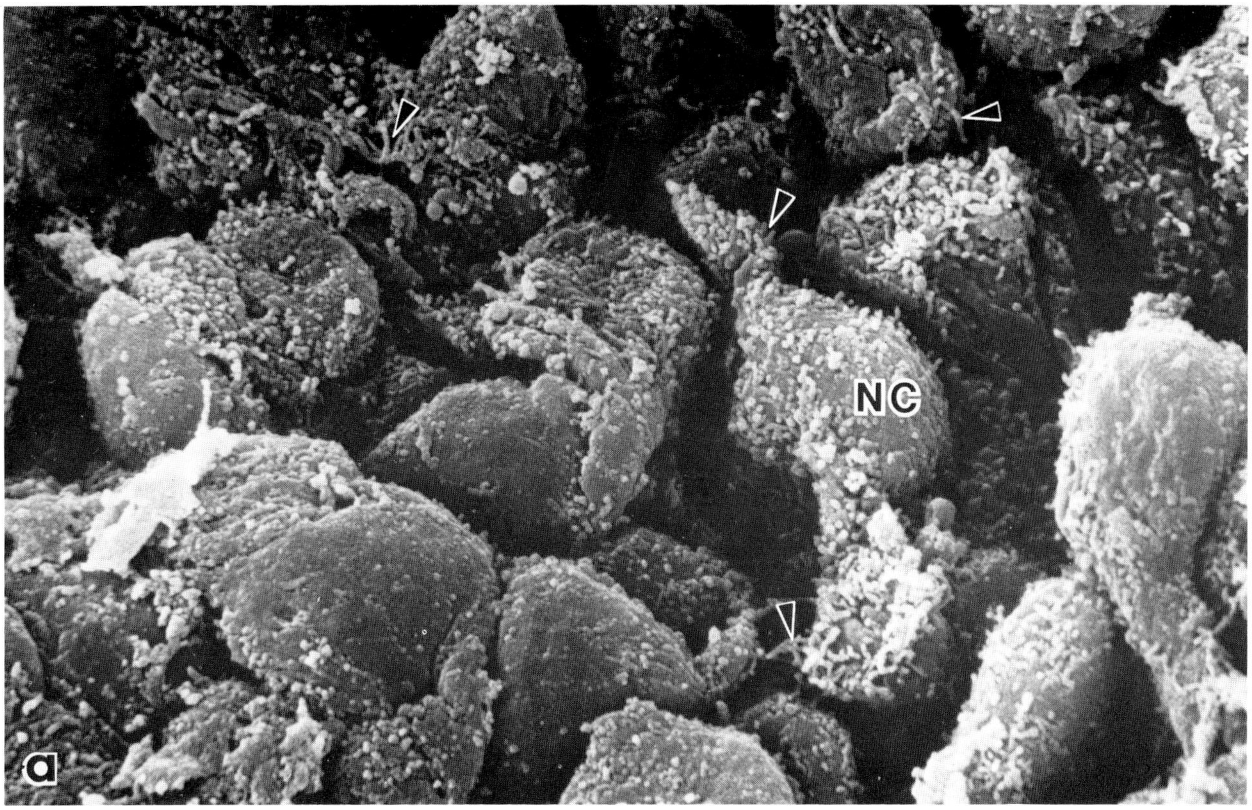

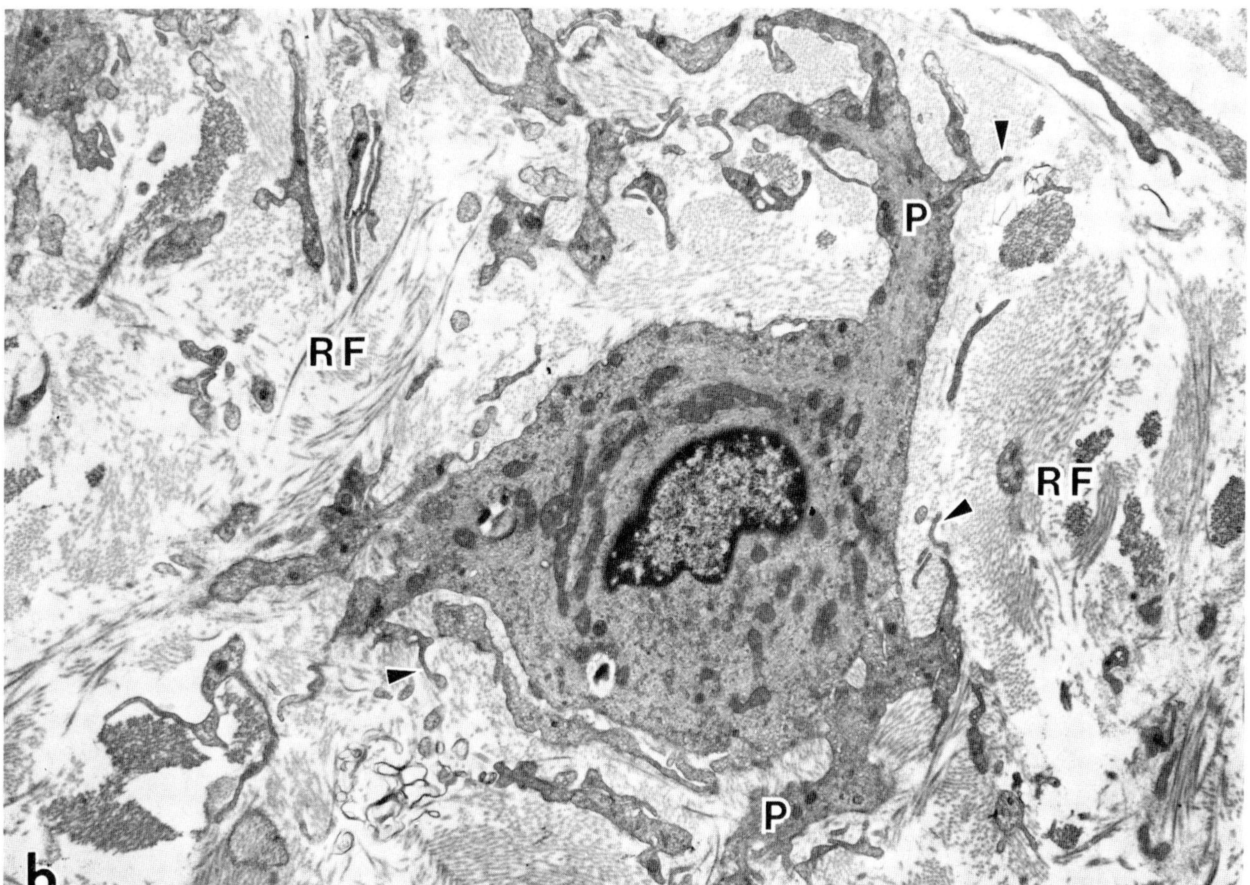

Figure 11–6. a. *Intradermal nevus, showing a nest of Type C cells (NC) in lower dermis. Most cells are spindle-shaped and have appendages (arrows).* × *6,000.*

b. *TEM, Type C nevus cell at the periphery of the nest in* a. *Most Type C cells have 2 to 3 major processes (P) from the cell body. These processes give rise to much smaller cytoplasmic processes (arrows) that correspond to the appendages observed by SEM. Reticular fibers (RF) are abundant at the nest's periphery and may permeate the nest to surround individual cells.* × *6,460.*

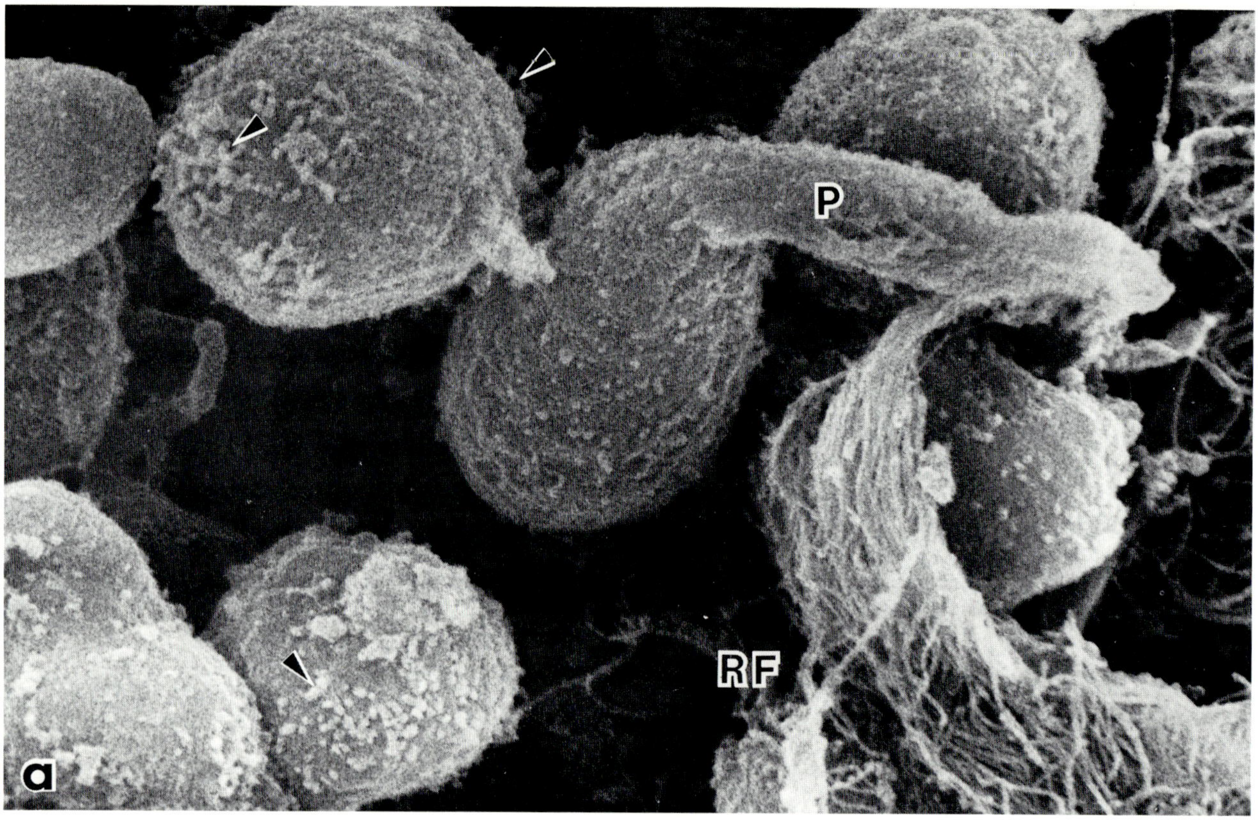
P
RF
a

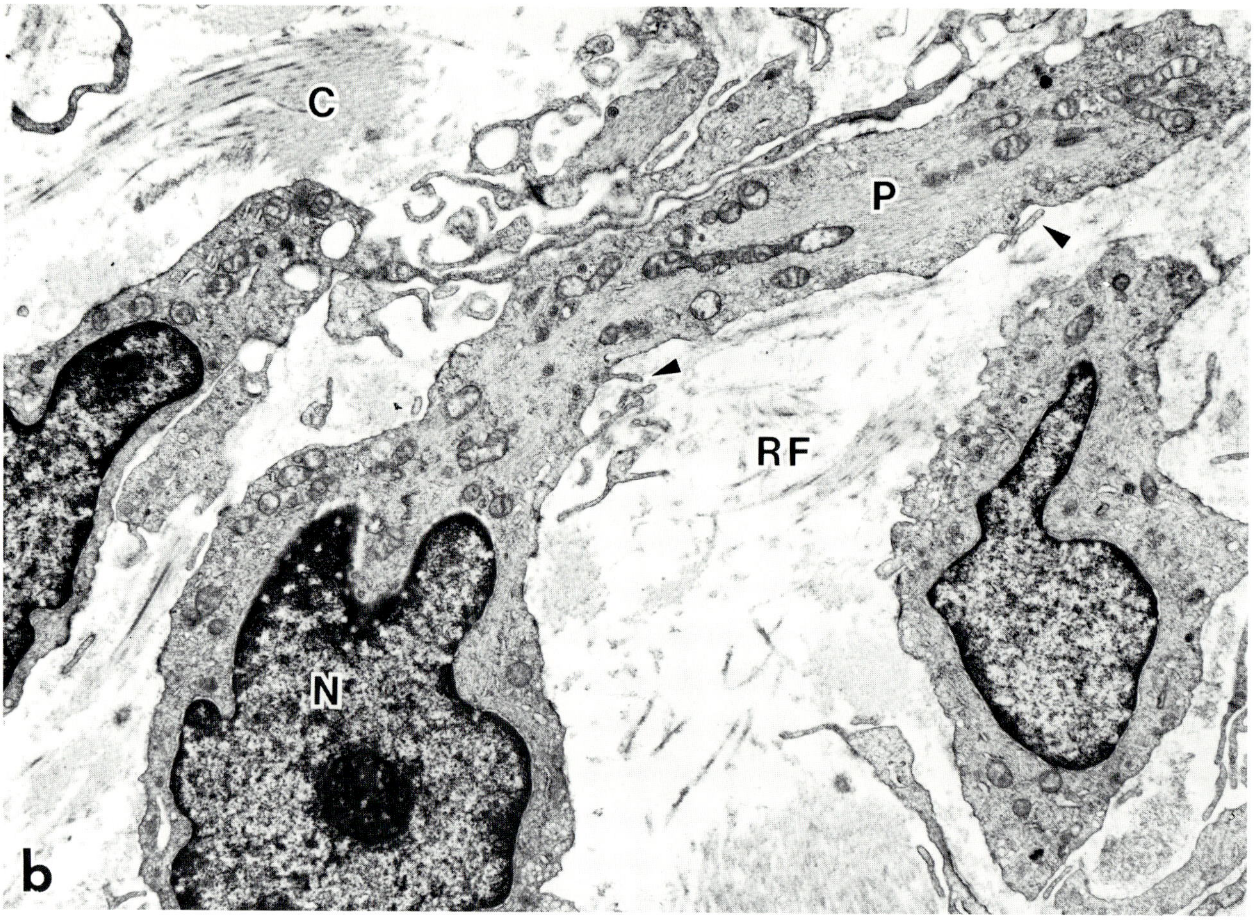
C
P
RF
N
b

Figure 11–7. a. *Type C cells in the deep dermis of an intradermal nevus. Type C cells occur in nests (Fig. 11–6), singly, and in groups of only a few cells. Cells in some nests are spindle-shaped. At other sites, they are flask-shaped, as shown here. One large or major process (P) extends from the cell body. Minor processes (arrows) are numerous. Reticular fibers (RF) and small bundles of collagen course between adjacent nevus cells. ×8,500.*

b. *TEM, depicting major process (P) of flask-shaped nevus cell in* a. *Note the processes (arrows). Nucleus (N), bundle of collagen (C), and reticular fibers (RF). ×8,100.*

Index